Clinical Electrocardiography

A SIMPLIFIED APPROACH

Clinical Electrocardiography

A SIMPLIFIED APPROACH

Ary L. Goldberger, M.D., F.A.C.C.

Associate Professor of Medicine, Harvard Medical School;
Director of Electrocardiography, Beth Israel Hospital
Boston, Massachusetts

Emanuel Goldberger, M.D., F.A.C.P.

FIFTH EDITION

 Mosby

St. Louis Baltimore Berlin Boston Carlsbad Chicago London Madrid
Naples New York Philadelphia Sydney Tokyo Toronto

Dedicated to Publishing Excellence

Acquisition Editor: Stephanie Manning
Assistant Editor: Carolyn Malik
Manuscript Editor: George B. Stericker, Jr.
Cover Design: G.W. Graphics & Publishing
Production: Teresa Breckwoldt
Manufacturing Supervisor: Theresa Fuchs

FIFTH EDITION
Copyright © 1994 by Mosby–Year Book, Inc.

Printed in the United States of America
Composition by Clarinda Company
Printing/Binding by R. R. Donnelley & Sons Company

Mosby–Year Book, Inc.
11830 Westline Industrial Drive
St. Louis, Missouri 63146

Library of Congress Cataloging-in-Publication Data
Goldberger, Ary Louis, 1949
    Clinical electrocardiography : a simplified approach / Ary L.
Goldberger, Emanuel Goldberger. — 5th ed.
      p. cm.
    Includes bibliographical references and index.
    1. Electrocardiography. I. Goldberger, Emanuel, 1913–
II. Title.
    [DNLM: 1. Electrocardiography. WG 140 G616c 1994]
    RC683.5.E5G593 1994
    616.1′207547—dc20
    DNLM/DLC   94-269
for Library of Congress   CIP

94 95 96 97 98 / 9 8 7 6 5 4 3 2 1

For

Ellen, Zach, and Lexy
(and sometimes Halley)

with love

Preface

This book is an introduction to electrocardiography. It is written particularly for medical students, nurses, and paramedical assistants, and assumes no previous instruction in ECG reading. It has been widely used in introductory courses on the subject. Physicians wishing to review basic electrocardiography have also found it useful. The text derives from the cumulative experience of both authors in the field of electrocardiography, beginning in 1944 with the invention of the aV_R, aV_L, and aV_F leads by one of us (E.G.). It is closely based on a series of lectures given over the past two decades by the other (A.G.) to physician associates, medical students, nurses, house officers, and specialists in emergency medicine.

We have divided the book into three sections. Part I covers the basic principles of electrocardiography, normal ECG patterns, and the major abnormal P-QRS-T patterns. Part II describes the major abnormalities of heart rhythm and conduction. Part III is an extensive collection of practice questions and problems for review. In addition, we have interspersed practice questions throughout the text. In reading ECGs, as in learning a new language, fluency is attained only with repetition and review.

The clinical applications of ECG reading have been stressed throughout the book. Each time an abnormal pattern is mentioned, there is a discussion of the conditions that might have produced it. Although this is not intended as a manual of therapeutics, general principles of treatment and clinical management are briefly discussed. Separate chapters are devoted to important special topics, including digitalis toxicity, cardiac arrest, the limitations and uses of the ECG, and pacemakers.

In addition, students are encouraged to approach ECGs in terms of a rational simple differential diagnosis, rather than through the tedium of rote memorization. It is comforting for most students to discover that the number of possible arrhythmias that can produce a heart rate of 170 beats per minute is limited to just a handful of choices. Only three basic ECG patterns are found with cardiac arrest. Similarly, there are only a few causes of low-voltage patterns, of patterns in which the QRS complex is abnormally wide, etc.

In approaching any given ECG, there are always three essential questions. First, what does the ECG show; second, what are the possible causes of this pattern; and, third, what if anything should be done about it? Most conventional ECG books focus on the first question, emphasizing pattern recognition. However, it is only a first step, for example, to diagnose the presence of atrial fibrillation on an ECG. More important questions are . . . what could have caused the arrhythmia and what adverse effects might follow it? Treatment, of course, will depend in part on the answers to these questions.

The aim of this book, therefore, is to present the ECG as it is used on the hospital wards, in the outpatient clinics, and in the intensive care units, where recognition of normal and abnormal patterns is only a starting point in patient management.

The fifth edition contains updated discussions on multiple topics, including arrhythmias and conduction disturbances, myocardial ischemia and infarction, and pacemakers. Furthermore, the review questions throughout the text and the self-assessment problems in Part III have been revised and expanded.

Ary L. Goldberger
Emanuel Goldberger

Contents

I

BASIC PRINCIPLES AND PATTERNS

1

Introductory Principles

DEFINITION

An *electrocardiogram* (ECG or EKG) records cardiac electrical currents (voltages, potentials) by means of metal *electrodes* placed on the surface of the body.* As described in Chapter 3, these metal electrodes are placed on the arms, legs, and chest wall (precordium).

BASIC CARDIAC ELECTROPHYSIOLOGY

Before discussing the basic ECG patterns, we will review some elementary aspects of cardiac electrophysiology. Fortunately, only certain simple principles are required for clinical interpretation of ECGs.

The function of the heart is to contract rhythmically and pump blood to the lungs for oxygenation and then to pump this oxygenated blood into the general (systemic) circulation. The signal for cardiac contraction is the spread of electrical currents through the heart muscle. These currents are produced both by pacemaker cells and specialized conducting tissue within the heart and by the heart muscle itself. The ECG records only the currents produced by the heart muscle.

Electrical Stimulation of the Heart

The electrical "wiring" of the heart is outlined in Figure 1-1. Normally the signal for cardiac electrical stimulation starts in the *sinus node* (also

---

*As discussed in Chapter 3, the electrocardiogram actually records the *differences* in potential between these electrodes.

called the sinoatrial or SA node). The sinus node is located in the right atrium near the opening of the superior vena cava. It is a small collection of specialized cells capable of automatically generating electrical stimuli (signals). From the sinus node, this electrical stimulus spreads first through the right atrium and then into the left atrium. Thus the sinus node functions as the normal *pacemaker* of the heart.

The first phase of cardiac activation consists of the electrical stimulation of right and left atria. This, in turn, signals the atria to contract and to pump blood simultaneously through the tricuspid and mitral valves into the right and left ventricles. The electrical stimulus then spreads to specialized conduction tissues in the *atrioventricular* (AV) *junction* (which includes the *AV node* and *bundle of His)* and then into the *left* and *right bundle branches,* which transmit the stimulus to the ventricular muscle cells.

The AV junction, which acts as a sort of electrical "bridge" connecting the atria and ventricles, is located at the base of the interatrial septum and extends into the interventricular septum (Fig. 1-1). It has two subdivisions: The upper (proximal) part is the AV node. (In some texts the terms "AV node" and "AV junction" are used synonymously.) The lower (distal) part is called the bundle of His, after the physiologist who described it. The bundle of His then divides into two main branches: the right bundle branch, which distributes the stimulus to the right ventricle, and the left bundle

CONDUCTION SYSTEM OF THE HEART

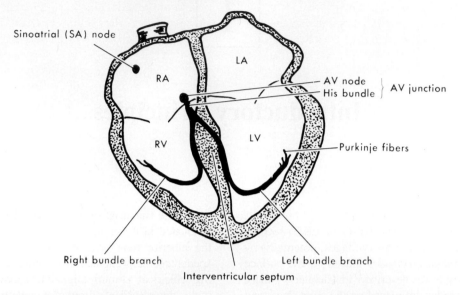

Fig. 1-1. Normally the cardiac stimulus is generated in the *SA node* (located in the right atrium, *RA*). It then spreads through the *RA* and *LA* (right and left atria). Next, it spreads through the *AV node* and *His bundle,* which comprise the *AV junction.* It then passes into the left and right ventricles *(LV* and *RV)* by way of the *left* and *right bundle branches,* which are continuations of the His bundle. Finally, it spreads to the ventricular muscle cells through the *Purkinje fibers.*

branch,* which distributes it to the left ventricle (Fig. 1-1).

The electrical stimulus spreads simultaneously down the left and right bundle branches into the ventricular muscle itself *(ventricular myocardium)* by way of specialized conducting cells, called *Purkinje fibers,* located in the ventricular myocardium.

Under normal circumstances, when the sinus node is pacing the heart (normal sinus rhythm), the AV junction appears to serve primarily as a shuttle, directing the electrical stimulus into the ventricles. However, under some circumstances the AV junction can also act as an independent pacemaker of the heart. For example, if the sinus node

---

*The left bundle branch divides into two major subbranches called *fascicles* (which are discussed in Chapter 7 along with the "hemiblocks").

fails to function properly, the AV junction can act as an *escape* pacemaker. In such cases an AV junctional rhythm (and *not* sinus rhythm) is present. This produces a distinct ECG pattern (described in Chapter 12).

Just as the spread of electrical stimuli through the atria leads to atrial contraction, so the spread of stimuli through the ventricles leads to ventricular contraction with pumping of blood to the lungs and into the general circulation.

Cardiac Conductivity and Automaticity

The speed with which electrical impulses are conducted through different parts of the heart varies. For example, conduction is *slowest* through the AV node and *fastest* through the Purkinje fibers. The relatively slow conduction speed through the AV node is of functional importance because it allows the ventricles time to fill with blood before the signal for cardiac contraction arrives.

In addition to *conductivity,* another major electrical feature of the heart is *automaticity.* Automaticity refers to the capacity of certain cardiac cells to function as pacemakers, to generate electrical impulses spontaneously that spread throughout the heart. Normally, as mentioned earlier, the sinus node is the primary pacemaker of the heart because of its inherent automaticity. Under special conditions, however, other cells outside the sinus node (in the atria, AV junction, or ventricles) can also act as independent pacemakers. For example, if the automaticity of the sinus node is depressed, the AV junction can act as a secondary or escape pacemaker.

The term "sick sinus syndrome" (Chapter 18) is used clinically to describe patients who have severe depression of sinus node function. Such individuals may experience light-headedness or even syncope (fainting) due to their excessive *bradycardia.* The sick sinus syndrome and other causes of bradycardia are discussed in Part II of this book, in the section on cardiac arrhythmias.

In other conditions the automaticity of pacemakers outside the sinus node may be abnormally increased, and these *ectopic* (non-sinus) pacemakers may compete with the sinus node for control of the heartbeat. A rapid run of ectopic beats results in an abnormal *tachycardia.* Ectopy is also discussed in detail in Part II of this book.

If you understand the normal physiologic stimulation of the heart, you have the basis for understanding the abnormalities of heart rhythm and conduction that produce distinctive ECG patterns. For example, failure of the sinus node to stimulate the heart properly can result in various rhythm disturbances associated with the sick sinus syndrome. Blockage of the spread of stimuli through the AV junction can produce various degrees of AV heart block (Chapter 15). Disease of the bundle branches can produce left or right bundle branch block (Chapter 7). Finally, any disease process that involves the ventricular muscle itself (e.g., destruction of the heart muscle by myocardial infarction) can produce marked changes in the normal ECG patterns.

The first part of this book therefore is devoted to explaining the basis of the normal ECG, followed by a detailed look at major conditions causing abnormal P, QRS, and T* patterns. The second part of the book is devoted to describing the various abnormal rhythms (arrhythmias) and AV conduction disturbances that can occur. The third part of the book is a collection of review questions and examples. A short selective bibliography is provided at the end of the text.

---

*P, QRS, and T are defined in Chapter 2.

REVIEW

An *electrocardiogram (ECG or EKG)* records the electrical voltages (potentials) produced in the heart. It does this by means of metal *electrodes* (connected to an electrocardiograph) placed on the patient's chest wall and extremities. The potentials recorded by the ECG are produced by the atrial and ventricular muscle fibers themselves.

Normally, the cardiac stimulus starts in pacemaker cells of the *sinus (sinoatrial or SA) node,* located high in the right atrium near the superior vena cava. From here it spreads downward and to the left, through the right and left atria, and reaches the *atrioventricular (AV) node,* located near the top of the interventricular septum (Fig. 1-1). After a delay, the stimulus spreads through the *AV junction (AV node* and *bundle of His).* The bundle of His then subdivides into *right* and *left bundle branches.* The *right* bundle branch runs down the interventricular septum and into the right ventricle. From there the small *Purkinje fibers* rapidly distribute the stimulus outward into the main muscle mass of the right ventricle. Simultaneously, the *left* main bundle branch carries the stimulus down the interventricular septum to the muscle mass of the left ventricle, also by way of the Purkinje fibers.

This repetitive sequence of stimulation of the heart is the normal basic process. Disturbances in it may produce abnormalities of heart rhythm (the cardiac *arrhythmias*).

Questions

1. Label the major parts of the cardiac conduction system in this diagram and then trace the spread of the normal cardiac stimulus from atria to ventricles.

2. What, essentially, is an electrocardiogram?

Answers

1. See Figure 1-1.
2. A graphical record of cardiac electrical activity obtained by means of electrodes placed on the surface of the body.

2

Basic ECG Waves

DEPOLARIZATION AND REPOLARIZATION

In Chapter 1 we used the general term "electrical stimulation" to refer to the spread of electrical stimuli through the atria and ventricles. The technical term for this cardiac electrical stimulation is *"depolarization."* The return of heart muscle cells to their resting state following stimulation (depolarization) is called *"repolarization."* These terms are derived from the fact that the normal "resting" myocardial cells (atrial and ventricular) are *polarized;* that is, they carry electrical charges on their surface. Figure 2-1, *A,* shows the resting polarized state of a normal atrial or ventricular heart muscle cell. Notice that the outside of the resting cell is positive and the inside is negative (about −90 mV).*

When a heart muscle cell is stimulated, it depolarizes. As a result the outside of the cell, in the area where the stimulation has occurred, becomes negative while the inside of the cell becomes positive. This produces a difference in electrical voltage on the outside surface of the cell between the stimulated depolarized area and the unstimulated polarized area (Fig. 2-1, *B*). As a result a small electrical current is formed that spreads along the

*Membrane polarization is due to differences in the concentration of ions inside and outside the cell. For references that present the electrophysiology of the *resting membrane potential* and *cellular depolarization and repolarization* (the action potential), refer to the Bibliography.

length of the cell as stimulation and depolarization occur until the entire cell is depolarized (Fig. 2-1, *C*). The path of depolarization can be represented by an arrow, as shown in Figure 2-1. For individual myocardial cells (fibers) depolarization and repolarization proceed in the same direction. However, for the entire myocardium depolarization proceeds from innermost layer (endocardium) to outermost layer (epicardium) while repolarization proceeds in the opposite direction. The mechanism of this difference is not well understood.

The depolarizing electrical current is recorded by the ECG as a *P wave* (when the atria are stimulated and depolarize) and as a *QRS complex* (when the ventricles are stimulated and depolarize).

After a time, the fully stimulated and depolarized cell begins to return to the resting state. This is known as repolarization. A small area on the outside of the cell becomes positive again (Fig. 2-1, *D*), and the repolarization spreads along the length of the cell until the entire cell is once again fully repolarized. Ventricular repolarization is recorded by the ECG as the *ST segment, T wave,* and *U wave.* (Atrial repolarization is usually obscured by ventricular potentials.)

The ECG records the electrical activity of a large mass of atrial and ventricular cells, not that of just a single cell. Since cardiac depolarization and repolarization normally occur in a synchronized fashion, the ECG is able to record these electrical currents as specific waves (P wave, QRS

POLARIZED RESTING CELL

DEPOLARIZING CELL

DEPOLARIZED CELL

REPOLARIZING CELL

Fig. 2-1. Depolarization and repolarization. The resting heart muscle cell, **A,** is polarized; that is, it carries an electrical charge, with the outside of the cell positively charged and the inside negatively charged. When the cell is stimulated *(S),* as in **B,** it begins to depolarize *(stippled area).* The fully depolarized cell, **C,** is positively charged on the inside and negatively charged on the outside. Repolarization, **D,** occurs when the stimulated cell returns to the resting state. The direction of depolarization and repolarization is represented by *arrows.* Depolarization (stimulation) of the atria produces the P wave on the ECG, whereas depolarization of the ventricles produces the QRS complex. Repolarization of the ventricles produces the ST-T complex.

complex, ST segment, T wave, and U wave).

To summarize: Regardless of whether the ECG is normal or abnormal, it records just two basic events: (1) depolarization, the spread of a stimulus through the heart muscle, and (2) repolarization, the return of the stimulated heart muscle to the resting state.

BASIC ECG COMPLEXES: P, QRS, ST, T, AND U WAVES

The spread of stimuli through the atria and ventricles followed by the return of stimulated atrial and ventricular muscle to the resting state produces the electrical currents recorded on the ECG. Furthermore, each phase of cardiac electrical activity produces a specific wave or complex (Fig. 2-2). These basic ECG waves are labeled alphabetically and begin with the P wave.

P wave:	atrial depolarization (stimulation)
QRS complex:	ventricular depolarization (stimulation)
ST segment ⎫	
T wave ⎬	ventricular repolarization
U wave ⎭	(recovery)

The P wave represents the spread of a stimulus through the atria (atrial depolarization). The QRS complex represents stimulus spread through the ventricles (ventricular depolarization). The ST segment and T wave represent the return of stimulated ventricular muscle to the resting state (ventricular repolarization). The U wave is a small deflection sometimes seen just after the T wave. It represents the final phase of ventricular repolarization, although its exact mechanism is not known.

You are probably wondering why there is no wave or complex representing the return of stimulated atria to their resting state. The answer is that the atrial ST segment (STa) and atrial T wave (Ta) are generally not observed on the normal ECG because of their low amplitudes. (An important exception is described in Chapter 10 in the discussion of pericarditis.) Similarly, the routine ECG is not sensitive enough to record any electrical activity during the spread of stimuli through the AV junction (AV node and bundle of His). The spread of electrical stimuli through the AV junction occurs between the beginning of the P wave and the

BASIC ECG COMPLEXES

Fig. 2-2. The P wave represents atrial depolarization. The PR interval is the time from initial stimulation of the atria to initial stimulation of the ventricles. The QRS represents ventricular depolarization. The ST segment, T wave, and U wave are produced by ventricular repolarization.

Fig. 2-3. Cardiac cycle. The basic cycle (P-QRS-T) repeats itself again and again.

beginning of the QRS complex. This interval, known as the PR interval, is a measure of the time it takes for the stimuli to spread through the atria and pass through the AV junction.

To summarize: The P-QRS-T sequence represents the repetitive cycle of the electrical activity in the heart, beginning with the spread of a stimulus through the atria (P wave) and ending with the return of stimulated ventricular muscle to its resting state (ST-T sequence). As shown in the rhythm strip in Figure 2-3, this cardiac cycle repeats itself again and again.

ECG PAPER

The P-QRS-T sequence is recorded on special ECG graph paper (Figs. 2-3 and 2-4). This paper is divided into gridlike boxes. Each of the small boxes is 1 millimeter square (1 mm^2). The paper usually moves at a speed of 25 mm/sec. Therefore, horizontally, each unit represents 0.04 second (25 mm/sec × 0.04 sec = 1 mm). Notice also that between every five boxes there are heavier lines, so each of the 5 mm units horizontally corresponds to 0.2 second (5 × 0.04 = 0.2).

The ECG can therefore be regarded as a mov-

Fig. 2-4. ECG paper is a graph divided into millimeter squares. Time is measured on the horizontal axis. With a paper speed of 25 mm/sec, each small (millimeter) box side equals 0.04 second and each larger (5 mm) box side equals 0.2 second. The amplitude of any wave is measured on the vertical axis in millimeters.

ing graph that horizontally corresponds to time, with 0.04 and 0.2 second divisions. Vertically the ECG graph measures the voltages, or amplitudes, of the ECG waves or deflections. The exact voltages can be measured because the electrocardiograph is standardized (calibrated) so a 1 millivolt signal produces a deflection of 10 mm amplitude (1 mV = 10 mm). (In most electrocardiographs the standardization can also be set at one-half or two times normal sensitivity.)

BASIC ECG MEASUREMENTS AND SOME NORMAL VALUES
Standardization Mark

The electrocardiograph must be properly calibrated so a 1 mV signal produces a 10 mm deflection. The unit may have a special standardization button that produces a 1 mV wave. As shown in Figure 2-5, the standardization mark (St) produced when the machine is correctly calibrated is a square wave 10 mm tall. If the machine is not standardized correctly, the 1 mV signal will produce a deflection either more or less than 10 mm

and the amplitudes of the P, QRS, and T deflections will be larger or smaller than they should. The standardization deflection is also important because standardization can be varied in most electrocardiographs (Fig. 2-5). When very large deflections are present (as occurs, for example, in some patients who have an electronic pacemaker that produces very large spikes), it may be advisable to take the ECG at half standardization to avoid damaging the stylus and to get the entire tracing on the paper. If the ECG complexes are very small, it may be advisable to double the standardization (e.g., to study a small Q wave more thoroughly). The standardization need be set only once on an ECG—just before the first lead is recorded.*

Because the ECG is calibrated, we can describe any part of the P, QRS, and T deflections in two

---

*Some electronic electrocardiographs do not display the calibration pulse. Instead, they print the paper speed and standardization at the bottom of the ECG paper (25 mm/sec, 10 mm/mV).

Fig. 2-5. Standardization mark. Before taking an ECG, the operator must check to see that the machine is properly calibrated such that the 1 mV standardization mark is 10 mm tall, **A.** Electrocardiographs can also be set at half standardization, **B,** or 2× standardization, **C.**

ways. We can measure the amplitude (voltage) of any of the deflections, and we can also measure the width (duration) of any of the deflections. We can therefore measure the amplitude and width of the P wave, the amplitude and width of the QRS complex, the amplitude of the ST segment deviation (if present), and the amplitude of the T wave. For clinical purposes, if the standardization is set at 1 mV = 10 mm, the height of a wave is usually recorded in millimeters and not in millivolts. For example, in Figure 2-3, the P wave is 1 mm in amplitude, the QRS complex is 8 mm, and the T wave is about 3.5 mm.

In describing the amplitude of any wave or deflection, it is also necessary to specify if it is positive or negative. By convention, an *upward* deflection or wave is called *positive*. A *downward* deflection or wave is called *negative*. A deflection or wave that rests on the baseline is said to be *isoelectric*. A deflection that is partly positive and partly negative is call *biphasic*. For example, in Figure 2-6 the P wave is positive, the QRS complex is biphasic (initially positive, then negative), the ST segment is isoelectric (flat on the baseline), and the T wave is negative.

In this chapter we look at the P, QRS, ST, T, and U waves in a general way and the measurement of heart rate, PR interval, QRS width, QT interval, and their normal values in detail.

P Wave

The P wave, which represents atrial depolarization, is a small positive (or negative) deflection be-

Fig. 2-6. Positive and negative complexes. The P wave here is positive (upward), and the T wave is negative (downward). The QRS complex is biphasic (partly positive, partly negative), and the ST segment isoelectric (neither positive nor negative).

fore the QRS complex. The normal values for P wave amplitude and width are described in Chapter 6.

PR Interval

The PR interval is measured from the beginning of the P wave to the beginning of the QRS complex (Fig. 2-7). The PR interval may vary slightly in different leads, and the shortest PR interval should be noted. The PR interval represents the time it takes for the stimulus to spread through the atria and to pass through the AV junction. (This physiologic delay allows the ventricles to fill fully

Fig. 2-7. Measurement of the PR interval. See text.

with blood before ventricular depolarization occurs.) *In adults the normal PR interval is between 0.12 and 0.2 second (three to five small box sides).* When conduction through the AV junction is impaired, the PR interval may become prolonged. Prolongation of the PR interval above 0.2 second is called *first-degree heart block* and is discussed in Chapter 15.

QRS Nomenclature

One of the most confusing aspects of electrocardiography for the beginning student is the nomenclature of the QRS complex. The QRS complex, as noted previously, represents the spread of a stimulus through the ventricles. However, not every QRS complex contains a Q wave, an R wave, and an S wave; hence the confusion. This bothersome but unavoidable nomenclature becomes understandable if you remember the following (Fig. 2-8): When the initial deflection of the QRS complex is negative (below the baseline), it is called a Q wave. The first positive deflection in the QRS complex is called an R wave. A negative deflection following the R wave is called an S wave. Thus this QRS complex $\left(\begin{array}{c}R\\ \bigwedge\\ Q\ \ S\end{array}\right)$ contains a Q wave, an R wave, and an S wave. This one $\left(\begin{array}{c}R\\ \bigwedge\\ S\end{array}\right)$ does

not. If the entire QRS complex is positive, it is simply called an R wave. However, if the entire complex is negative, it is termed a QS wave (not just a Q wave as you might expect). Occasionally the QRS complex will contain more than two or three deflections, and in such cases the extra waves are called R′ (R prime) waves if they are positive and S′ (S prime) waves if they are negative. Fig. 2-8 shows the various possible QRS complexes and the nomenclature of the respective waves. Notice that capital letters (QRS) are used to designate waves of relatively large amplitude while small letters (qrs) label relatively small waves (Fig. 2-8).

This nomenclature is confusing at first, but it allows you to describe any QRS complex over the phone and to evoke in the mind of the trained listener an exact mental picture of the complex named. For example, in describing an ECG you might say that lead V_1 showed an rS complex $\left(\begin{array}{c}r\\ \bigvee\\ S\end{array}\right)$ ("small r, capital S") while lead aV_F showed a QS wave $\left(\begin{array}{c}\bigvee\\ QS\end{array}\right)$.

QRS Width (Interval)

The QRS width (Fig. 2-9) represents the time required for a stimulus to spread through the ventricles (ventricular depolarization) and is normally

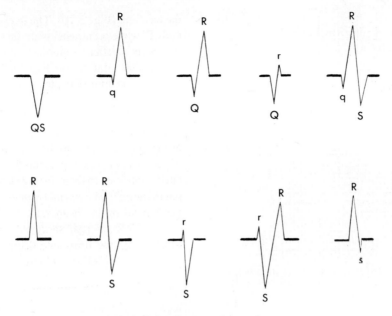

Fig. 2-8. QRS nomenclature. See text.

0.1 second or less. If the spread of stimulus through the ventricles is slowed, for example, by a block in one of the bundle branches, the QRS width will be prolonged. (The full differential diagnosis of a wide QRS is discussed on page 140.)

ST Segment

The ST segment is that portion of the ECG cycle from the end of the QRS complex to the beginning of the T wave (Fig. 2-10). It represents the beginning of ventricular repolarization. The normal ST segment is usually *isoelectric* (i.e., flat on the baseline, neither positive nor negative), but it may be slightly elevated or depressed normally (usually by less than 1 mm). Some pathologic conditions, such as myocardial infarction, produce characteristic abnormal deviations of the ST segment. The very beginning of the ST segment (actually the junction between the end of the QRS complex and the beginning of the ST segment) is

Fig. 2-9. Measurement of the QRS width. See text.

Fig. 2-10. Characteristics of the normal ST segment and T wave. *J,* Junction, marks the beginning of the ST segment.

Fig. 2-11. ST segments. **A,** Normal. **B,** Abnormal elevation. **C,** Abnormal depression.

sometimes called the J point. Figure 2-10 shows the J point and the normal shape of the ST segment. Figure 2-11 compares a normal isoelectric ST segment with abnormal ST segment elevation and ST segment depression. ·

T Wave

The T wave represents part of ventricular repolarization. A normal T wave has an asymmetric shape; that is, its peak is closer to the end of the wave than to the beginning (Fig. 2-10). When the T wave is positive, it normally rises slowly and then abruptly returns to the baseline.* When it is negative, it descends slowly and abruptly rises to

*The exact point at which the ST segment ends and the T wave begins is arbitrary and sometimes impossible to define.

the baseline (Fig. 2-10). The *asymmetry* of the normal T wave contrasts with the symmetry of T waves in certain abnormal conditions, such as myocardial infarction (Chapters 8 and 9) and high serum potassium (Chapter 10).

QT Interval

The QT interval is measured from the beginning of the QRS complex to the end of the T wave (Fig. 2-12). It primarily represents the return of stimulated ventricles to their resting state (ventricular repolarization). The normal values for the QT interval depend on the heart rate. As the heart rate increases (RR interval shortens), the QT normally shortens; as the heart rate decreases (RR interval lengthens), the QT lengthens.

The QT should be measured in ECG leads (Chapter 3) that show the largest-amplitude T waves. You should measure several intervals and use the average value. The QT is often difficult to measure when it is long because the end of the T wave may merge imperceptibly with the U wave. As a result you may be measuring the QU interval rather than the QT.

Table 2-1 shows the upper normal limits for the QT interval with different heart rates. Unfortunately, there is no simple rule for calculating the normal limits of the QT interval.

Because of this problem, another index of the QT has been devised. It is the *rate-corrected* QT or QT_c. The rate-corrected QT is obtained by dividing the actual QT by the square root of the RR interval (both measured in seconds):

$$QT_c = \frac{QT}{\sqrt{RR}}$$

Normally the QT_c is less than or equal to 0.44 second.

There are a number of factors that can abnormally prolong the QT interval (Fig. 2-13). For example, certain drugs (e.g., quinidine, procainamide, disopyramide, sotalol, amiodarone) and electrolyte disturbances (a low serum potassium or low serum calcium) can prolong it. Hypothermia also prolongs it, by slowing the repolarization of myocardial cells. The QT may be prolonged with myocardial ischemia and infarction and with subarachnoid hemorrhage. QT prolongation may predispose patients to potentially lethal ventricular arrhythmias. (See the discussion of torsade de pointes, Chapter 14.)

The QT interval may also be shortened, for example, by digitalis in therapeutic doses or by hypercalcemia. The lower limits of normal for the QT have not been well defined, so only the upper limits are given in Table 2-1.

U Wave

The U wave is a small rounded deflection sometimes seen after the T wave (Fig. 2-2). As noted previously, its exact significance is not known. Functionally U waves represent the last phase of ventricular repolarization. Prominent U waves are characteristic of hypokalemia (Chapter 10). Very prominent U waves may also be seen in other settings, for example, in patients taking drugs such as quinidine or one of the phenothiazines, or sometimes after a cerebrovascular accident. The appearance of very prominent U waves in such settings, with or without actual QT prolongation, may also predispose patients to ventricular arrhythmias (p. 188).

Normally the direction of the U wave is the same as that of the T wave. Negative U waves sometimes appear with positive T waves. This is abnormal and has been noted in left ventricular hypertrophy and myocardial ischemia.

Calculation of Heart Rate

There are two simple methods for measuring the heart rate (number of heartbeats per minute) from the ECG.

1. The easier way, when the heart rate is regular, is to count the number of large (0.2 sec) boxes between two successive QRS complexes and

Table 2-1. QT Interval: Upper Limits of Normal

Measured RR Interval (sec)	Heart Rate (per min)	QT Interval Upper Normal Limits (sec)
1.50	40	0.50
1.20	50	0.45
1.00	60	0.42
0.86	70	0.40
0.80	75	0.38
0.75	80	0.37
0.67	90	0.35
0.60	100	0.34
0.50	120	0.31
0.40	150	0.25

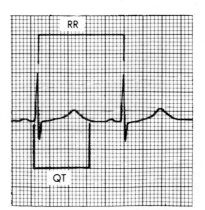

Fig. 2-13. Abnormal QT prolongation in a patient taking quinidine. The QT interval (0.6 sec) is markedly prolonged for the heart rate (65/min). See Table 2-1. The rate-corrected QT (normally 0.44 or less) is also prolonged (0.63).*

Fig. 2-12. Measurement of the QT interval. *RR* is the interval between two consecutive QRS complexes. See text.

*In Figure 2-13, find the QT_c:

$$\frac{QT}{\sqrt{RR}} = \frac{0.60}{\sqrt{0.92}} = 0.63$$

Fig. 2-14. Measurement of heart rate (beats per minute) by counting the number of large (0.2 sec) time boxes between two successive QRS complexes and dividing 300 by this number. In this example the heart rate is $300 \div 4 = 75$ beats/min.

divide a constant (300) by this. (The number of large time boxes is divided into 300, because $300 \times 0.2 = 60$ and we are calculating the heart rate in beats per minute or 60 seconds.)

For example, in Figure 2-14 the heart rate is 100 beats/min, since there are three large time boxes between successive R waves ($300 \div 3 = 100$). Similarly, if there are two large time boxes between successive R waves, the heart rate is 150 beats/min. If there are five intervening large time boxes, the heart rate is 60 beats/min.

When it is necessary to measure the heart rate very accurately from the ECG, you can use the following modification of the above rule: Count the number of small (0.04 sec) boxes between successive R waves and divide a constant (1500) by this number. In Figure 2-14 there are 15 small time boxes between QRS complexes. Therefore the heart rate is $1500 \div 15 = 100$ beats/min. (The constant 1500 is used since $1500 \times 0.04 = 60$ and we are calculating the heart rate in beats per 60 seconds.)

2. If the heart rate is irregular, the first method will not be accurate since the intervals between QRS complexes will vary from beat to beat. In such cases an average rate can be determined simply by counting the number of cardiac *cycles* every 6 seconds and multiplying this number by 10 (Fig. 2-15). (A cardiac cycle is the interval be-

tween two successive R waves.) Counting the number of cardiac cycles every 6 seconds can be easily done because the top of the ECG paper, as shown in Figure 2-14, is generally scored with vertical marks every 3 seconds.

By definition, a heart rate exceeding 100 beats/min is termed "tachycardia" (*tachys,* Greek, swift) while one slower than 60 beats/min is called "bradycardia" (*bradys,* slow). Thus, during exercise you probably develop a sinus tachycardia but during sleep or relaxation your pulse rate may drop into the 50s, or even lower, indicating a sinus bradycardia.

THE ECG AS A COMBINATION OF ATRIAL AND VENTRICULAR ELECTROCARDIOGRAMS

The ECG we have been discussing really consists of two separate but normally related parts: an atrial ECG, represented by the P wave, and a ventricular ECG, represented by the QRS-T sequence. With normal sinus rhythm, when the sinus node is pacing the heart, the P wave (atrial stimulation or depolarization) will always precede the QRS complex (ventricular stimulation or depolarization) because the atria are first to be electrically stimulated. Therefore we normally consider the P-QRS-T cycle as a unit. However, as we shall see later on, in some abnormal conditions the atria and the ventricles can be stimulated by separate pacemakers. For example, suppose that the AV junction is diseased and stimuli cannot pass from the atria to the ventricles. In such cases a new (subsidiary) pacemaker located below the level of the block in the AV junction may take over the task of pacing the ventricles while the sinus node continues to pace the atria. In this case, stimulation of the atria is independent of stimulation of the ventricles, and the P waves and QRS complexes have no relation to each other. This type of arrhythmia is called *complete heart block* and is described in detail in Chapter 15. Figure 15-5 shows an example of this abnormal condition, in which the atrial and ventricular ECGs are independent of each other.

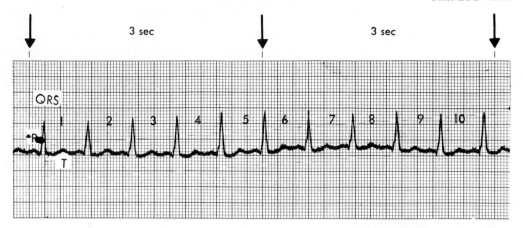

Fig. 2-15. Measurement of heart rate (beats per minute) by counting the number of cardiac cycles in a 6-second interval and multiplying by 10. In this example there are 10 cardiac cycles/6 sec. Therefore the heart rate is 10 × 10 = 100 beats/min.

THE ECG IN PERSPECTIVE

Up to this point we have considered only the basic components of the ECG. Several general items need to be emphasized before we proceed with our discussion of actual ECG patterns:

First, it is always necessary to remember that the ECG is a recording of cardiac *electrical* activity. It does not directly measure the *mechanical* function of the heart, that is, how well the heart is contracting and performing as a pump. Thus a patient with acute pulmonary edema may have a normal ECG. Conversely, a patient with a grossly abnormal ECG may have normal cardiac function.

Furthermore, the ECG does not directly depict abnormalities in cardiac structure, such as ventricular septal defects or abnormalities of the heart valves. It only records the electrical changes produced by structural defects. However, in some cases we can infer a specific structural diagnosis such as mitral stenosis, pulmonary embolism, or myocardial infarction from the ECG because typical electrical abnormalities may develop in such patients.

Finally, it is necessary to remember that the ECG does not record *all* the heart's electrical activity. The electrodes placed on the surface of the body record only those currents transmitted to the area of electrode placement. Therefore there are actually "silent" electrical areas of the heart. For example, the ECG is not sensitive enough to record depolarization of pacemaker cells *in* the sinus node occurring just before the P wave. Repolarization of the atria, as noted earlier, is generally not recorded by the conventional electrocardiograph. (See page 131 for an important exception.) Also the spread of stimuli through the AV junction is not detected by the conventional ECG. The electrical activity of the AV junction can be recorded using a special apparatus and a special electrode placed in the heart *(His bundle electrogram)*. In addition, remember that the ECG records the summation of electrical potentials produced by innumerable cardiac muscle cells. Therefore the presence of a normal ECG does not necessarily mean that all these heart muscle cells are being depolarized and repolarized in a normal way.

For these reasons the ECG must be regarded as any other laboratory test, with proper consideration for both its uses and its limitations. (See Chapter 19.)

In Chapter 3 we will look first at the 12 ECG leads and then proceed with a discussion of normal and abnormal ECG patterns.

REVIEW

The ECG, whether normal or abnormal, records the following two basic physiologic processes: (1) *Depolarization* (the spread of stimulus through the heart muscle) produces the P wave from the atria and the QRS complex from the ventricles. (2) *Repolarization* (the return of stimulated muscle to the resting state) produces the atrial ST segment and T wave (which are ordinarily not seen on the ECG) and the ventricular ST segment, T wave, and U wave.

ECGs are recorded on special paper that is divided into gridlike boxes (Fig. 2-4). Each small box is 1 mm^2. Each millimeter horizontally represents 0.04 second. Each 0.2 second is denoted by a heavier vertical line. ECG deflections are usually standardized so a 1 mV signal produces a 10 mm deflection. Therefore, each millimeter vertically represents 0.1 mV. Each 5 mm interval is denoted by a heavier horizontal line.

Four basic intervals are measured on the ECG:

1. *PR interval*. The PR interval is measured from the beginning of the P wave to the beginning of the QRS complex. The normal PR interval varies from 0.12 to 0.2 second.
2. *QRS interval*. The normal QRS width is 0.1 second or less. Description of the QRS complex is shown in Fig. 2-8.
3. *QT interval*. The QT interval is measured from the beginning of the QRS complex to the end of the T wave. It varies with the heart rate, becoming shorter as the heart rate increases.
4. *Heart rate (based on R-R intervals)*. The heart rate can be calculated in two ways:

    METHOD 1. Count the number of large (0.2 sec) time boxes between two successive R waves and divide the constant 300 by this number (Fig. 2-14). If you want a more accurate measurement of the rate, divide the constant 1500 by the number of small (0.04 sec) time boxes between two successive R waves.

    METHOD 2. Count the number of cardiac cycles that occur every 6 seconds and multiply this number by 10 (Fig. 2-15). A vertical mark may be present on the top of the ECG paper every 3 seconds. A cardiac cycle is the interval between two successive QRS complexes.

A heart rate slower than 60 beats/min is called *bradycardia;* a rate faster than 100 beats/min is called *tachycardia*.

Questions

1. Calculate the heart rate in each of the following examples:

A

2. Name the major abnormality in each example.

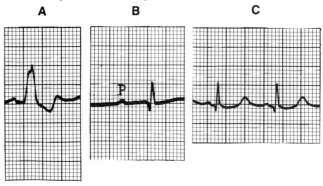

3. A block in the AV node is most likely to do which of the following?
   a. Prolong the PR
   b. Prolong the QRS
   c. Prolong the QT
   d. None of the above

4. A block in the left or right bundle branch is most likely to do which of the following?
   a. Prolong the PR
   b. Prolong the QRS
   c. Shorten the QT
   d. None of the above

5. Name the component waves of the QRS complexes shown below.

6. Name four factors that may prolong the QT interval.

Answers

1. a. 50 beats/min.
   b. 150 beats/min.
   c. 60 beats/min.
   d. Approximately 160 beats/min. (There are 16 QRS cycles in 6 seconds.*)

2. a. Abnormally wide QRS complex (0.14 sec).
   b. Abnormally long PR interval (approximately 0.3 sec).
   c. Abnormally long QT interval (0.4 sec). The RR measures 0.6 second, and the heart rate is 100 beats/min. (See Table 2-1.) The rate-corrected QT ($QT_c = QT/\sqrt{RR}$ is also prolonged, at 0.77 (0.4/0.6). Normal is ≤ 0.44.

3. a.

4. b

5. a. R wave.
   b. qRS complex.
   c. QS complex
   d. RSR′ complex.
   e. QR complex.

6. Drugs (quinidine, procainamide, disopyramide, sotalol, amiodarone), electrolyte abnormalities (hypocalcemia, hypokalemia), hypothermia, myocardial infarction.

---

*Notice the irregularity of the QRS complexes and the absence of P waves. This rhythm is *atrial fibrillation* (Chapter 13).

3

ECG Leads

In Chapter 1 we saw that the heart produces electrical currents similar to the familiar dry cell battery. The strength or voltage of these currents and the way they are distributed throughout the body can be measured by a suitable recording instrument, such as an electrocardiograph.

The body acts as a conductor of electricity. Therefore recording electrodes placed at some distance from the heart, such as on the arms, legs, or chest wall, are able to detect the voltages of the cardiac currents conducted to these locations. The usual way of recording these voltages from the heart is with the 12 standard ECG *leads*. The leads actually show the *differences* in voltage (potential) between electrodes placed on the surface of the body.

Taking an ECG is like drawing a picture or taking a photograph of a person. If we want to know what a person's face really looks like, for example, we have to draw it or take photographs from the front, side, and back. One view is not enough. Similarly, it is necessary to record multiple ECG leads to be able to describe the electrical activity of the heart adequately. Figure 3-1 shows the various ECG patterns that are obtained when electrodes are placed at varying points on the chest. Notice that each lead presents a different pattern.

Figure 3-2 is an ECG illustrating the 12 leads. The leads can be subdivided into two groups: the six *extremity* (limb) leads (shown in the left two columns) and the six chest (precordial) leads (shown in the right two columns).

The six extremity leads—I, II, III, aV_R, aV_L, and aV_F—record voltage differences by means of electrodes placed on the limbs. They can be further divided into two subgroups: the *bipolar* extremity leads (I, II, and III) and the *unipolar* extremity leads (aV_R, aV_L, and aV_F).

The six chest leads—V_1, V_2, V_3, V_4, V_5, and V_6—record voltage differences by means of electrodes placed at various positions of the chest wall.

The 12 ECG leads can also be viewed as 12 "channels." However, in contrast to television channels (which can be tuned to different events), the 12 ECG channels (leads) are all tuned to the *same* event (the P-QRS-T cycle), with each lead viewing the event from a different angle.

EXTREMITY (LIMB) LEADS
Bipolar Leads (I, II, and III)

We will begin with the extremity leads, since they are recorded first. In connecting a patient to an electrocardiograph, first place metal electrodes on the arms and legs. The right leg electrode functions solely as an electrical ground, so you need concern yourself with it no further. As shown in Figure 3-3, the arm electrodes are attached just above the wrist and the leg electrodes above the ankles.

The electrical voltages of the heart are conducted through the torso to the extremities. Therefore an electrode placed on the right wrist will detect electrical voltages equivalent to those recorded below the right shoulder. Similarly, the voltages

Fig. 3-1. Multiple chest leads give a three-dimensional view of cardiac electrical activity.

detected at the left wrist or anywhere else on the left arm will be equivalent to those recorded below the left shoulder. Finally, voltages detected by the left leg electrode will be comparable to those at the left thigh or near the groin. In clinical practice the electrodes are attached to the wrists and ankles simply for convenience.*

As mentioned, the extremity leads consist of two groups: the bipolar (I, II, and III) and the unipolar (aV_R, aV_L, and aV_F) leads. The bipolar leads are so named because the differences in electrical voltage between two extremities are recorded by them.

Lead I, for example, records the difference in voltage between the left arm (LA) and right arm (RA) electrodes.

$$\text{Lead I} = \text{LA} - \text{RA}$$

*Obviously, if you are taking an ECG on an amputee or someone with a cast, you will have to place the electrodes below or near the shoulders or groin depending on the circumstance.

Fig. 3-2. A, Sample ECG showing the 12 standard leads. **B,** A lead II rhythm strip. What is the approximate heart rate? (Answer: 55-60/min.)

Lead II records the difference between the left leg (LL) and right arm (RA) electrodes.

Lead II = LL − RA

Lead III records the difference between the left leg (LL) and left arm (LA) electrodes.

Lead III = LL − LA

Consider then what happens when you turn on the electrocardiograph to lead I. The LA electrode detects the electrical voltages of the heart transmitted to the left arm. The RA electrode detects the voltages transmitted to the right arm. Inside the electrocardiograph the RA voltages are subtracted from the LA voltages and the difference appears at lead I. When lead II is recorded, a similar situation occurs between the voltages of LL and RA. When lead III is recorded, the same occurs between the voltages of LL and LA.

Leads I, II, and III can be represented schematically in terms of a triangle, called *Einthoven's triangle* (after the Dutch physician who invented the electrocardiograph in the early 1900s). At first the ECG consisted only of recordings from leads I, II, and III. Einthoven's triangle (Fig. 3-4) shows the spatial orientation of the three bipolar extremity leads (I, II, and III). As you can see, lead I points horizontally. Its left pole (LA) is positive and its right pole (RA) is negative. Therefore lead I = LA − RA. Lead II points diagonally downward. Its lower pole (LL) is positive and its upper pole (RA) is negative. Therefore lead II = LL − RA. Lead III also points diagonally downward. Its lower pole (LL) is positive and its upper pole (LA) is negative. Therefore lead III = LL − LA.

Einthoven, of course, could have hooked the leads up differently; but because of the way he arranged them, the bipolar leads are related by the following simple equation:

Lead I + Lead III = Lead II

In other words, add the voltage in lead I to that in lead III and you get the voltage in lead II.* You can test this equation by looking at Figure 3-2. Add the voltage of the R wave in lead I (+9 mm) to the voltage of the R wave in lead III (+4 mm)

Fig. 3-3. Metal electrodes strapped on the patient to take an ECG. The right leg *(RL)* electrode functions solely as ground to prevent alternating current interference.

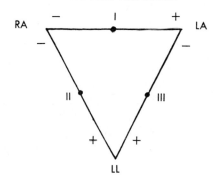

Fig. 3-4. Orientation of leads I, II, and III. Lead I records the difference in electrical potentials between the left arm and the right arm. Lead II records it between the left leg and the right arm. Lead III records it between the left leg and left arm.

---

*This rule is only approximate. It is exact when the three bipolar extremity leads are recorded simultaneously, using a three-channel electrocardiograph, because the peaks of the R waves in the three leads do *not* occur simultaneously. The exact rule is as follows: the voltage at the peak of the R wave (or at any point) in lead II equals the sum of the voltages in leads I and III at points occurring simultaneously.

and you get +13 mm, the voltage of the R wave in lead II. You can do the same with the voltages of the P waves and T waves.

It is a good custom to scan leads I, II, and III rapidly when you first look at a mounted ECG. If the R wave in lead II does not seem to be the sum of R waves in leads I and III, this may be a clue that the leads have been either recorded incorrectly or mounted improperly.

Einthoven's equation is simply the result of the way the bipolar leads are recorded. (The LA is positive in lead I and negative in lead III and thus cancels out when the two leads are added.)

$$I = L\!\!\!/A - RA$$
$$III = LL - L\!\!\!/A$$
$$I + III = LL - RA = II$$

In electrocardiography, therefore, one plus three equals two.

To summarize: The first three leads (I, II, and III) are bipolar extremity leads, which historically were the first invented. These leads record the differences in electrical voltage between extremities.

In Figure 3-5 the Einthoven triangle has been redrawn so leads I, II, and III all intersect at a common central point. This was done simply by sliding lead I downward, lead II rightward, and lead III leftward. The result is the *triaxial* diagram in Figure 3-5, *B*. This diagram is a useful way of representing the three bipolar leads and will be employed later (in Chapter 5).

Unipolar Extremity Leads (aV_R, aV_L, and aV_F)

Following the invention of the three bipolar extremity leads nine additional leads were added. In the 1930s Dr. Frank N. Wilson and his colleagues at the University of Michigan invented the unipolar limb leads and introduced the six unipolar chest leads, V_1 through V_6. Shortly after this, one of the authors of this text (E.G.) invented the three augmented unipolar extremity leads, aV_R, aV_L, and aV_F. The abbreviation *a* refers to *augmented; V, voltage; R, L,* and *F, right arm, left arm,* and *left foot* (leg) respectively. So, today, 12 leads are routinely employed.

A unipolar lead records the electrical voltages at one location relative to zero potential, rather than relative to the voltages at another extremity, as in the case of the bipolar extremity leads. The zero potential is obtained inside the electrocardiograph by joining the three extremity leads to a central terminal. Since the sum of the voltages of RA, LA, and LL equals zero, the central terminal has a zero voltage. The aV_R, aV_L, and aV_F leads are derived in a slightly different way, because the voltages recorded by the electrocardiograph have been augmented 50% over the actual voltages detected at each extremity. This augmentation is also done electronically inside the electrocardiograph.*

---

*Augmentation was developed to make the complexes more readable.

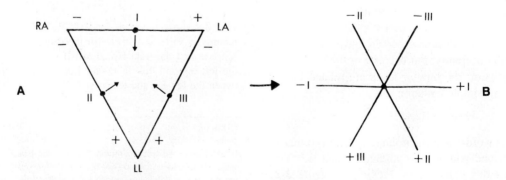

Fig. 3-5. Einthoven's triangle, **A,** has been converted to a triaxial diagram, **B.** This is done simply by shifting leads I, II, and III so they intersect at a common point.

Just as we used Einthoven's triangle to represent the spatial orientation of the three bipolar extremity leads, so we can use the diagram in Figure 3-6 to represent the spatial orientation of the three unipolar extremity leads. Notice that each of the unipolar leads can also be represented by a line (axis) with a positive and a negative pole.* Since the diagram has three axes, it is also called a *triaxial* diagram.

The positive pole of lead aV_R, the right arm lead, points upward and to the patient's right arm as you would expect. The positive pole of lead aV_L points upward and to the patient's left arm. The positive pole of lead aV_F points downward toward the patient's left foot.

Furthermore, just as leads I, II, and III are related by Einthoven's equation, so leads aV_R, aV_L, and aV_F are related:

$$aVR + aVL + aVF = 0$$

In other words, when the three unipolar extremity leads are recorded, their voltages should total zero. Thus the sum of the P wave voltages is zero, the sum of the QRS voltages is zero, and the sum of the T wave voltages is zero. Go back to Figure 3-2 and test this equation by adding the QRS voltages in the three unipolar extremity leads (aV_R, aV_L, and aV_F).

It is also a good custom to scan aV_R, aV_L, and aV_F rapidly when you first look at a mounted ECG. If the sum of the waves in these three leads does not equal zero, this may also be a clue that the leads have been either recorded incorrectly or mounted improperly.

The ECG leads, both bipolar and unipolar, have two major features, which have already been described. They have both a specific *orientation* and a specific *polarity*.

Thus the axis of lead I is oriented horizontally while the axis of lead aV_R points diagonally downward. The orientation of the bipolar leads is shown in Einthoven's triangle (Fig. 3-5) while that of the unipolar extremity leads is diagrammed in Figure 3-6.

The second major feature of the ECG leads, their polarity, can be represented by a line (axis) with a positive and a negative pole, as shown before. The polarity and spatial orientation of the leads are discussed further in Chapters 4 and 5 (when we consider the normal ECG patterns seen in each of the leads and the concept of electrical axis).

Do not be confused by the difference in meaning between ECG electrodes and ECG leads. An *electrode* is simply the metal plate used to detect the electrical currents of the heart in any location. An ECG *lead* shows the differences in voltage detected by these electrodes. (For instance, lead I presents the differences in voltage detected by the left and right arm electrodes.) Therefore, a lead is a means of recording the differences in cardiac voltages obtained by different electrodes.

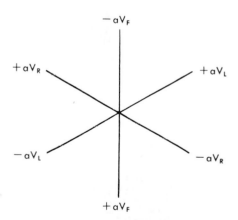

Fig. 3-6. Triaxial lead diagram showing the relationship of the three augmented unipolar leads: aV_R, aV_L, and aV_F. Notice that these leads are represented by axes with both a positive and a negative pole. *Unipolar* means that the leads record the voltage in one location relative to zero potential.

---

*Although unipolar leads (like bipolar leads) are represented by axes with positive and negative poles, the term "unipolar" does not refer to these poles; rather it refers to the fact that unipolar leads record the voltage in *one* location relative to zero potential.

Relationship Between Unipolar and Bipolar Extremity Leads

The Einthoven triangle (Fig. 3-4) shows the relationship of the three bipolar extremity leads (I, II, and III). Similarly the triaxial diagram in Figure 3-7 shows the relationship of the three unipolar extremity leads (aV_R, aV_L, and aV_F). For convenience, we can combine these two diagrams so the axes of all six extremity leads intersect at a common point. The result is the *hexaxial* lead diagram shown in Figure 3-7. The hexaxial diagram shows the spatial orientation of the six extremity leads (I, II, III, aV_R, aV_L, and aV_F).

The exact relationships among the three unipolar extremity leads and the three bipolar extremity leads can also be described mathematically. However, for present purposes, the following simple guidelines allow you to get an overall impression of the similarities between these two sets of leads.

As you might expect by looking at the hexaxial diagram, the pattern in lead aV_L usually resembles that in lead I. The positive poles of lead aV_R and lead II, on the other hand, point in opposite directions. Therefore the P-QRS-T pattern recorded by lead aV_R is generally the reverse of that recorded

qR $\left(\begin{smallmatrix} R \\ \wedge \\ q \end{smallmatrix} \right)$

by lead II. (For example, when lead II shows a qR

rS $\left(\begin{smallmatrix} r \\ \vee \\ S \end{smallmatrix} \right)$

pattern lead aV_R usually shows an rS pattern.) Finally, the pattern shown by lead aV_F usually but not always resembles that shown by lead III.

CHEST (PRECORDIAL) LEADS

The chest leads (V_1 to V_6) show the electrical currents of the heart detected by electrodes placed at different positions on the chest wall. The chest leads used today are also unipolar leads in that they measure the voltage in any one location relative to zero potential. By convention the six leads are placed as follows*:

Lead V_1 is recorded with the electrode in the fourth intercostal space just to the right of the sternum.

Lead V_2 is recorded with the electrode in the fourth intercostal space just to the left of the sternum.

Lead V_3 is recorded on a line midway between V_2 and V_4.

Lead V_4 is recorded in the midclavicular line in the fifth interspace.

Lead V_5 is recorded in the anterior axillary line at the same level as V_4.

Lead V_6 is recorded in the midaxillary line at the same level as V_4.

The chest leads are recorded simply by means of electrodes (usually attached to suction cups to hold them in place on the chest) at six designated locations on the chest wall (Fig. 3-8).

Two points are worth mentioning here:

First, how do you locate the fourth intercostal space? Start by placing your finger at the top of the sternum and moving it slowly downward. After moving down about 1½ inches, you will feel a slight horizontal ridge. This is called the *angle of Louis* (Fig. 3-8), where the manubrium joins the body of the sternum. The second intercostal space is just below and lateral to this point. Move down two more spaces and you are in the fourth interspace and ready to place lead V_4.

Second, in females the situation is complicated by breast tissue, which may result in misplacement of the chest leads. In taking ECGs on women you

---

*Sometimes, in special circumstances (e.g., a patient with suspected congenital heart disease or right ventricular infarction), additional leads are placed on the right side of the chest. For example, lead V_{3R} is equivalent to V_3 but the electrode is placed to the right of the sternum.

DERIVATION OF HEXAXIAL LEAD DIAGRAM

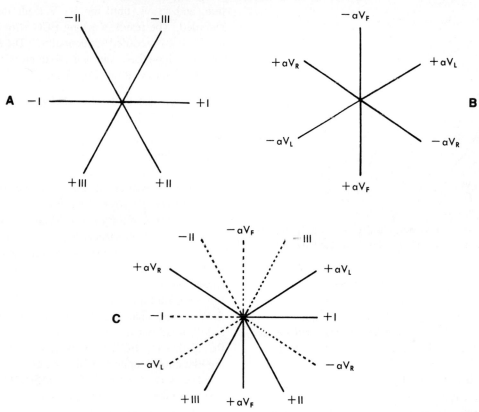

Fig. 3-7. Triaxial diagrams of the bipolar leads (I, II, and III), **A,** and the unipolar leads (aV_R, aV_L, and aV_F), **B,** can be combined into a hexaxial diagram, **C,** showing the relationship of all six extremity leads. The negative pole of each lead is now indicated by a *dashed line*.

CHEST LEAD PLACEMENT

Fig. 3-8. Locations of the electrodes for the chest (precordial) leads.

ORIENTATION OF CHEST LEADS

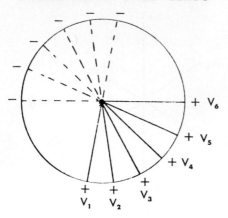

Fig. 3-9. The positive poles of the chest leads point anteriorly, and the negative poles (indicated by *dashed lines*) point posteriorly.

must remember to place the electrode *under* the breast for leads V_3 to V_6. If, as often happens, the electrode is placed *on* the breast, you will be recording electrical voltages from higher interspaces.

(*Never* use the nipples to locate the position of any of the chest lead electrodes, even in men, because nipple location varies greatly in different persons.)

The chest leads, like the six extremity leads, can be represented diagrammatically as shown in Figure 3-9. Like the other leads, each of the chest leads has a positive and a negative pole. The positive pole of each chest lead points anteriorly, toward the front of the chest. The negative pole of the chest leads points posteriorly, toward the back (*dashed lines* in Fig. 3-9).

TAKING AN ECG

Now you are ready to take an ECG. The extremity electrodes are attached to the patient. First, the machine is standardized (p. 10). Then the dial on the electrocardiograph is turned to lead I. Several P-QRS-T cycles are run. Next, the dial is advanced to lead II and the ECG records a few more cycles. This is repeated for leads III, aV_R, aV_L, and aV_F. Next the dial is turned to the position for the chest

leads. The suction cup is placed in the V_1 position, and so on, until the six V leads have been recorded. The result is a long ECG strip showing the 12 leads recorded sequentially.* The ECGs in this book have been cut and mounted in the usual way for interpretation (Fig. 3-2).

THE 12-LEAD ECG: FRONTAL AND HORIZONTAL PLANE LEADS

You may now be wondering why we use 12 leads in clinical electrocardiography; why not 10 or 22? The reason for exactly 12 leads is partly historical, a matter of the way the ECG has evolved over the years since Einthoven's original three bipolar extremity leads. There is nothing sacred about the electrocardiographer's dozen. In some cases, for example, we do record additional leads by placing the chest electrode at different positions on the chest wall. There are good reasons for using multiple leads. The heart, after all, is a three-dimensional structure and its electrical currents spread out in all directions across the body. Recall that the ECG leads were described as being like photographs by which we can see the electrical activity of the heart from different locations. To a certain extent, the more points we record from the more accurate will be our representation of the heart's electrical activity.

The importance of multiple leads is illustrated in the diagnosis of myocardial infarction (MI). An MI typically affects one localized portion of either the anterior or the inferior portion of the left ventricle. The ECG changes produced by an anterior MI are usually best shown by the chest leads, which are close to and face the injured anterior surface of the heart. The changes seen with an inferior MI usually appear only in leads such as II, III, and aV_F, which face the injured inferior surface of the heart. (We discuss this further in Chapters 8 and 9.) The 12 leads therefore provide a three-

---

*Many of the modern electrocardiographs have been designed to record three ECG leads simultaneously; thus four groups of three leads (I, II, III), (aV_R, aV_L, aV_F), (V_1 to V_3), and (V_4 to V_6) can be recorded at the same time. (For example, see Figure 3-2.)

FRONTAL PLANE LEADS

HORIZONTAL PLANE LEADS

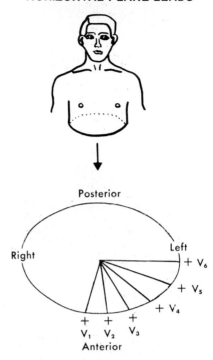

Fig. 3-11. Spatial relationships of the six chest (horizontal plane) leads.

Fig. 3-10. Spatial relationships of the six extremity (frontal plane) leads.

dimensional view of the electrical activity of the heart.

Specifically, the six extremity leads (I, II, III, aV$_R$, aV$_L$, aV$_F$) will record electrical voltages transmitted onto the *frontal* plane of the body (Fig. 3-10) while the six precordial leads record voltages transmitted onto the *horizontal* plane. For example, if you walk up to and face a large window, the window will be parallel to the frontal plane of your body. Similarly heart voltages directed upward and downward and to the right and left will be recorded by the frontal plane leads.

The chest leads (V$_1$ through V$_6$) record heart voltages from a different viewpoint, on the *horizontal* plane of the body, as shown in Figure 3-11. The horizontal plane cuts your body into an upper and a lower half. Similarly the chest leads record heart voltages directed anteriorly (front), posteriorly (back), and to the right and left.

We therefore have two sets of ECG leads: the six *extremity* leads (three unipolar and three bipolar), which record voltages on the frontal plane of the body, and the six *chest* (precordial) leads, which record voltages on the horizontal plane. Together these 12 leads provide a three-dimensional picture of atrial and ventricular depolarization and repolarization.

Fig. 3-12. Rhythm strips from a cardiac monitor taken moments apart. Notice that **A** is completely the opposite of **B.** This is because the polarity of the electrodes in **B** was reversed.

Fig. 3-13. Monitor lead. A chest electrode ($+$) is placed at the V_1 position (between the fourth and fifth ribs on the right side of the sternum). The right shoulder acts as a negative ($-$) electrode. A ground electrode *(G)* is placed at the left shoulder.

CARDIAC MONITORS AND MONITOR LEADS
Bedside Cardiac Monitors

Up to now, we have considered only the standard 12 lead ECG. However, it is not always necessary or feasible to record a full 12-lead ECG. For example, patients in coronary care units require continuous monitoring. In such settings special cardiac monitors are used to give a continuous beat-to-beat record of cardiac activity from one monitor lead.

Figure 3-12 is a rhythm strip recorded from a monitor lead obtained by means of three disk electrodes on the chest wall. As shown in Figure 3-13, one of these electrodes (the positive one) is usually pasted in the V_1 position. The other two are placed near the right and left shoulders. One serves as the negative electrode, the other as ground.

When the location of the electrodes on the chest wall is varied, the resultant ECG patterns will also vary. In addition, if the polarity of the electrodes changes (e.g., connecting the negative electrode to the V_1 position and the positive electrode to the right shoulder), the ECG will show a completely opposite pattern (Fig. 3-12).

Ambulatory (Holter) Monitors

The cardiac monitors just described are useful in patients confined to bed or chair, but sometimes it is essential to record the heartbeat in ambulatory patients over longer periods. A special portable ECG system, designed in 1961 by N.J. Holter, records the cardiac activity of patients as they go about their daily activities. The Holter monitor currently in use consists of electrodes placed on the chest wall and lower abdomen and a special portable tape recorder to record the ECG. The patient can then be monitored over a long period (e.g., 24 hours). Usually two ECG leads are recorded. The tape is played back, and the P-QRS-T complexes are displayed on a special screen. Printouts of any portion of the ECG can be obtained for further study and permanent records.

Holter monitors are invaluable in many settings. For example, in evaluating patients with unexplained *syncope,* they may reveal serious arrhythmias that are intermittent and may not have been seen on a routine ECG. Holter monitors are also useful for establishing the diagnosis of the *brady-tachy syndrome* (Chapter 18), in which periods of bradycardia alternate with periods of tachycardia. A Holter monitor may be useful in detecting ST segment shifts associated with *myocardial ischemia* in selected patients (Chapter 9).

For subjects with very intermittent symptoms, portable *patient-activated* monitors are now available. Some of these event recorders are designed with replaceable electrodes so a patient can be monitored for several weeks.

Special ECG Recordings

To help diagnose arrhythmias, special ECG electrodes have been developed for recording inside the esophagus (esophageal leads) or inside the right atrium and right ventricle (intracardiac leads). Discussion of these topics, however, is beyond the scope of this introductory text.

REVIEW

The electrical currents produced during atrial and ventricular depolarization and repolarization are detected by electrodes placed on the extremities and chest wall.

Twelve leads are usually recorded.

1. The six *extremity* (limb) leads record voltages from the heart directed onto the frontal plane of the body. (This divides the body into front and back halves.) These six leads consist of the three bipolar extremity leads (I, II, and III) and three augmented unipolar extremity leads (aV_R, aV_L, and aV_F).

   A *bipolar* lead records the difference between voltages from the heart detected at two extremities. A *unipolar* lead records voltages at one point relative to zero potential. The bipolar extremity leads can be represented by Einthoven's triangle (Fig. 3-4). They are related by the equation II = I + III. The unipolar extremity leads can also be represented by a triaxial diagram (Fig. 3-6). They are related by the equation $aV_R + aV_L + aV_F = 0$.

   The three unipolar extremity leads and the three bipolar extremity leads can be shown on the same diagram so the axes of all six leads intersect at a common point, producing the *hexaxial lead diagram.*

   As a general rule, the P-QRS-T pattern in lead I resembles that in lead aV_L. Leads aV_R and II usually show reverse patterns. Lead aV_F usually resembles lead III.

2. The six *chest* (precordial) leads (V_1 to V_6) record voltages from the heart directed onto the horizontal plane of the body (dividing the body into an upper and a lower half). They are taken with electrodes in specific anatomic locations (Fig. 3-8).

In addition to the 12 conventional leads, ECGs can be taken in special ways: In cardiac care units (CCUs), monitor leads, in which electrodes are placed on the chest, are generally used. Figure 3-13 shows the usual location of the chest electrodes for a monitor lead. Continuous ECGs are often recorded with the Holter apparatus for a period of 24 or more hours in ambulatory patients who have a transient or unpredictable arrhythmia. Sporadic symptoms can be correlated with ECG rhythm changes by using patient-activated event recorders.

Questions

1. Leads I and II are shown below. Draw the P-QRS-T pattern in lead III.

2. Leads I, II, and III are shown below. What is wrong with them?

3. Draw the hexaxial lead diagram showing the six frontal plane (extremity) leads.
4. Why does the P-QRS-T pattern in lead aV_R usually show a reverse of the pattern in lead II?

Answers

1. Since lead II = lead I + lead III, then according to Einthoven's equation lead III = lead II −
   lead I as shown below:

III

   Notice that the voltages of the P wave, QRS complex, and T wave in lead II are equal to the sum
   of the P, QRS, and T voltages in leads I and III.
2. The voltages in lead II here do *not* equal those in leads I and III. The reason is that leads II and
   III were mislabeled. Reverse the labels; now the voltage in II will equal the voltages in I and III.
3. See Figure 3-7, *C*.
4. The positive poles of lead aV_R and lead II point in opposite directions (Fig. 3-7).

4

The Normal ECG

We have reviewed the cycle of atrial and ventricular depolarization and repolarization detected by the ECG as well as the 12 lead system used to record this electrical activity. This chapter describes the P-QRS-T patterns seen normally in each of the 12 leads. Fortunately, this does not require memorization of 12 or more separate patterns. Rather, knowledge of a few basic ECG principles and understanding of the sequence of atrial and ventricular depolarization will enable us to predict the normal ECG patterns in each lead.

As you can see from the sample ECG in Figure 3-2, each of the 12 leads appears to be different from the next. In some leads, for example, the P waves are positive (upward); in others they are negative (downward). In some leads the QRS complexes are represented by an rS wave; in other leads they are represented by RS or qR waves. Finally, in some leads the T waves are positive, and in others negative. What determines this variety in the appearance of ECG complexes in the different leads, and how does the repetitive cycle of cardiac electrical activity produce such different patterns in these leads?

THREE BASIC "LAWS" OF ELECTROCARDIOGRAPHY

Answering the preceding questions requires understanding of the following three basic ECG "laws" (Fig. 4-1):

1. A *positive* (upward) *deflection* will appear in any lead if the wave of depolarization spreads toward the positive pole of that lead. Thus, if the path of atrial stimulation is directed downward and to the patient's left, toward the positive pole of lead II, a positive (upward) P wave will be seen in lead II (Figs. 4-2 and 4-3). Similarly, if the ventricular stimulation path is directed to the left, a positive deflection (an R wave) will be seen in lead I (Fig. 4-1, *A*).

2. A *negative* (downward) *deflection* will appear in any lead if the wave of depolarization spreads toward the negative pole of that lead (or away from the positive pole). Thus, if the atrial stimulation path spreads downward and to the left, a negative P wave will be seen in lead aV_R (Figs. 4-2 and 4-3). If the ventricular stimulation path is directed entirely away from the positive pole of any lead, a negative QRS complex (QS deflection) will be seen (Fig. 4-1, *B*).

3. If the mean depolarization path is directed at right angles (perpendicular) to any lead, you will usually see a small *biphasic deflection* (consisting of positive and negative deflections of equal size). If the atrial stimulation path spreads at right angles to any lead, you will see a biphasic P wave in that lead. If the ventricular stimulation path spreads at right angles to any lead, then the QRS complex will be biphasic (Fig. 4-1, *C*). A biphasic QRS complex may consist of either an RS pattern or a QR pattern.

• • •

To summarize: When the mean depolarization wave spreads toward the positive pole of any lead, it produces a positive (upward) deflection. When

THREE BASIC "LAWS" OF ELECTROCARDIOGRAPHY

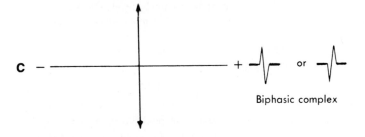

Fig. 4-1. A, A positive complex will be shown in any lead if the wave of depolarization spreads toward the positive pole of that lead. **B,** A negative complex will be shown if the depolarization wave spreads toward the negative pole (away from the positive pole) of the lead. **C,** A biphasic (partly positive, partly negative) complex will be seen if the mean direction of the wave is at right angles (perpendicular) to the lead. These three basic laws apply to both the P wave (atrial depolarization) and the QRS complex (ventricular depolarization).

DIRECTION OF ATRIAL DEPOLARIZATION WITH NORMAL SINUS RHYTHM

Fig. 4-2. With normal sinus rhythm the atrial depolarization wave *(arrow)* spreads from the right atrium downward toward the AV junction and left leg.

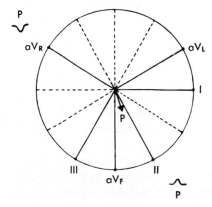

Fig. 4-3. With sinus rhythm the normal P wave is negative (downward) in lead aV_R and positive (upward) in lead II. Recall that with normal atrial depolarization the arrow points down toward the patient's left (Fig. 4-2), away from the positive pole of aV_R and toward the positive pole of II.

it spreads toward the negative pole (away from the positive pole) of any lead, it produces a negative (downward) deflection. When it spreads at right angles to any lead axis, it produces a biphasic deflection.

Mention of repolarization—the return of stimulated muscle to the resting state—has deliberately been omitted. The subject will be touched upon later in this chapter in discussing the normal T wave.

With these three basic ECG laws in mind, all you need to know is the direction in which depolarization spreads through the heart at any time to predict what the P waves and the QRS complexes will look like in any lead.

THE NORMAL P WAVE

Let us begin our description of the normal ECG with the first waveform seen in any cycle, the P wave, which represents atrial depolarization. Atrial depolarization is initiated by the sinus node, in the right atrium (Fig. 1-1). The atrial depolarization path therefore spreads from right to left and downward toward the AV junction. We can represent the spread of atrial depolarization by an arrow* that points downward and to the patient's left (Fig. 4-2).

Now go back to the diagram we drew in Chapter 3 showing the spatial relationship of the six frontal plane (extremity) leads. This diagram is redrawn in Figure 4-3. Notice that the positive pole of lead aV$_R$ points upward in the direction of the right shoulder. The normal path of atrial depolarization, as described, spreads downward toward the left leg (away from the positive pole of aV$_R$). *Therefore, with normal sinus rhythm, lead aV$_R$ will always show a negative P wave.* Conversely, lead II is oriented with its positive pole pointing downward in the direction of the left leg (Fig. 4-3). Therefore the normal atrial depolarization path will

---

*The arrows used to represent cardiac electrical potentials have both specific direction and specific magnitude and are, therefore, "vectors." The details of *vectorcardiography* lie outside the scope of this book, although vectorial principles are used throughout the discussions.

DIRECTION OF ATRIAL DEPOLARIZATION WITH AV JUNCTIONAL RHYTHM

Fig. 4-4. When the AV junction acts as the cardiac pacemaker (junctional rhythm), the atria are depolarized in a retrograde (backward) fashion. An *arrow* representing atrial depolarization in such cases will point upward toward the right atrium, just opposite the pattern seen with sinus rhythm.

be directed toward the positive pole of that lead. *When normal sinus rhythm is present, lead II will always record a positive (upward) P wave.*

To summarize: When normal sinus rhythm is present, the P wave will always be negative in lead aV$_R$ and positive in lead II.

Using the same principles of analysis, can you predict what the P wave will look like in leads II and aV$_R$ if the heart is being paced not by the sinus node but by the AV junction (AV junctional rhythm)? When the AV junction (or an "ectopic" pacemaker in the lower part of either atrium) is pacing the heart, atrial depolarization will have to spread up the atria in a *retrograde* direction, just the opposite of what happens with normal sinus rhythm. Therefore an arrow representing the spread of atrial depolarization with AV junctional rhythm will point upward and to the right (Fig. 4-4), just the opposite of what occurs with normal sinus rhythm. Spread of atrial depolarization upward and to the right will result in a positive P wave in lead aV$_R$, since the stimulus is spreading toward the positive pole of that lead (Fig. 4-5). Conversely, lead II will show a negative P wave.

ORIENTATION OF P WAVES WITH AV JUNCTIONAL RHYTHM

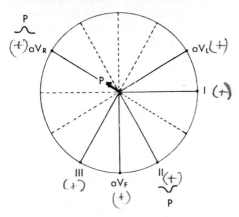

Fig. 4-5. With AV junctional rhythm the P waves are upward (positive) in lead aV_R and downward (negative) in lead II.

AV junctional rhythms are considered in detail in Part II. The topic was introduced here simply to show how the polarity of the P waves in lead aV_R and lead II depends on the direction of atrial depolarization and how the patterns can be predicted using simple basic principles.

You need not be concerned at this point with the polarity of P waves in the other 10 leads. You can usually get all the clinical information you need to determine whether the sinus node is pacing the atria by simply looking at the P waves in leads II and aV_R. Their size and shape in other leads may be of importance in determining whether left or right atrial enlargement is present (which will be discussed in Chapter 6).

THE NORMAL QRS COMPLEX

The same principles as those used above can be applied in deducing the shape of the QRS waveform in the various leads. The QRS, which represents ventricular depolarization, is somewhat more complex than the P wave, but the same basic ECG rules apply to both.

To predict what the QRS will look like in the different leads, you must first know the direction of ventricular depolarization. Although the spread of atrial depolarization can be represented by a single arrow, the spread of ventricular depolarization consists of two major sequential phases:

The *first* phase is of relatively brief duration (shorter than 0.04 sec) and small amplitude. It results from stimulus spread through the interventricular septum. The septum is the first part of the ventricles to be stimulated. Furthermore, the left side of the septum is stimulated first (by a branch of the left bundle of His); thus depolarization spreads from the left ventricle to the right across the septum. Phase one of ventricular depolarization, septal stimulation, can therefore be represented by a small arrow pointing from the left septal wall to the right (Fig. 4-6, *A*).

The *second* phase of ventricular depolarization involves simultaneous stimulation of the main mass of both the left and the right ventricles from the inside (endocardium) to the outside (epicardium) of the heart muscle. In the normal heart the left ventricle is electrically predominant. In other words, it electrically overbalances the right ventricle. Therefore an arrow representing phase two of ventricular stimulation will point toward the left ventricle (Fig. 4-6, *B*).

To summarize: The ventricular depolarization process can be divided into two main phases: stimulation of the interventricular septum (represented by a short arrow pointing through the septum into the right ventricle) and simultaneous left and right ventricular stimulation (represented by a larger arrow pointing through the left ventricle and toward the left chest).

Now that the ventricular stimulation sequence has been outlined, we can begin to predict what types of QRS patterns this sequence will produce in the different leads. For the moment, we will discuss only the QRS patterns normally seen in the chest leads (the horizontal plane leads).

Chest Leads

We will talk first about leads V_1 and V_6. As discussed in Chapter 3, lead V_1 shows voltages detected by an electrode placed on the right side of the sternum (fourth intercostal space). Lead V_6, a

NORMAL VENTRICULAR DEPOLARIZATION

Fig. 4-6. Ventricular depolarization consists of two major sequential phases. Phase one, **A,** proceeds from the left wall of the septum to the right. An *arrow* representing this phase points through the septum from the left to the right side. Phase two, **B,** is depolarization of the main bulk of the ventricles. The *arrow* points through the left ventricle, because this is normally electrically predominant. The two phases will produce an rS complex in the right chest lead (V_1) and a qR complex in the left chest lead (V_6).

left chest lead, shows voltages detected in the left midaxillary line (Fig. 3-8). What will the QRS complex look like in these leads (Fig. 4-6)?

The first phase of ventricular stimulation, septal stimulation, is represented by an arrow pointing to the right, reflecting the left-to-right spread of depolarization stimulus through the septum (Fig. 4-6,

A). This small arrow will point toward the positive pole of lead V_1. Therefore the spread of stimulation to the right during the first phase produces a small positive deflection (r wave) in lead V_1. What will lead V_6 show? The left-to-right spread of septal stimulation will produce a small negative deflection (q wave) in lead V_6. Thus the same electrical event, septal stimulation, produces a small positive deflection (or r wave) in lead V_1 and a small negative deflection (q wave) in the left precordial lead like V_6. (This situation is analogous to the one described for the P wave, which is normally positive in lead II but always negative in lead aV_R.)

The second phase of ventricular stimulation is represented by an arrow pointing in the direction of the left ventricle (Fig. 4-6, *B*). This arrow will point away from the positive pole of lead V_1 and toward the negative pole of V_6. Therefore the spread of stimulation to the left during the second phase results in a negative deflection in the right precordial leads and a positive deflection in the left precordial leads. Lead V_1 will show a deep negative (S) wave, lead V_6 a tall positive (R) wave.

To summarize what we have learned about the normal QRS patterns in leads V_1 and V_6: Normally lead V_1 shows an rS type of complex. The small initial r wave represents the left-to-right spread of septal stimulation. This wave is sometimes referred to as the *septal r wave* because it reflects septal stimulation. The negative (S) wave reflects the spread of ventricular stimulation forces during phase two, away from the right and toward the dominant left ventricle. Conversely, the same electrical events, septal and ventricular stimulation, viewed from an electrode in the V_6 position will produce a qR pattern. The q wave is a *septal q wave,* reflecting the left-to-right spread of the stimulus through the septum away from lead V_6. The positive (R) wave reflects the leftward spread of ventricular stimulation voltages through the left ventricle.

Once again, to reemphasize, the same electrical event, whether depolarization of the atria or depolarization of the ventricles, will produce very different-looking waveforms in different leads be-

NORMAL R WAVE PROGRESSION

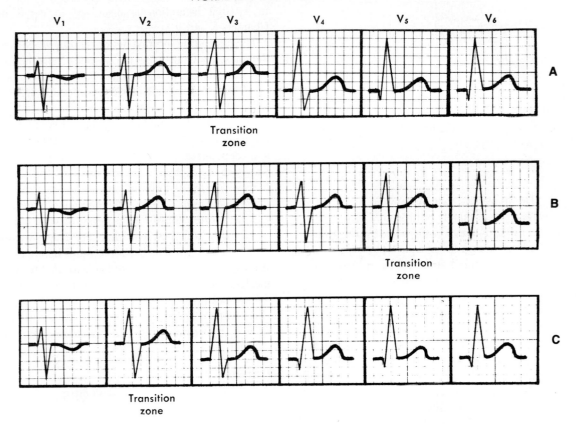

Fig. 4-7. Normally R waves in the chest leads become relatively taller from lead V_1 to the left chest leads. **A,** Notice the transition in lead V_3. **B,** Somewhat delayed R wave progression, with the transition in lead V_5. **C,** Early transition in lead V_2.

cause the spatial orientation of the leads is different.

We have discussed the patterns normally seen in leads V_1 and V_6. What happens *between* these leads? The answer is that as you move across the chest (in the direction of the electrically predominant left ventricle) the R wave tends to become relatively larger and the S wave becomes relatively smaller. This increase in height of the R wave, which usually reaches a maximum around lead V_4 or V_5, is called *normal R wave progression*. Figure 4-7 shows examples of normal R wave progression.

At some point, generally around the V_3 or V_4 position, the R/S ratio becomes 1. This point, where the amplitude of the R wave equals that of the S wave, is called the *transition zone* (Fig. 4-7). In some normal people the transition may be seen as early as lead V_2. This is called *early transition*. In other cases the transition zone may not appear until leads V_5 and V_6. This is called *delayed transition*.

Examine the set of normal chest leads in Figure 4-8. Notice the rS complex in lead V_1 and the qR complex in lead V_6. The R wave tends to get gradually larger here as you move toward the left chest

Fig. 4-8. Normal chest leads. The transition is in lead V_4. Notice the normal septal r wave in lead V_1 (as part of an rS complex) and the normal septal q in lead V_6 (part of a qR complex).

leads. The transition zone, where the R wave and S wave are about equal, is in lead V_4. In normal chest leads the R wave voltage need not get literally larger as you go from leads V_1 and V_6. However, the overall trend should show a relative increase. For example, notice that in this example there is not much difference between the complexes in leads V_2 and V_3, and that the R wave in lead V_5 is taller than the R wave in lead V_6.

In summary: The normal chest lead ECG shows an rS-type complex in lead V_1 with a steady increase in the relative size of the R wave toward the left chest and a decrease in S wave amplitude. Leads V_5 and V_6 generally show a qR-type complex.*

The concept of *normal R wave progression* is key in distinguishing normal and abnormal ECG patterns. For example, imagine the effect that an anterior wall myocardial infarction would have on normal R wave progression. Anterior wall infarction results in the death of myocardial cells and the loss of normal positive (R wave) voltages. Therefore one of the major ECG signs of an anterior wall infarction will be the loss of normal R

---

*Normal chest lead patterns may show slight variation from the patterns we have been discussing. For example, some people will have a QS and not an rS pattern in lead V_1. In other cases the septal q wave in the left chest leads may not be seen and thus leads V_5 and V_6 will show an R wave and not a qR complex. On other normal ECGs, leads V_5 and V_6 may show a narrow qRs complex as a normal variant (Fig. 3-2, lead V_4) and lead V_1 may show a narrow rSr'.

wave progression in the chest leads. (The topic of myocardial infarction is discussed in detail in Chapters 8 and 9.)

Understanding normal R wave progression in the chest leads also sets the basis for recognizing other basic ECG abnormalities. For example, consider the effect of left or right ventricular hypertrophy (enlarged muscle mass) on the chest lead patterns. As mentioned before, the left ventricle is normally electrically predominant; and left ventricular depolarization produces deep (negative) S waves in the right chest leads with tall (positive) R waves in the left chest leads. With left ventricular hypertrophy, these left ventricular voltages will be further increased, resulting in very tall R waves in the left chest leads and very deep S waves in the right chest leads. On the other hand, right ventricular hypertrophy would be expected to shift the balance of electrical forces to the right, producing tall positive waves (R waves) in the right chest leads. (These patterns of left and right ventricular hypertrophy are described in detail in Chapter 6.)

Extremity Leads

We have discussed the normal QRS patterns in the chest leads. All that remains is to describe the normal QRS patterns in the extremity leads: I, II, III, aV_R, aV_L, and aV_F.

We will begin with lead aV_R, which is the easiest to visualize. The positive pole of lead aV_R is oriented upward and toward the right shoulder. The ventricular stimulation forces are oriented primarily toward the left ventricle. Therefore lead aV_R normally shows a predominantly negative QRS complex. You may see any of the QRS-T complexes shown in Figure 4-9 in lead aV_R. In all cases the QRS is predominantly negative. The T wave in lead aV_R is also normally negative. The QRS patterns in the other five extremity leads are somewhat more complicated. The reason is that there is considerable normal variation in the QRS patterns seen in the extremity leads. For example, some normal people will have an ECG that shows one pattern (Fig. 4-10). In the extremity leads (qR-type complexes in I and aV_L, rS-type complexes

LEAD aV_R: NORMAL PATTERNS

Fig. 4-9. Normally lead aV_R shows one of three basic negative patterns: an rS complex, a QS complex, or a Qr complex. The T wave also is normally negative.

NORMAL HORIZONTAL QRS AXIS

Fig. 4-10. With a horizontal QRS position (axis) leads I and aV_L show qR complexes while lead II shows RS and leads III and aV_F show rS complexes.

NORMAL VERTICAL QRS AXIS

Fig. 4-11. With a vertical QRS position (axis) leads II, III, and aV_F show qR complexes while lead aV_L (and sometimes lead I) shows an RS complex. This is just the reverse of the pattern with a normal horizontal axis.

in III and aV_F) while other people will have just the opposite picture (Fig. 4-11) (qR complexes in II, III, and aV_F, RS complexes in aV_L and sometimes I).

How can we account for this marked normal variability in the QRS patterns shown in the extremity leads? The patterns seen depend on the *electrical position* of the heart. The term "electrical position" is virtually synonymous with *"mean QRS axis,"* which is described in greater detail in Chapter 5.

In simplest terms the electrical position of the heart may be described as either *horizontal* or *vertical*.

1. When the heart is electrically horizontal *(horizontal QRS axis)*, ventricular depolarization is directed mainly horizontally and to the left in the frontal plane. Looking at the frontal plane diagram (Fig. 3-10), you can see that the positive poles of leads I and aV_L are oriented horizontally and to the left. Therefore, when the heart is electrically horizontal, the QRS voltages will be directed toward leads I and aV_L, producing a tall R wave (usually as part of a qR complex) in these leads.

2. When the heart is electrically vertical *(vertical QRS axis)*, ventricular depolarization is directed mainly downward. Looking at the frontal plane diagram (Fig. 3-10), you can see that the positive poles of leads II, III, and aV_F are oriented downward. Therefore, when the heart is electrically vertical, the QRS voltages will be directed toward leads II, III, and aV_F, producing a tall R wave (usually as part of a qR complex) in these leads.

The concepts of electrically horizontal and electrically vertical heart positions can be expressed in another way. When the heart is electrically horizontal, leads I and aV_L will show qR complexes similar to the qR complexes seen normally in the left chest leads (V_5 and V_6). Leads II, III, and aV_F will show rS or RS complexes similar to those seen in the right chest leads normally. Therefore, when the heart is electrically horizontal, the patterns in

leads I and aV_L will resemble those in V_5 and V_6 while the patterns in II, III, and aV_F resemble those in the right chest leads. Conversely, when the heart is electrically vertical, just the opposite patterns will be seen in the extremity leads. With a vertical heart II, III, and aV_F will show qR complexes, similar to those seen in the left chest leads, while I and aV_L show rS-type complexes, resembling those in the right chest leads.

Dividing the electrical position of the heart into vertical and horizontal variants is obviously an oversimplification. For example, look at Figure 4-12. Here leads I, II, aV_L, and aV_F all show positive QRS complexes. Therefore, this tracing has features of *both* the vertical and the horizontal variants. (Sometimes this pattern is referred to as an "intermediate" heart position.)

For present purposes, however, you can regard the QRS patterns in the extremity leads to be basically variants of either the horizontal or the vertical QRS patterns described.

To summarize: The extremity leads in normal people can show a variable QRS pattern. Lead aV_R normally always records a predominantly negative QRS complex (Qr, QS, or rS). The QRS patterns in the other extremity leads will vary depending on the "electrical position" (QRS axis) of the heart. With an electrically vertical axis, leads II, III, and aV_F will show qR type complexes. With an electrically horizontal axis, leads I and aV_L will show qR complexes. Therefore it is not possible to define a single normal ECG pattern; rather, there is a normal variability. Students and clinicians must familiarize themselves with the normal variants in both the chest leads and the extremity leads.

THE NORMAL ST SEGMENT

As noted in Chapter 2, the normal ST segment, representing the early phase of ventricular repolarization, is usually isoelectric (flat on the baseline). Slight deviations (generally of less than 1 mm) may be seen normally. As described in Chapter 10, certain normal people will have more marked ST segment elevations as a normal variant (early repolarization pattern). Finally, examine the ST segments in the right chest leads (V_1 to V_3) of Fig-

NORMAL INTERMEDIATE QRS AXIS

Fig. 4-12. Sometimes extremity leads show patterns that are hybrids of vertical and horizontal variants, with R waves in leads I, II, III, aV_L, and aV_F. This represents an intermediate QRS axis and is also a normal variant.

ures 3-2 and 6-10. Notice that they are short and the T waves appear to take off almost from the J point (junction of the QRS complex and the ST segment). This pattern of an early takeoff of the T wave in the right chest leads is not an uncommon finding in normal persons.

THE NORMAL T WAVE

Up to this point, we have deferred discussion of ventricular repolarization—the return of stimulated muscle to the resting state, which produces the ST segment, T wave, and U wave. Deciding whether the T wave in any lead is normal or not is generally straightforward. As a rule, the T wave follows the direction of the main QRS deflection. Thus, when the main QRS deflection is positive (upright), the T wave is normally positive. We can also make some more specific rules about the direction of the normal T wave.

The normal T wave in lead aV_R is always negative, while in lead II it is always positive. Left-sided chest leads, such as V_4 to V_6, normally always show a positive T wave.

The T wave in the other leads may be variable. In the right chest leads (V_1 and V_2) it may be normally negative, isoelectric, or positive but it is almost always positive by lead V_3.* Furthermore, if the T wave is positive in any chest lead, it must remain positive in all chest leads to the left of that lead. Otherwise, it is abnormal. For example, if the T wave is negative in V_1 and V_2 and becomes positive in V_3, it should normally remain positive in V_4 to V_6.

The polarity of the T wave in the extremity leads depends on the electrical position of the heart. With a horizontal heart the main QRS deflection is positive in I and aV_L and the T wave is also positive in these leads. With an electrically vertical heart the QRS is positive in II, III, and aV_F and the T wave is also positive in these leads. However, on some normal ECGs with a vertical axis the T wave may be negative in lead III.

*In children and in some normal adults, a downward T wave may extend as far left as V_3 or V_4. This is known as the *juvenile T wave pattern*.

REVIEW

The three basic "laws" of electrocardiography are as follows:

1. A positive *(upward)* deflection will be seen in any lead if depolarization spreads toward the positive pole of that lead.
2. A negative *(downward)* deflection will be seen if depolarization spreads toward the negative pole (or away from the positive pole) of any lead.
3. If the mean depolarization path is directed at right angles *(perpendicular)* to any lead, a small biphasic (RS or QR) deflection will be seen.

Atrial depolarization starts in the sinus node and spreads downward and to the patient's left, toward the positive pole of lead II and away from the positive pole of lead aV_R. Therefore, with normal sinus rhythm, the P wave will always be positive in lead II and negative in lead aV_R.

Ventricular depolarization consists of two sequential phases:

1. The first phase is stimulation of the ventricular septum from left to right. This produces a small (septal) r wave in the right chest leads and a small (septal) q wave in the left chest leads.
2. During the second major phase of ventricular depolarization, the stimulus spreads simultaneously outward through the right and left ventricles. Since the mass of the normal left ventricle overbalances the mass of the right ventricle, the spread of depolarization through the left ventricle predominates on the normal ECG. This spread of stimulus through the left ventricle produces a tall R wave in the left chest leads (e.g., V_5 and V_6) (in association with a small initial q wave) and a deep S wave in the right chest leads (V_1 and V_2) (associated with a small initial r wave).

Chest leads between these extreme positions show a relative increase in R wave amplitude and a decrease in S wave amplitude.

In the extremity leads the shape of the QRS complex varies with the electrical position (axis) of the heart:

1. When the heart is electrically horizontal, leads I and aV_L show a qR pattern.
2. When the heart is electrically vertical, leads II, III, and aV_F show a qR pattern.

The normal T wave generally follows the direction of the main deflection of the QRS complex in any lead. In the chest leads the T may normally be negative in leads V_1 and V_2. In most adults it becomes positive by lead V_2 and remains positive in the left chest leads. In the extremity leads the T wave is always positive in lead II and negative in lead aV_R. When the heart is electrically horizontal, the QRS and the T are positive in leads I and aV_L. When the heart is electrically vertical, the QRS and T are positive in leads II, III, and aV_F.

Questions

1. Examine the following 12-lead ECG and lead II rhythm strip. Then answer these questions:
   a. Is normal sinus rhythm present?
   b. In the extremity leads, is the QRS axis electrically vertical or electrically horizontal?
   c. In the chest leads, where is the transition zone?
   d. Is the PR interval normal?
   e. Is the QRS interval normal?
   f. Are the T waves in the chest leads normal?

2. On the following ECG, is sinus rhythm present?

Answers

1. a. Yes. The P waves are positive (upright) in lead II and negative in aV_R, with a rate of about 75/min.
    b. Electrically vertical. The R waves are most prominent in leads II, III, and aV_F.
    c. The transition zone is in lead V_3. Notice that the RS complexes have the R wave approximately equal to the S wave.
    d. The PR interval is about 0.16 second. This is within normal range (0.12 to 0.2 sec).
    e. The QRS width is 0.08 second. This is normal (less than or equal to 0.1 sec).
    f. Yes.
2. No. Although there is a P wave before each QRS complex, notice that it is negative in lead II. With sinus rhythm the P should be positive (upright) in lead II. Thus in this patient the pacemaker must be outside the sinus node (ectopic), probably in a low atrial focus, near the AV junction. Inverted P waves such as these are called *retrograde* because the atria are depolarized in the opposite direction from normal, that is, from the bottom to the top rather than from the top (sinus node) to the bottom (AV junction). See also Chapters 11 and 12.

5

Electrical Axis and Axis Deviation

In the previous chapter we discussed normal ECG patterns in the chest and extremity leads. The general terms *"horizontal heart"* (or horizontal QRS axis) and *"vertical heart"* (or vertical QRS axis) were used to describe the normal variations in QRS patterns seen in the extremity leads. In this chapter we will refine this concept of electrical axis and see how the electrical axis of the QRS pattern can be quickly estimated in a simple way.

MEAN QRS AXIS: DEFINITION

The depolarization stimulus spreads through the ventricles in different directions from instant to instant. For example, it may be directed toward lead I at one moment and toward lead III the next. We can also talk about the mean direction of the QRS complex, or *mean QRS electrical axis*. If you could draw an arrow to represent the overall, or mean, direction in which the QRS complex is pointed *in the frontal plane* of the body, you would be drawing the electrical axis of the QRS complex.

The term *"mean QRS axis"* therefore describes the general direction in the frontal plane toward which the QRS complex is predominantly pointed.

Since we are defining the QRS axis in the frontal plane, we are describing the QRS only in reference to the six extremity leads (the six frontal plane leads). (See Figure 5-1.) Therefore the scale of reference used to measure the mean QRS axis is the diagram of the frontal plane leads (described in Chapter 3). We also discussed the Einthoven triangle in Chapter 3 and saw how the triangle can

easily be converted into a triaxial lead diagram by simply having the three axes (leads I, II, and III) intersect at a central point (Fig. 5-1, *A*). Similarly we saw how the axes of the three unipolar extremity leads (aV_R, aV_L, and aV_F) also form a triaxial lead diagram (Fig. 5-1, *B*). These two triaxial lead diagrams were combined to produce a hexaxial lead diagram (Fig. 5-1, *C*). This is the lead diagram we will use in determining the mean QRS axis and in describing axis deviation.

As noted in Chapter 3, each of the leads has a positive and a negative pole (Fig. 5-1, *C*). As a wave of depolarization spreads toward the positive pole, an upward (positive) deflection occurs. As a wave spreads toward the negative pole, a downward (negative) deflection is inscribed.

Finally, to determine or calculate the mean QRS axis, we need a scale. By convention, the positive pole of lead I is said to be at 0°; all points below the lead I axis are positive; all points above that axis are negative (Fig. 5-2). Thus, as we move toward the positive pole of lead aV_L ($-30°$), the scale becomes negative; and as we move downward toward the positive poles of leads II, III, and aV_F, the scale becomes more positive—lead II at $+60°$, lead aV_F at $+90°$, lead III at $+120°$.

Figure 5-2 is the completed hexaxial diagram used to measure the QRS axis. By convention again, we can say that an electrical axis that points toward lead aV_L is *leftward* or *horizontal*. An axis that points toward leads II, III, and aV_F is *rightward* or *vertical*.

47

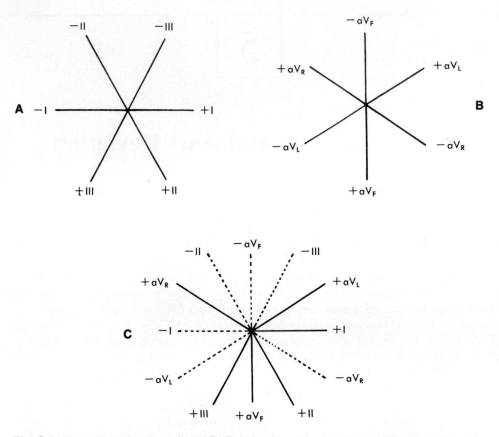

Fig. 5-1. Hexaxial lead system. **A** and **B,** Relationship of leads I, II, and III and of aV$_R$, aV$_L$, and aV$_F$. **C,** These diagrams have been combined to form a hexaxial lead diagram. Notice that each lead has both a positive and a negative pole (the latter designated by *dashed lines*).

Fig. 5-2. Hexaxial lead diagram. Notice that each lead has an angular designation—with the positive pole of lead I at 0° and all leads above it having negative angular values while those below it have positive values.

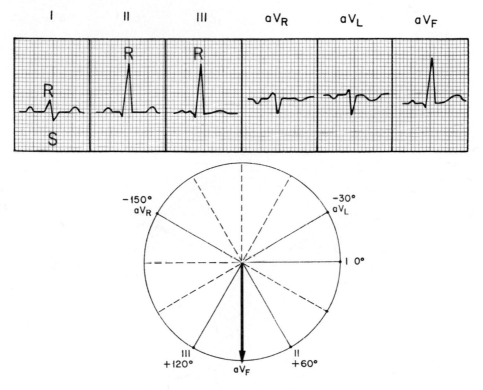

Fig. 5-3. Mean QRS axis of +90°. See text.

MEAN QRS AXIS: CALCULATION

In calculating the mean QRS axis you are answering the question: in what general direction or toward which lead axis is the QRS complex predominantly oriented? For example, consider Figure 5-3. Notice that there are tall R waves in leads II, III, and aV$_F$, indicating that the heart is electrically vertical (vertical electrical axis). Furthermore, the R wave is equally tall in leads II and III.* Therefore, by simple inspection, the mean electrical QRS axis can be seen to be directed between leads II and III and toward aV$_F$. Lead aV$_F$ on the hexaxial diagram is at +90°.

As a general rule: *The mean QRS axis will point midway between any two leads that show tall R waves of equal height.*

In the preceding example the mean electrical axis could have been calculated a second way. Recall from Chapter 3 that if a wave of depolarization is oriented at right angles to any lead axis a biphasic complex (RS or QR) will be recorded in that lead. Reasoning in a reverse manner, if you find a biphasic complex in any of the extremity leads, then the mean QRS axis must be directed at 90° to that lead. Now look at Figure 5-3 again. Are there any biphasic QRS complexes? Obviously lead I is biphasic and shows an RS pattern. Therefore, the mean electrical axis must be directed at right angles to lead I. Since lead I on the hexaxial lead scale is at 0°, the mean electrical axis must be at right angles to 0° or at either −90° or +90°. If the axis were −90°, then the depolariza-

---

*In this case there are actually three leads (II, III, and aV$_F$) with R waves of equal height. In such cases the electrical axis will point toward the middle lead, that is, toward aV$_F$ or at +90°.

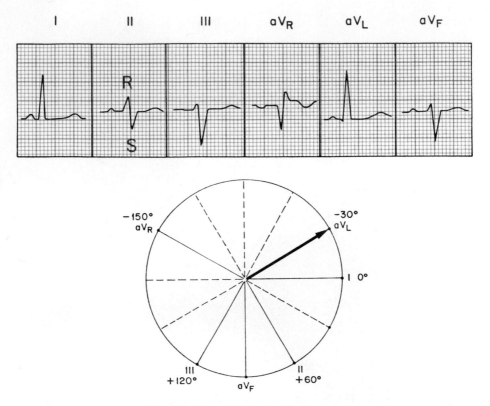

Fig. 5-4. Mean QRS of −30°. See text.

tion forces would be oriented away from the positive pole of lead aV_F and that lead would show a negative complex. In this case lead aV_F shows a positive complex (tall R wave), so the axis must be +90°.

Figure 5-4 presents another example. In this case, by inspection, the mean QRS axis is obviously horizontal since leads I and aV_L are positive and leads II, III, and aV_F are predominantly negative. The precise electrical axis can be calculated by looking at lead II, which shows a biphasic RS complex. Therefore, using the same logic as before, we can say that the axis must be at right angles to lead II. Since lead II is at +60° on the hexaxial scale (Fig. 5-2), the axis must be either −30° or +150°. If it were +150°, then leads II, III, and aV_F would be positive. Clearly in this case the axis is −30°.

Another example is given in Figure 5-5. The QRS complex is positive in leads II, III, and aV_F. Therefore we can say that the axis is relatively vertical. Since the R waves are of equal magnitude in leads I and III, the mean QRS axis must be oriented between these two leads, or at +60°.

Alternatively, we could have calculated the axis by looking at lead aV_L (in Fig. 5-5), which shows a biphasic RS-type complex. The axis must be at right angles to lead aV_L (−30°), that is, either −120° or +60°. Obviously, in this case the answer is +60°. The electrical axis must be oriented toward lead II, which shows a tall R wave.

We can now describe a second general rule: *The mean QRS axis will be oriented at right angles to any lead showing a biphasic complex. In such cases the mean QRS axis will point in the direction of leads showing tall R waves.*

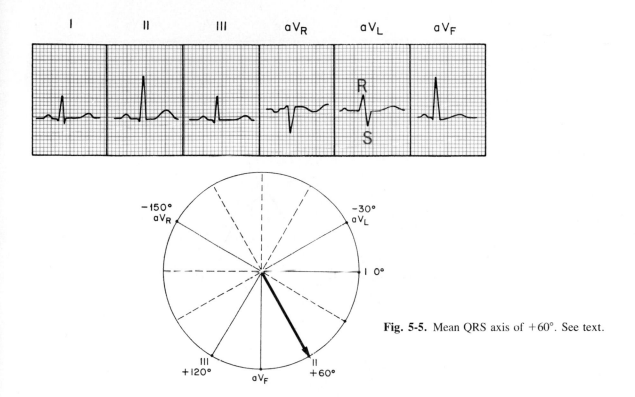

Fig. 5-5. Mean QRS axis of +60°. See text.

Fig. 5-6. Mean QRS axis of +90°. See text.

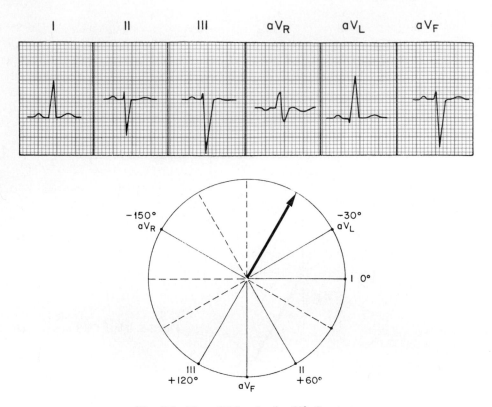

Fig. 5-7. Mean QRS axis of −60°. See text.

Still another example is given in Figure 5-6. By inspection, the electrical axis can be seen to be oriented away from leads II, III, and aV$_F$ and toward leads aV$_R$ and aV$_L$, which show positive complexes. Since the R waves are of equal magnitude in leads aV$_R$ and aV$_L$, the axis must be oriented precisely between these leads, or at −90°. Alternatively, look at lead I, which shows a biphasic RS complex. In this case the axis must be directed at right angles to lead I (0°); that is, it must be either −90° or +90°. Since the axis is oriented away from the positive pole of lead aV$_F$ and toward the negative pole of that lead, it must be −90°.

Again, look at Figure 5-7. There are two ways of approaching the calculation of the mean QRS in this case. Since lead aV$_R$ shows a biphasic RS-type complex, the electrical axis must be at right angles to the axis of that lead; and since the axis of aV$_R$ is at −150°, the electrical axis in this case must be either −60° or +120°. Clearly it is −60° since aV$_L$ is positive and III shows a negative complex.*

These basic examples should establish the ground rules for calculating the mean QRS axis. It is worth emphasizing that such calculations are generally only an estimate or a near approximation. An error of 10° or 15° is not clinically significant. Thus it is perfectly acceptable to calculate the axis from leads in which the QRS is nearly

---

*The QRS axis can also be calculated by looking at lead I, in Figure 5-7. It shows an R wave of equal amplitude with the S wave in lead II. The mean QRS axis must be oriented between the positive pole of lead I (0°) and the negative pole of lead II (−120°). Therefore it must be −60°.

biphasic or from two leads where the R (or S) waves are of approximately equal amplitude.*

To summarize: The mean QRS axis can be determined on the basis of one or both of the following rules:

1. It will point midway between the axes of two extremity leads that show tall R waves of equal amplitude.
2. It will point at 90° (right angles) to any extremity lead that shows a biphasic (QR or RS) type complex and in the direction of leads showing relatively tall R waves.

AXIS DEVIATION

The mean QRS axis is a basic measurement that should be made on every ECG. In most normal people it will lie between −30° and +100°. An axis of −30° or more negative is described as *left axis deviation (LAD),* and one that is +100° or more positive *right axis deviation (RAD).* In other words, LAD is abnormal extension of the mean QRS axis found in persons with an electrically horizontal heart while RAD is abnormal extension of the mean QRS axis in persons with an electrically vertical heart.

The mean QRS axis is determined by two major factors: (1) the anatomic position of the heart and (2) the direction in which the stimulus spreads through the ventricles (i.e., the direction of ventricular depolarization).

The influence of *cardiac anatomic position* on the electrical axis can be illustrated by the effects of respiration. When a person breathes in, the diaphragm descends and the heart becomes more vertical in the chest cavity. This change generally shifts the QRS electrical axis vertically (to the right). (Patients with emphysema and chronically hyperinflated lungs will usually have anatomically vertical hearts and electrically vertical QRS axes.) Conversely, when the person breathes out, the diaphragm ascends and the heart assumes a more horizontal position in the chest. This generally shifts the QRS electrical axis horizontally (to the left).

The influence of the *direction of ventricular depolarization* can be illustrated by left anterior hemiblock (Chapter 7), in which the spread of stimuli through the more superior and leftward portions of the left ventricle is delayed and the mean QRS axis shifts to the left. By contrast, with right ventricular hypertrophy the QRS axis shifts to the right.

Recognition of right and left axis deviation is quite simple.

RAD exists if the QRS axis is found to be +100° or more positive.

Recall that if leads II and III show tall R waves of equal height then the axis must be +90°. As an approximate rule: *If leads II and III show tall R waves and the R wave in lead III exceeds that in lead II then right axis deviation is present.* In addition, lead I will show an RS pattern with the S wave deeper than the R wave is tall (Figs. 5-8 and 5-10).

LAD exists if the QRS axis is found to be −30° or more negative.

Figure 5-4 presents an ECG in which the QRS axis is exactly −30°. Notice that lead II shows a biphasic (RS) complex. Remember that the location of lead II is aligned at +60° (Fig. 5-2) and a biphasic complex indicates that the electrical axis must be at right angles to that lead (at either −30° or +150°). Thus, with an axis of −30°, lead II will show an RS complex with the R and S of equal amplitude. *If the electrical axis is more negative than −30° (LAD) then lead II will show an RS complex with the S wave deeper than the R wave is tall* (Figs. 5-9 and 5-11).

---

*For example, when the R (or S) waves in two leads have similar but not identical voltages, the mean QRS axis will not lie exactly between these two leads. Instead, it will point more toward the lead with the larger amplitude.

Similarly, if a lead shows a biphasic (RS or QR) deflection with the R and S (or Q and R) waves *not* of identical amplitude, then the mean QRS axis will *not* be pointed exactly perpendicular to that lead. If the R wave is larger than the S (or Q) wave, the axis will point slightly less than 90° away from the lead. If the R wave is smaller than the S (or Q) wave, the axis will point slightly more than 90° away from that lead.

RIGHT AXIS DEVIATION

LEFT AXIS DEVIATION

Fig. 5-8. Right axis deviation (RAD)—mean QRS axis more positive than +100°—can be determined by simple inspection of leads I, II, and III. Notice that lead III shows an R wave taller than the R wave in lead II.

Fig. 5-9. Left axis deviation (LAD)—mean QRS axis more negative than −30°—can also be determined by simple inspection of leads I, II, and III. Notice that lead II shows an rS complex (with the S wave of greater amplitude than the r wave).

RIGHT AXIS DEVIATION

Fig. 5-10. Notice the R waves in leads II and III, with the one in lead III greater than the one in lead II, from a patient with RAD.

LEFT AXIS DEVIATION

Fig. 5-11. Notice the rS complex in lead II from a patient with LAD.

The rules for recognition of axis deviation can be summarized as follows:

1. *Right axis deviation* is present if the R wave in lead III is taller than the R wave in lead II. Notice that with right axis deviation lead I shows an RS-type complex with the S wave deeper than the R wave is tall (Figs. 5-8 and 5-10).

2. *Left axis deviation* is present if lead I shows a tall R wave, lead III shows a deep S wave, and lead II shows a biphasic S complex (with the amplitude of the S wave exceeding the height of the r wave) (Figs. 5-9 and 5-11) or a QS complex. Leads I and aV_L will both show R waves.

In Chapter 3 the terms *"electrically vertical"* and *"electrically horizontal"* heart positions (mean QRS axes) were introduced. Now in this chapter *"left axis deviation"* and *"right axis deviation."* have been added. What is the difference between these terms? "Electrically vertical" and "electrically horizontal" heart positions are qualitative. With an electrically vertical mean QRS axis, leads II, III, and aV_F will show tall R waves. With an electrically horizontal mean QRS axis, leads I and aV_L will show tall R waves. With an electrically vertical heart, the actual mean QRS axis may be normal (e.g., $+80°$) or abnormally rightward (e.g., $+120°$). Similarly, with an electrically horizontal heart, the actual axis may be normal ($0°$) or abnormally leftward ($-50°$).

RAD, therefore, is simply an extreme form of a vertical mean QRS axis (Fig. 5-12). LAD, similarly, is an extreme form of a horizontal mean QRS axis (Fig. 5-13). Saying that the patient has an electrically vertical or horizontal mean QRS axis does not, in fact, tell whether actual axis deviation is present.

Clinical Significance

Right and left axis deviations may be encountered in a variety of settings:

RAD, with the mean QRS axis $+100°$ or more, is sometimes seen in normal people. Right ventricular hypertrophy (Chapter 6) is an important cause

of RAD. Another cause is myocardial infarction of the lateral wall of the left ventricle. Loss of the normal leftward depolarization forces in this setting may lead "by default" to a rightward axis (Fig. 8-11). Left posterior hemiblock (Chapter 7) is a much rarer cause of RAD. Patients with chronic lung disease (emphysema or chronic bronchitis) often have electrocardiograms showing RAD. Finally, a sudden shift in the mean QRS axis to the right (not necessarily causing actual RAD) may occur with acute pulmonary embolism (Chapter 10).

LAD, with the mean QRS axis $-30°$ or more, may also be seen in several settings. Patients with left ventricular hypertrophy (Chapter 6) sometimes, but not always, have it. Left anterior hemiblock (Chapter 7) is a fairly common cause of marked deviation (more negative than $-45°$). LAD may be seen in association with left bundle branch block (Chapter 7). It may even occur in the absence of apparent cardiac disease.

However, axis deviation, right or left, does not necessarily imply significant underlying heart disease. Nevertheless, its recognition (Fig. 5-14) often provides supportive evidence for left or right ventricular hypertrophy, ventricular conduction disturbance (left anterior or posterior hemiblock), or one of the other disorders just listed.

Finally, it should be realized that the limits for left and right axis deviation ($-30°$ to $+100°$) used in this book are necessarily arbitrary. Some authors use different criteria (e.g., $0°$ to $+90°$). These apparent discrepancies reflect the important fact that there are no absolute parameters in clinical electrocardiography. The best we can do is apply general criteria. The same problems will be found in the next chapter, on left and right ventricular hypertrophy, in which different voltage criteria have been described by different authors.

On rare occasion, all six extremity leads will show biphasic (QR or RS) complexes, making it impossible to calculate the mean frontal plane QRS axis. In such cases the term *"indeterminate axis"* is used (Fig. 5-15). An indeterminate QRS axis may occur as a normal variant or be seen in a variety of pathologic settings.

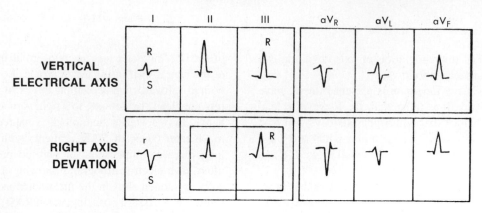

Fig. 5-12. Comparison of a normal vertical axis with actual RAD. See text.

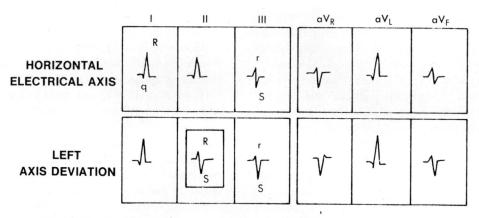

Fig. 5-13. Comparison of a normal horizontal axis with actual LAD. See text.

Fig. 5-14. Normal QRS axis and axis deviation. Most electrocardiograms show either a normal axis or left or right axis deviation. (Occasionally the QRS axis will be between $-90°$ and $180°$. Such an extreme shift may be caused by marked left or marked right axis deviation.)

Fig. 5-15. Indeterminate axis. Notice the biphasic complexes (RS or QR) in all six frontal plane leads.

MEAN ELECTRICAL AXIS OF THE P WAVE AND T WAVE

Up to now, only the mean electrical axis of the QRS complex in the frontal plane has been considered. Using the same principles, we can also discuss the mean electrical axes of the P wave and T wave in the frontal plane.

For example, when sinus rhythm is present, the normal P wave is always negative in lead aV_R and positive in lead II. Therefore, normally, the P wave is generally directed toward lead II (Fig. 4-3), making the normal mean P wave axis about $+60°$. On the other hand, if the AV junction (and not the sinus node) is pacing the heart, then the atria will be stimulated in a retrograde way. When AV junctional rhythm is present, atrial depolarization spreads upward, toward lead aV_R and away from lead II (Fig. 4-5). In such patients lead aV_R may show a positive P wave and lead II a negative P wave, and the mean P wave axis may be about $-150°$.

Using the same principles, we can also calculate the mean electrical axis of the T wave in the frontal plane. As a rule the mean T wave axis and the mean QRS axis normally point in the same general (but not identical) direction. In other words, when the electrical position of the heart is horizontal, the T waves will normally be positive in leads I and aV_L, in association with tall R waves in those leads; and when the electrical position is vertical, the T waves will normally be positive in leads II, III, and aV_F, in association with tall R waves in those leads. (However, the T wave is often negative in lead III normally, regardless of the electrical position of the heart.)

To summarize: The concept of mean electrical axis can be applied to the QRS complex, P wave, or T wave. In each case the mean electrical axis describes the general or overall direction in which depolarization or repolarization is directed in the frontal plane.

REVIEW

The term *"mean QRS axis"* describes the general direction toward which the QRS axis is directed in the frontal plane of the body. Therefore the mean QRS axis is measured in reference to the six extremity (frontal plane) leads. These leads can be arranged in the form of a hexaxial (six axes) diagram (Fig. 5-1, *C*).

The approximate mean QRS axis can be determined by using one of the following rules:
1. The axis will be pointed midway between any two leads that show tall R waves of equal height.
2. The axis will be pointed at right angles (perpendicular) to any lead showing a biphasic complex and toward other leads showing tall R waves.

The normal mean QRS axis lies between $-30°$ and $+100°$. An axis more negative than $-30°$ is defined as *left axis deviation* (LAD). An axis more positive than $+100°$ is defined as *right axis deviation* (RAD). LAD is an extreme form of a "horizontal" electrical axis. RAD is an extreme form of a "vertical" electrical axis.

LAD can be readily recognized if *lead II* shows an RS complex in which the S wave is deeper than the R wave is tall. In addition, *lead I* will show a tall R wave and *lead III* a deep S wave. LAD can be seen in cases of left ventricular hypertrophy, left anterior hemiblock, and other pathologic conditions and is sometimes seen in normal people.

RAD is present if the R wave in *lead III* is taller than the R wave in *lead II*. In addition, *lead I* will show an rS complex. RAD can be seen in several conditions, including right ventricular hypertrophy, lateral wall myocardial infarction, chronic lung disease, and left posterior hemiblock, and sometimes in normal people.

In rarer cases the QRS will be biphasic in all six extremity leads, making the mean electrical axis *indeterminate*.

The mean electrical axis of the P wave and T wave can also be estimated in the same manner as the mean QRS axis. With normal sinus rhythm the normal P wave will be about $+60°$ (positive P wave in lead II). Normally the T wave axis in the frontal plane will be similar to the QRS axis, so the T waves will normally be positive in leads with a predominantly positive QRS complex.

Questions

1. The six extremity leads (I, II, III, aV_R, aV_L, and aV_F) from a patient are shown. What is the approximate mean QRS axis?

2. *A, B,* and *C* are, in mixed order, leads I, II, and III from a patient with a mean QRS axis of −30°. This information should allow you to sort out which lead is which.

A   **B**   **C**

Answers

1. The QRS axis is roughly +60°. Notice that the QRS complex in lead aV$_L$ is biphasic. Therefore the mean QRS axis must point at a right angle to −30°. In this case the axis is obviously about +60° since leads II, III, and aV$_F$ are positive. Note that the R wave in III is slightly taller than the R wave in II. If the axis were exactly +60°, these waves would be equally tall. Thus the axis must be somewhat more positive than +60°, probably around +70°. Estimating the QRS axis to within 10° or 20° is usually quite adequate for clinical diagnosis.

2. *A,* lead II; *B,* lead I; *C,* lead III. Explanation: You are told that the mean QRS axis is −30°. Therefore, you know that the QRS axis is pointed toward lead I (which is at 0°) and away from lead III (which is at +120°). Obviously lead I must be *B* and lead III must be *C*. Lead II is *A*, which is biphasic. Lead II is at +60° on the hexaxial diagram; and if the mean QRS axis is −30°, then lead II will have to show a biphasic complex since the mean QRS axis is at right angles to that lead.

6

Atrial and Ventricular Enlargement

The basics of the normal ECG have been described in the first five chapters. From this point on, we will be concerned primarily with abnormal ECG patterns, beginning in this chapter with a consideration of the effects on the ECG of enlargement of the four cardiac chambers.

Two basic terms must first be defined. "Cardiac enlargement" refers to either *dilation* of a heart chamber or *hypertrophy* of the heart muscle.

In dilation of a chamber the heart muscle is *stretched* and the chamber becomes enlarged. For example, with congestive heart failure due to acute aortic valve regurgitation, dilation of the left ventricle occurs.

In cardiac hypertrophy the heart muscle fibers actually *increase in size,* with resulting enlargement of the chamber. For example, aortic stenosis, which obstructs the outflow of blood from the left ventricle, leads to hypertrophy of the left ventricular muscle. The atria and the right ventricle can also become hypertrophied in other situations (described later in this chapter). When cardiac hypertrophy occurs, the total number of heart muscle fibers does not increase; rather, each individual fiber becomes larger. One predictable ECG effect of cardiac hypertrophy will be an increase in voltage or duration of the P wave or QRS complex. Not uncommonly hypertrophy and dilation occur together.

Both dilation and hypertrophy usually result from some type of chronic pressure or volume load on the heart muscle. We will proceed with a discussion of the ECG patterns seen with enlargement of each of the four cardiac chambers, beginning with the right atrium.

RIGHT ATRIAL ENLARGEMENT (RAE)

Enlargement of the right atrium (either dilation or actual hypertrophy) may increase the voltage of the P wave. To recognize a large P wave, you must know the dimensions of the normal P wave.

When the P wave is positive, its amplitude is measured in millimeters from the upper level of the baseline, where the P wave begins, to the peak of the P wave. A negative P wave is measured from the lower level of the baseline to the lowest point of the P wave (Fig. 6-1). Measurement of the width of the P wave is also shown in Figure 6-1.

Normally the P wave in every lead is less than or equal to 2.5 mm (0.25 mV) in amplitude and less than 0.12 second (three small boxes) in width. A P wave exceeding either of these dimensions in any lead is abnormal.

Enlargement of the right atrium may produce an abnormally tall P wave (greater than 2.5 mm). However, because pure RAE does not generally increase the total duration of atrial depolarization, the width of the P wave will be normal (less than 0.12 sec) (Fig. 6-2). The abnormal P wave in RAE is sometimes referred to as *P pulmonale* because the atrial enlargement that it signifies is often seen with severe pulmonary disease. Figure 6-3 shows

Fig. 6-1. The normal P wave does not exceed 2.5 mm in height and is less than 0.12 second in width.

P pulmonale

Fig. 6-2. Tall narrow P waves indicate right atrial enlargement (P pulmonale pattern).

Fig. 6-3. Notice the tall P waves *(arrow)* in leads II, III, aV$_F$, and V$_1$, from a patient with chronic lung disease. This is the *P pulmonale* pattern.

an actual example of RAE with a P pulmonale pattern.

The tall narrow P waves characteristic of RAE can usually be seen best in leads II, III, aV$_F$, and sometimes V$_1$. The ECG diagnosis of P pulmonale can be made by finding a P wave exceeding 2.5 mm in any of these leads. *Echocardiographic* evidence, however, suggests that the finding of a tall peaked P wave does not consistently correlate with RAE. On the other hand, patients may have RAE and not tall P waves. In other words, tall peaked

P waves are of limited sensitivity and specificity (Chapter 19) in the diagnosis of right atrial enlargement.

RAE can be seen in a variety of clinical settings. Usually it is associated with right ventricular enlargement. Two of the most common clinical causes of RAE are pulmonary disease and congenital heart disease. The pulmonary disease may be either acute (bronchial asthma, pulmonary embolism) or chronic (emphysema, bronchitis). Congenital heart lesions producing RAE include pulmonic valve stenosis, atrial septal defects, Ebstein's anomaly of the tricuspid valve, and tetralogy of Fallot.

LEFT ATRIAL ENLARGEMENT (LAE); LEFT ATRIAL ABNORMALITY (LAA)

Enlargement of the left atrium (either by dilation or by actual hypertrophy) also produces predictable changes in the P wave. Normally the left atrium depolarizes after the right atrium. Thus left atrial enlargement should prolong the total duration of atrial depolarization, indicated by an abnormally wide P wave. LAE characteristically produces a wide P wave of 0.12 second (three small boxes) or more duration. The amplitude (height) of the P wave with LAE may be either normal or increased.

Figure 6-4 illustrates the characteristic P wave changes seen in LAE. Sometimes, as shown, the P wave will have a distinctive "humped" or "notched" appearance (Fig. 6-4, *A*). The second hump corresponds to the delayed depolarization of the left atrium. These humped P waves are usually best seen in one or more of the extremity leads (Fig. 6-5). The term *"P mitrale"* is sometimes used to describe wide P waves seen with LAE because they were first described in patients with rheumatic mitral valve disease.

In cases of LAE, lead V_1 sometimes shows a distinctive biphasic P wave (Figs. 6-4, *B*, and 6-6).

This wave has a small initial positive deflection and a prominent wide negative deflection. The negative component will be of >0.04 second duration or ≥ 1 mm depth. The prominent negative deflection corresponds to the delayed stimulation of the enlarged left atrium. Remember that, anatomically, the left atrium is situated posteriorly, up against the esophagus, whereas the right atrium lies anteriorly, against the sternum. The initial positive deflection of the P wave in lead V_1 therefore indicates right atrial depolarization whereas the deep negative deflection is a result of left atrial depolarization voltages directed posteriorly (away from the positive pole of lead V_1).

In some cases of LAE you will see both the broad often humped P waves in leads I and II and the biphasic P wave in lead V_1. In other cases only the broad notched P waves will be seen. Sometimes a biphasic P wave in lead V_1 will be the only ECG evidence of left atrial enlargement.

Clinically LAE may occur in a variety of settings including

1. Valvular heart disease, particularly aortic stenosis, aortic regurgitation, mitral regurgitation, and mitral stenosis (With mitral stenosis there is valvular obstruction to the emptying of the left atrium into the left ventricle. This will eventually result in a backup of pressure through the pulmonary vessels to the right ventricle. Therefore with advanced mitral stenosis

LEFT ATRIAL ENLARGEMENT (ABNORMALITY)

Fig. 6-4. Left atrial enlargement may produce, **A,** wide sometimes notched P waves in one or more extremity leads (*P mitrale* pattern) and/or, **B,** wide biphasic P waves in lead V_1.

Fig. 6-5. Broad humped P waves from a patient with left atrial enlargement.

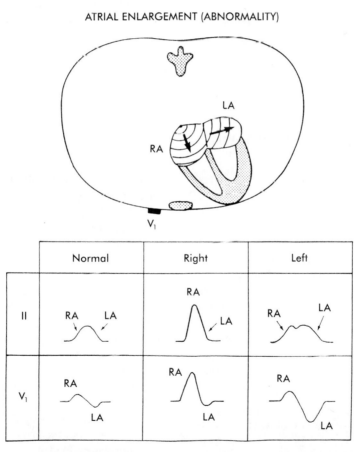

Fig. 6-6. Right atrial *(RA)* overload may cause tall peaked P waves in the limb or precordial leads. Left atrial *(LA)* abnormality may cause broad, often notched, P waves in the limb leads and a biphasic P in V_1 with a prominent negative component representing delayed depolarization of the left atrium. (Modified from Park MK, Guntheroth WG: *How to read pediatric ECGs*, ed 2, St Louis, 1987, Mosby.)

the ECG may show a combination of LAE with signs of right ventricular hypertrophy, as depicted in Figure 19-1.)

2. Hypertensive heart disease, which causes left ventricular enlargement and eventually LAE
3. Cardiomyopathies
4. Coronary artery disease

Some patients, particularly those with coronary artery disease, may have broad P waves without detectable enlargement of the left atrium. The abnormal P waves in these cases probably represent an atrial conduction delay in a normal-sized chamber. Therefore the more general term *"left atrial abnormality"* is increasingly being used in preference to left atrial "enlargement" to describe these abnormally broad P waves.

The patterns of left and right atrial enlargement (abnormality) are summarized schematically in Figure 6-6. Patients with enlargement of both atria (biatrial enlargement) may show a combination of patterns (e.g., tall and wide P waves).

RIGHT VENTRICULAR HYPERTROPHY (RVH)

Although atrial enlargement (dilation or hypertrophy) may produce prominent changes in the P wave, the QRS complex will be modified primarily by ventricular *hypertrophy*. The effects to be described indicate actual hypertrophy of the ventricular muscle and not simply ventricular dilation.

The ECG changes produced by both right and left ventricular hypertrophy can be predicted on the basis of what you already know about the normal QRS patterns. Normally (as described in Chapter 4) the left and right ventricles depolarize simultaneously and the left ventricle is electrically predominant because it has greater mass. As a result, leads placed over the right side of the chest (such as V_1) will record rS-type complexes $\left(\bigvee_{S}^{r} \right)$, in which the deep negative S wave indicates the spread of depolarization voltages away from the right and toward the left side. Conversely, leads placed over the left chest (such as V_5 or V_6) will record a qR-type complex $\left(\bigwedge_{q}^{R} \right)$, in which the tall positive R wave indicates the predominant depolarization voltages that point to the left generated by the left ventricle.

Now, if the right ventricle becomes sufficiently hypertrophied, this normal electrical predominance of the left ventricle can be overcome. In such cases, what type of QRS complex might you expect to see in the right chest leads? With RVH, the right chest leads will show tall R waves, indicating the spread of positive voltages from the hypertrophied right ventricle toward the right (Fig. 6-7). Figures 6-8 and 6-9 show actual examples of RVH. Instead of the rS complex normally seen in lead V_1, we now see a tall positive (R) wave, indicating marked hypertrophy of the right ventricle.

How tall an R wave in lead V_1 do you have to see to make a diagnosis of RVH? As a general rule the normal R wave in lead V_1 in adults will be smaller than the S wave in that lead. An R wave exceeding the S wave in lead V_1 is suggestive, but not diagnostic, of RVH. Sometimes, as shown in Figure 6-8, a small q wave will precede the tall R wave in lead V_1 in cases of RVH.

Along with tall right chest R waves, RVH often produces two additional ECG signs: right axis deviation and right ventricular "strain" T wave inversions.

As noted in Chapter 5, the normal mean QRS axis in adults lies approximately between $-30°$ and $+100°$. A mean QRS axis of $+100°$ or more is called *right axis deviation*. One of the most common causes of right axis deviation is RVH. Therefore, whenever you see an ECG with right axis deviation, you should search carefully for other signs or confirmatory evidence of RVH (Figs. 6-8 and 6-9).

RVH, however, not only produces depolariza-

QRS IN HYPERTROPHY

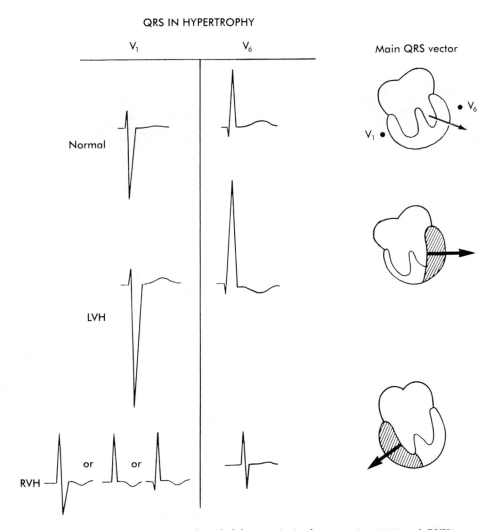

Fig. 6-7. The QRS patterns with left and right ventricular hypertrophy *(LVH* and *RVH)* can be anticipated based on the abnormal physiology. Notice that LVH exaggerates the normal pattern, causing deeper right precordial S waves and taller left precordial R waves. By contrast, RVH shifts the QRS vector to the right, causing increased right precordial R waves.

RIGHT VENTRICULAR HYPERTROPHY

Fig. 6-8. Notice the tall R wave in lead V_1 (with an inverted T wave caused by right ventricular strain). There is also right axis deviation (R wave in lead III taller than that in lead II). This patient has tetralogy of Fallot.

tion (QRS) changes, it also affects repolarization (the ST-T complex). For reasons not fully understood, hypertrophy of the heart muscle alters the normal sequence of repolarization. With RVH the characteristic repolarization change is the appearance of inverted T waves in the right and middle chest leads, as shown in Figures 6-8 and 6-9. These right chest T wave inversions are referred to as a right ventricular *strain* pattern. (Strain is a descriptive term. The exact mechanism for the strain pattern is not understood.)

To summarize: With RVH, the ECG may show tall R waves in the right chest leads, with the R wave greater than the S wave in lead V_1.* Right

axis deviation and right ventricular strain T wave inversions are also often present. Some cases of RVH are more subtle, and the ECG may show only one of these patterns. The appearance of all three patterns (tall right precordial R waves, right axis deviation, and right ventricular "strain"), however, firmly establishes the diagnosis of RVH, although the absence of these patterns does not necessarily exclude RVH.

RVH may occur in a variety of clinical settings. An important cause is congenital heart disease (e.g., pulmonic stenosis, atrial septal defect,* tetralogy of Fallot, or the Eisenmenger syndrome). Patients with long-standing severe pulmonary disease may have pulmonary artery hypertension and RVH. Mitral stenosis, as mentioned previously, can produce a combination of LAE and RVH.

---

*With RVH the chest leads to the left of leads showing tall R waves may show a variable pattern: Sometimes the middle and left chest leads show poor R wave progression, with rS or RS complexes all the way to lead V_6 (Fig. 6-9). In other cases normal R wave progression is preserved and the left chest leads also show R waves (Fig. 6-8).

---

*Patients with right ventricular enlargement from the atrial septal defect often exhibit a right bundle branch block pattern (RSR′ in lead V_1) with a vertical or rightward QRS axis.

RIGHT VENTRICULAR HYPERTROPHY

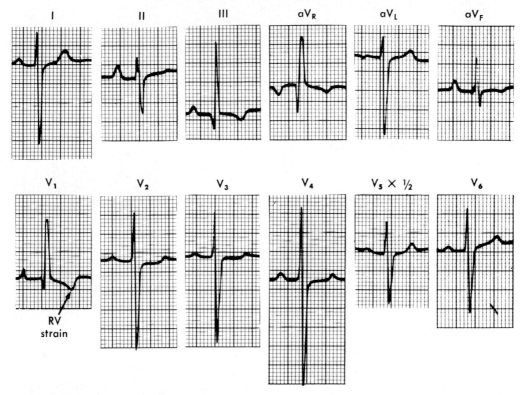

Fig. 6-9. Sometimes lead V_1 will show a tall R wave as part of the qR complex. Notice the peaked P waves (leads II, III, and V_1) because of right atrial enlargement. The T wave inversion in V_1 and ST depressions in V_2 and V_3 are due to right ventricular "strain." There is also a prolonged PR interval (0.24 sec), indicating first-degree AV block.

Right ventricular "strain" T wave inversions (in V_1 to V_3) may also occur without other ECG signs of RVH, as in acute pulmonary embolism (Chapter 10).

In patients with RVH associated with emphysema the ECG may not show any of the patterns just described. Instead of tall R waves in the right precordial leads, there will be poor R wave progression. Right axis deviation is also commonly present. (See Figure 10-17.)

LEFT VENTRICULAR HYPERTROPHY (LVH)

The ECG changes produced by LVH, like those from RVH, are predictable (Fig. 6-7). Normally the left ventricle is electrically predominant over

the right ventricle, producing prominent S waves in the right chest leads and tall R waves in the left chest leads. When LVH is present, the balance of electrical forces is tipped even further to the left. Thus, when LVH is present, abnormally tall R waves will be seen in the left chest leads with abnormally deep S waves in the right chest leads.

The following criteria and guidelines have been established to help in the ECG diagnosis of LVH:

1. If the depth of the S wave in lead V_1 (S_{V_1}) added to the height of the R wave in either lead V_5 or V_6 (R_{V_5} or R_{V_6}) exceeds 35 mm (3.5 mV), then consider LVH (Fig. 6-10).

2. You should also realize that high voltage in the chest leads is commonly seen as a normal finding, particularly in young adults with

LEFT VENTRICULAR HYPERTROPHY

Fig. 6-10. This patient has severe hypertension. Notice the pattern of left ventricular hypertrophy: tall voltage in the chest leads and aV_L (R = 16 mm) with "strain" pattern in these leads. In addition, there is the pattern of left atrial enlargement, including a biphasic P wave in lead V_1 and a broad notched P wave in lead II.

Fig. 6-11. Tall voltage in the chest leads (R_{V_1} + S_{V_5} = 36 mm) in a 20-year-old man. This is a normal variant caused by the patient's thin chest wall. The ST-T complexes are normal, without evidence of left ventricular "strain."

LEFT VENTRICULAR "STRAIN" PATTERN

Fig. 6-12. Notice the characteristic wavy ST-T pattern with T wave inversion in leads showing tall R waves. These repolarization abnormalities associated with LVH are often referred to as the "strain" pattern, an imprecise but commonly used term.

thin chest walls. Consequently, high voltage in the chest leads ($S_{V_1} + R_{V_5}$ or $R_{V_6} > 35$ mm) is not a *specific* indicator of LVH (Fig. 6-11).

3. In some cases LVH will produce tall R waves in lead aV_L. An R wave of 11 to 13 mm or more in lead aV_L (Fig. 6-9) is another sign of LVH.* Sometimes a tall R wave in lead aV_L will be the only ECG sign of LVH and the voltage in chest leads will be normal. In other cases the chest voltages will be abnormally high, with a normal R wave in lead aV_L.

4. Furthermore, just as RVH is associated with a right ventricular "strain" pattern, so left ventricular strain ST-T changes are often seen in LVH. Figure 6-12 illustrates the characteristic shape of the ST-T complex with left ventricular strain. Notice that it has a distinctively asymmetric appearance, with slight ST segment depression followed by a broadly inverted T wave. In some cases these T wave inversions will be very deep. The left ventricular "strain" pattern is seen in leads with tall R waves (Fig. 6-10).

5. With LVH the electrical axis is usually horizontal. Actual left axis deviation (axis $-30°$ or more negative) may also be seen. In addition, the QRS complex may become wider. Not uncommonly patients with LVH may eventually develop a left bundle branch block–type pattern. (See Chapter 7.)

6. Finally, the signs of LAE (broad P waves in the extremity leads or wide biphasic P waves in V_1) are often seen in patients with ECG evidence of LVH. Most conditions that lead to LVH ultimately produce left atrial overload as well.

A variety of clinical conditions may be associated with LVH. In adults three of the most common are (1) valvular heart disease (particularly aortic stenosis, aortic regurgitation, or mitral regurgitation), (2) systemic hypertension, and (3) cardiomyopathies (p.136).

To summarize: The diagnosis of LVH can be made with reasonable certainty from the ECG if you find high QRS voltages with characteristic ST-T changes ("strain" pattern). Signs of left atrial abnormality are also often present. High voltage in the chest or extremity leads can sometimes be seen in normal subjects, so the diagnosis of LVH should not be made on this finding alone.* T wave inversion resulting from left ventricular overload can also occur without other evidence of LVH.

THE ECG IN CARDIAC ENLARGEMENT: A PERSPECTIVE

The ECG findings associated with enlargement of each of the four cardiac chambers have been presented. In some cases combined patterns will be seen on the same tracing (e.g., LAE and RVH in cases of mitral stenosis or LAE and LVH with hypertension). You may be wondering what the ECG shows if both left and right ventricles become hypertrophied (biventricular hypertrophy). In such cases it usually shows mainly evidence of LVH.

Finally, always remember that in the assessment of cardiac size the ECG is only an indirect laboratory test and not an absolute measurement. A person may have underlying cardiac enlargement that does not show up on the ECG. Conversely, high voltage may be present in normal persons without cardiac enlargement. When the presence or degree of cardiac chamber enlargement must be determined with more precision, an *echocardiogram* should be obtained. (For further discussion of the diagnostic limitations of the ECG, see Chapter 19.)

---

*Occasionally LVH develops with an electrically vertical axis. In such cases a qR pattern with a tall R wave (exceeding 20 mm) may appear in lead aV_F.

*The voltage criteria used here for diagnosing LVH in the chest and extremity leads are by no means absolute numbers. Some authors use slightly different voltage criteria.

REVIEW

Cardiac *dilation* refers to stretching of muscle fibers, with enlargement of one or more of the cardiac chambers. Cardiac *hypertrophy* refers to an abnormal increase in the actual size of the heart muscle fibers. The ECG can indicate either right or left atrial dilation or hypertrophy but generally only right or left ventricular hypertrophy.

Right atrial enlargement may be associated with tall peaked P waves *(P pulmonale pattern)* exceeding 2.5 mm in height, usually best seen in leads II, III, aV_F, and sometimes V_1 or V_2.

Left atrial enlargement (abnormality) is manifested by wide, sometimes notched, P waves *(P mitrale pattern)* of 0.12 second or more duration in one or more of the extremity leads. A biphasic P wave with a prominent wide negative deflection may be seen in lead V_1.

Right ventricular hypertrophy may produce any or all of the following:
1. Tall R wave in lead V_1, equal to or larger than the S wave in that lead
2. RAD often present
3. Right ventricular strain pattern (T wave inversions in the right to middle chest leads)

Left ventricular hypertrophy may produce any or all of the following:
1. The voltage of the S wave in lead V_1 plus the voltage of the R wave in lead V_5 or V_6 exceeding 35 mm ($S_{V_1} + R_{V_5}$ or $R_{V_6} > 35$ mm)
2. A high-voltage R wave in lead aV_L (11 to 13 mm or more) when the heart is electrically horizontal (When the axis is vertical, lead aV_F may show a tall R wave [>20 mm] as part of a qR complex.)
3. A left ventricular strain pattern (inverted T waves in leads with a qR pattern)

The diagnosis of LVH should *not* be made solely on the basis of high voltage in the chest leads, since this may occur normally, particularly in young adults and thin-chested people. In addition, enlargement of any of the four cardiac chambers can be present without diagnostic ECG changes.

Questions

1. Answer these questions about the ECG to the right:
   a. What is the approximate heart rate?
   b. Is sinus rhythm present?
   c. Where is the transition zone in the chest leads?
   d. Mention three signs of LVH.

2. In the ECG on page 72
   a. What is the heart rate?
   b. Name two abnormal findings.

Answers

1. a. About 75 beats/min.
   b. The PR interval is prolonged (about 0.22 sec) because of first-degree AV block (Chapter 15). Also, the P wave in lead II is abnormally wide and notched (notice the two humps) as a result of left atrial enlargement (abnormality).

2. a. About 100 beats/min.
   b. No. Notice the retrograde P waves, positive in lead aV_R and negative in lead II, owing to an AV junctional (or ectopic atrial) rhythm.
   c. Between leads V_4 and V_5.
   d. Tall voltage in chest leads ($S_{V_1} + R_{V_6} > 35$ mm); tall voltage in lead aV_L (R wave > 13 mm); left ventricular strain pattern in leads I, aV_L, and V_5 and V_6.

7

Ventricular Conduction Disturbances

BUNDLE BRANCH BLOCKS

Recall that in the normal process of ventricular activation (Chapter 4) the electrical stimulus reaches the ventricles from the atria by way of the AV junction. The first part of the ventricles stimulated (depolarized) is the left side of the ventricular septum. Soon after, the depolarization spreads to the main mass of the left and right ventricles by way of the left and right bundle branches. Normally the entire process of ventricular depolarization is completed within about 0.1 second (100 msec). This is the reason why the normal width of the QRS complex is less than or equal to 100 msec (two and a half small boxes on the ECG graph paper). Any process that interferes with the normal stimulation of the ventricles may prolong the QRS width. In this chapter we will be concerned primarily with the effects of blocks within the bundle branch system on the QRS complex.

RIGHT BUNDLE BRANCH BLOCK (RBBB)

Consider, first, the effect of cutting (or markedly slowing conduction in) the right bundle branch. Obviously this will delay right ventricular stimulation and widen the QRS complex. Furthermore, the shape of the QRS with a right bundle branch block (RBBB) can be predicted on the basis of some familiar principles.

Normally the *first* part of the ventricles to be depolarized is the interventricular septum (Fig. 4-6,

A). The left side of the interventricular septum is stimulated first (by a branch of the left bundle). This septal depolarization produces the small septal r wave in lead V_1 and the small septal q wave in V_6 seen on the normal ECG (Fig. 7-1, A). Clearly, RBBB should not affect this first septal phase of ventricular stimulation, since the septum is stimulated by a part of the left bundle.

The *second* phase of ventricular stimulation is the simultaneous depolarization of the left and right ventricles (Fig. 4-6, B). RBBB should not affect this phase either, since the left ventricle is normally electrically predominant, producing deep S waves in the right chest leads and tall R waves in the left chest leads (Fig. 7-1, B). The change in the QRS complex produced by RBBB is a result of the delay in the total time needed for stimulation of the right ventricle. This means that following the completion of left ventricular depolarization, the right ventricle continues to depolarize.

This delayed right ventricular depolarization produces a *third* phase of ventricular stimulation. The electrical voltages in the third phase are directed to the right, reflecting the delayed depolarization and slow spread of the depolarization wave outward through the right ventricle. Therefore a lead placed over the right side of the chest (e.g., V_1) will record this third phase of ventricular stimulation as a positive wide deflection (R′ wave).

RIGHT BUNDLE BRANCH BLOCK

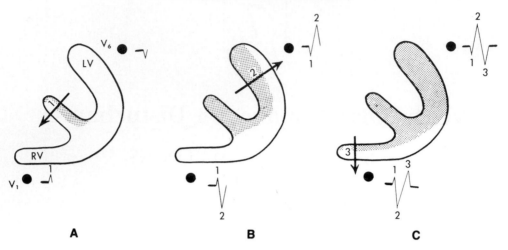

Fig. 7-1. Step-by-step sequence of ventricular depolarization in RBBB. See text.

The same delayed and slow right ventricular depolarization voltages spreading to the right will produce a wide negative (S wave) deflection in the left chest leads (e.g., V_6) (Fig. 7-1, *C*).

Putting together in step-by-step fashion what has been explained, we can now derive the pattern seen in the chest leads with RBBB. Lead V_1 will show an rSR′ complex with a broad R′ wave. Lead V_6 will show a qRS-type complex with a broad S wave. The tall wide R wave in the right chest leads and the deep terminal S wave in the left chest leads represent the same event viewed from opposite sides of the chest—the slow spread of delayed depolarization voltages through the right ventricle.

To make the initial diagnosis of RBBB, look at leads V_1 and V_6 in particular. The characteristic appearance of QRS complexes in these leads makes the diagnosis simple.

Figure 7-1 shows how the delay in ventricular depolarization with RBBB produces the characteristic ECG patterns we have been discussing.

To summarize: In RBBB the ventricular stimulation process can be divided into three phases. The first two consist of normal septal and left ventricular depolarization. The third phase is delayed stimulation of the right ventricle. These three phases of ventricular stimulation with RBBB are represented on the ECG by the triphasic complexes seen in the chest leads—V_1 showing an rSR′ complex with a wide R′ wave, V_6 showing a qRS pattern with a wide S wave.

We have seen that with an RBBB the QRS complex in lead V_1 generally shows an rSR′ pattern. Occasionally, however (Fig. 7-3), the S wave never quite makes its way below the baseline, giving the complex in lead V_1 the appearance of a large notched R wave.

Figures 7-2 and 7-3 show some typical examples of RBBB. Do you notice anything abnormal about the ST-T complexes in these tracings? If you look carefully, you will see that the T waves in the right leads are inverted. Right chest lead T wave inversions are a characteristic finding with RBBB. They are referred to as *secondary changes* because they reflect just the delay in ventricular stimulation. By contrast, *primary T wave abnormalities* reflect an actual change in repolarization, independent of any QRS change. For example, T wave inversions resulting from ischemia (Chapters 8 and 9), hypokalemia (Chapter 10), or drugs such as digitalis (Chapter 10) are all examples of primary T wave abnormalities.

RIGHT BUNDLE BRANCH BLOCK

Fig. 7-2. Notice the wide rSR′ complex in lead V_1 and the qRS complex in lead V_6. Inverted T waves in the right precordial leads (in this case V_1 to V_3) are common with RBBB and are called *secondary* T wave inversions.

RIGHT BUNDLE BRANCH BLOCK

Fig. 7-3. Sometimes, with RBBB, instead of the classic rSR′ pattern, the right precordial leads show a wide notched R wave (seen here in leads V_1 to V_3). Notice the *secondary* T wave inversions in leads V_1 to V_3, II, III, and aV_F, all of which show rSR′-type complexes. However, the abnormal ST-T changes in V_4 and V_5 are *primary* since they are present in leads without an R′ wave.

Some ECGs will show both primary and secondary ST-T changes. In Figure 7-3 the T wave inversions in leads V_1 to V_3 and in II, III, and aV_F can be explained solely on the basis of the RBBB since they occur in leads with an rSR'-type complex. However, the T wave inversions or ST depressions in other leads (V_4 and V_5) represent a primary change, perhaps resulting from ischemia or a drug effect.

Complete vs Incomplete RBBB

RBBB can be subdivided into complete and incomplete forms depending on the width of the QRS complex. Complete RBBB is defined by a QRS that is 0.12 second or more in duration with an rSR' in lead V_1 and a qRS in V_6. Incomplete RBBB shows the same QRS patterns, but its duration is between 0.1 and 0.12 second.

Clinical Significance

RBBB may be caused by a number of factors. First, some normal people will have this finding without any underlying heart disorder. Therefore RBBB per se is not necessarily abnormal. In many people, however, it is associated with organic heart disease. It may occur with virtually any condition that affects the right side of the heart (atrial septal defect with left-to-right shunting of blood, chronic pulmonary disease with pulmonary artery hypertension, or a valvular lesion like pulmonic stenosis). In some individuals (particularly older people) it is related to chronic degenerative changes in the conduction system. It may also occur with myocardial ischemia or infarction.

Pulmonary embolism, which produces acute right-sided heart overload, may cause a right ventricular conduction delay. When RBBB occurs following coronary artery bypass graft surgery, it does not seem to have any special clinical implications.

RBBB may be permanent or transient. Sometimes it appears only when the heart rate exceeds a certain critical value (rate-related RBBB).

Blockage of the right bundle branch does not, by itself, require any specific treatment. However, in patients with acute anterior wall infarction a new RBBB may indicate increased risk of complete heart block (see Chapter 15), particularly when associated with left anterior or posterior hemiblock.

LEFT BUNDLE BRANCH BLOCK (LBBB)

Left bundle branch block (LBBB) also produces a pattern with a widened QRS complex. However, the QRS with LBBB is very different from that with RBBB. The major reason for this difference is that RBBB affects mainly the terminal phase of ventricular activation while LBBB affects the early phase as well.

Recall that the first phase of ventricular stimulation—depolarization of the left side of the septum—is started by a branch of the left bundle. LBBB therefore will block this normal pattern. When LBBB is present, the septum depolarizes from *right* to *left* and not from left to right. Thus the first major change on the ECG produced by LBBB will be a loss of the normal septal r wave in lead V_1 and the normal septal q wave in lead V_6 (Fig. 7-4, *A*). Furthermore, the total time for left ventricular depolarization will be prolonged with LBBB, resulting in an abnormally wide QRS complex. Lead V_6 will show a wide, entirely positive, (R) wave (Fig. 7-4, *B*). The right chest leads (e.g., V_1) record a negative QRS (QS) complex because the left ventricle is still electrically predominant with LBBB and therefore produces greater voltages than the right ventricle. The major change is that the total time for completion of left ventricular depolarization is delayed. Therefore, with LBBB the entire process of ventricular stimulation is oriented toward the left chest leads—the septum depolarizing from right to left, with stimulation of the electrically predominant left ventricle prolonged. Figure 7-4 illustrates the sequence of ventricular activation in LBBB.*

---

*A variation of this pattern that sometimes occurs is for lead V_1 to show an rS complex with a very small r wave and a wide S wave. This superficially suggests that the septum is being stimulated normally from left to right. However, lead V_6 in such cases will show an abnormally wide and notched R wave *without* an initial q wave.

LEFT BUNDLE BRANCH BLOCK

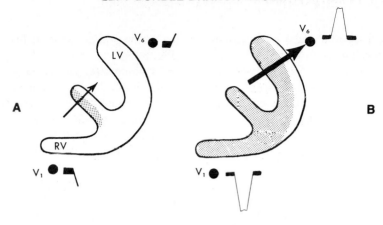

Fig. 7-4. The sequence of ventricular depolarization in LBBB produces a wide QS complex in lead V_1 and a wide R wave in V_6.

LEFT BUNDLE BRANCH BLOCK

Fig. 7-5. Notice the characteristic wide QS complex in lead V_1 and the wide R wave in lead V_6 with slight notching at the peak. The inverted T waves in V_5 and V_6 are also characteristic of LBBB (secondary T wave inversions).

Sometimes the QS wave in lead V_1 with LBBB will show a small notching at its point, giving it a characteristic W shape. Similarly the R wave in lead V_6 may show a notching at its peak, giving it a distinctive M shape. An actual example of an LBBB pattern is shown in Figure 7-5.

Just as there are *secondary* T wave inversions with RBBB, so there are also secondary T wave inversions with LBBB. As you can see from Figure 7-5, the T waves in the leads with tall R waves are inverted (e.g., the left precordial leads), characteristic of LBBB. However, T wave inversions in the right precordial leads cannot be explained solely on the basis of LBBB and, if present, re-

flect some *primary* abnormality, such as ischemia (Fig. 8-21).

To summarize: The diagnosis of LBBB can be made simply by inspection of leads V_1 and V_6. Lead V_1 usually shows a wide, entirely negative, QS complex (rarely a wide rS complex) whereas V_6 shows a wide tall R wave without a q wave. You should have no problem differentiating left and right bundle branch block patterns. Figure 7-6 compares the complexes seen. Occasionally an ECG will show wide QRS complexes that are not typical of an RBBB or LBBB pattern. In such cases the general term *"intraventricular delay"* is used (Fig. 7-7).

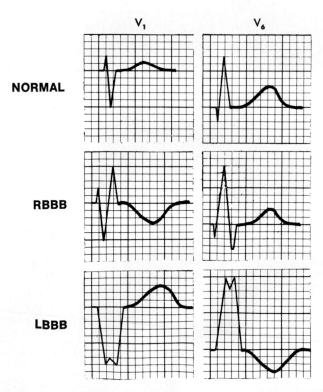

Fig. 7-6. Comparison of leads V_1 and V_6, with normal conduction, right bundle branch block, and left bundle branch block. Normally V_1 shows an rS complex and V_6 a qR complex. With RBBB, lead V_1 shows a wide rSR′ complex and V_6 a qRS complex. With LBBB, lead V_1 shows a wide QS complex and V_6 a wide R wave.

Complete vs Incomplete LBBB

As with RBBB, there are complete and incomplete forms of LBBB. With complete LBBB the QRS complex has the characteristic appearance described previously and is 0.12 second or wider. With incomplete LBBB the QRS is between 0.1 and 0.12 second wide.

Clinical Significance

Unlike RBBB, which is occasionally seen in normal people, LBBB is usually a sign of organic heart disease. It may develop in patients with long-standing hypertensive heart disease, a valvular lesion (e.g., calcification of the mitral annulus, aortic stenosis or aortic regurgitation), or different types of cardiomyopathy (p. 136). It is also seen in patients with coronary artery disease. Most patients with LBBB have underlying left ventricular hypertrophy (Chapter 6). In rare instances some otherwise normal individuals will have an LBBB pattern.

Like RBBB, LBBB may be a permanent condi-

Fig. 7-7. Nonspecific intraventricular conduction delay. The QRS here is abnormally wide (0.11 sec). However, such a pattern is not typical of LBBB or RBBB. In this case it was caused by a lateral wall myocardial infarction. (See Chapter 8.)

tion or transient. It also may appear only when the heart rate exceeds a certain critical value (rate-dependent LBBB). In some cases its presence may be the first clue to previously undiagnosed but clinically important abnormalities—for example, coronary artery disease, valvular heart disease, hypertensive heart disease, or cardiomyopathy.

PACEMAKER PATTERNS

Pacemakers are battery-operated devices designed to stimulate the heart electrically. They are used primarily when the patient's own heart rate is not adequate (e.g., in complete heart block or "sick sinus syndrome"). In most cases the pacemaker electrode is inserted into the right ventricle. Therefore the ECG will show an LBBB pattern, reflecting delayed activation of the left ventricle. Figure 7-8 is an example of a pacemaker tracing.

The vertical spike preceding each QRS complex is the pacemaker spike, followed by a wide QRS with an LBBB morphology (QS in lead V_1 with a wide R wave in V_6). Pacemakers are discussed in greater detail in Chapter 20.

Up to this point, we have considered major causes of a very wide QRS complex: RBBB, LBBB, and pacemaker patterns. Later (p. 140) the list will be expanded to include hyperkalemia, the Wolff-Parkinson-White preexcitation syndrome, and toxicity due to certain drugs (e.g., quinidine or procainamide).

HEMIBLOCKS (FASCICULAR BLOCKS)

A slightly more complex but important topic is the hemiblocks. Up to now we have discussed the left bundle branch system as if it were a single pathway. Actually it has been known for many

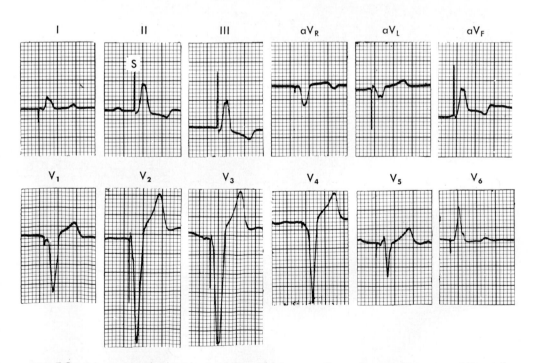

Fig. 7-8. A pacemaker inserted in the right ventricle generally produces a pattern resembling that of LBBB, with a wide QS in lead V_1 and a wide R wave in V_6, caused by delayed depolarization of the left ventricle. Notice the pacemaker spike in each lead preceding the QRS complex. In some leads (e.g., II) the spike *(S)* is positive; in others (V_1 to V_6) it is negative.

years to be subdivided into two major branches, or *fascicles* (*fasciculus,* Latin, small bundle). It consists of an anterior fascicle and a posterior fascicle. The right bundle branch, by contrast, is a single pathway and consists of just one main fascicle or bundle.

This revised concept of the bundle branch system as a trifascicular highway (one right lane, two left) is illustrated in Figure 7-9.

To summarize: The bundle of His divides into a right bundle branch and a left main bundle branch. The left main bundle branch then subdivides into an anterior and a posterior fascicle.

It makes sense to suppose that a block can occur at any single point (or at multiple points) in this trifascicular system. We have already seen the ECG pattern with a block in the right bundle branch. The pattern of LBBB can obviously occur in one of two ways: by a block in the left main bundle before it divides or by blocks in both subdivisions (anterior and posterior fascicles).

The next question is, what happens if a block occurs in just the anterior or just the posterior fascicle of the left bundle? A block in either fascicle of the left bundle branch system is called a *hemiblock* or *fascicular block.* Recognition of

hemiblocks on the ECG is intimately related to the subject of axis deviation, presented in Chapter 5. Somewhat surprisingly, a hemiblock (unlike a full left or right bundle branch block) does not widen the QRS complex markedly. It has been found experimentally that the main effect of cutting these fascicles is to change the QRS axis. Specifically, *left anterior* hemiblock results in marked left axis deviation ($-45°$ or more); *left posterior* hemiblock produces right axis deviation ($+120°$ or more).*

To summarize: Hemiblocks are partial blocks in the left bundle branch system and involve either the anterior or the posterior fascicle. The diagnosis of a hemiblock is made from the mean QRS axis in the extremity (frontal plane) leads. This is in contrast to the diagnosis of complete (or incomplete) right or left bundle branch block, which is made primarily from the QRS patterns in the chest (horizontal plane) leads. Complete bundle branch

---

*Left anterior hemiblock shifts the QRS axis to the left by delaying activation of the more superior and leftward portions of the left ventricle. Left posterior hemiblock shifts it to the right by delaying activation of the more inferior and rightward portions of the left ventricle. In both cases therefore the QRS axis is shifted *toward* the direction of delayed activation.

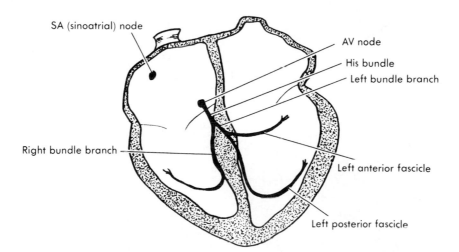

Fig. 7-9. Trifascicular conduction system. Notice that the left bundle branch subdivides into a left anterior fascicle and a left posterior fascicle. This diagram is a revision of the original drawing of the conduction system (Fig. 1-1).

blocks, unlike hemiblocks, do not cause a characteristic shift in the mean QRS axis.

Left anterior hemiblock. Isolated left anterior hemiblock is diagnosed by finding a mean QRS axis of $-45°$ or more and a QRS width of less than 0.12 second. A mean QRS axis of $-45°$ or more can be easily recognized because the S wave in lead aV_F equals or exceeds the R wave in lead I (Fig. 7-10).

Left posterior hemiblock. Isolated left posterior hemiblock (Fig. 9-8, *B*) is diagnosed by finding a mean QRS axis of $+120°$ or more, with a QRS width of less than 0.12 second. *However, the diagnosis of left posterior hemiblock can be considered only if other, more common, causes of right axis deviation* (e.g., right ventricular hypertrophy, normal variant, emphysema, lateral wall infarction [Fig. 8-11], and pulmonary embolism) *are first excluded*.

Although left anterior hemiblock is relatively common, isolated left posterior hemiblock is rare. In general, the finding of *isolated* left anterior or left posterior hemiblock is not of much clinical significance.

We will consider the hemiblocks and *bifascicular* and *trifascicular* blocks further in the section on complete heart block (Chapter 15).

DIAGNOSIS OF HYPERTROPHY IN THE PRESENCE OF BUNDLE BRANCH BLOCKS

The ECG diagnosis of hypertrophy (Chapter 6) in the presence of bundle branch blocks may pose special problems. Therefore a few general guidelines will be discussed.

When right ventricular hypertrophy (RVH) occurs with RBBB, right axis deviation is often present. A tall peaked P wave with RBBB should also suggest underlying RVH.

The usual voltage criteria for left ventricular hypertrophy (LVH) can be used in the presence of RBBB. Unfortunately, RBBB often masks these typical voltage increases.

The finding of LBBB, regardless of the QRS voltage, is highly suggestive of underlying LVH. Finding LBBB with prominent QRS voltages (pp. 67-70) *and* evidence of left atrial abnormality (p. 62) virtually assures the diagnosis of LVH.

Fig. 7-10. Left anterior hemiblock. Notice the marked left axis deviation, without significant widening of the QRS duration. Compare this with Figure 9-8, *B*, showing left posterior hemiblock.

Finally, it should be emphasized that the *echocardiogram* is much more accurate than the ECG in the diagnosis of cardiac enlargement. (See page 70.)

DIAGNOSIS OF MYOCARDIAL INFARCTION IN THE PRESENCE OF BUNDLE BRANCH BLOCKS

The ECG diagnosis of myocardial infarction in the presence of bundle branch blocks is discussed in Chapter 8.

REVIEW

RBBB shows the following characteristic patterns: an rSR' with a prominent wide final R' wave in V_1, a qRS with a wide final S wave in V_6, and a QRS width of 0.12 second (three small time boxes) or more. *Incomplete RBBB* shows the same chest lead patterns, but the QRS width is between 0.1 and 0.12 second.

LBBB shows the following characteristic patterns: a deep wide QS (occasionally an rS with a wide S wave) in V_1, a prominent (often notched) R wave *without* a preceding q wave in V_6, and a QRS width of 0.12 second or more. *Incomplete LBBB* shows the same chest lead patterns as LBBB, but the QRS width is between 0.1 and 0.12 second.

Pacemaker patterns produced by an electrode in the right ventricle generally resemble LBBB but have a pacemaker spike before each QRS complex.

Hemiblocks can occur because the left bundle splits into two subdivisions (fascicles): the left anterior fascicle and the left posterior fascicle. Conduction through either or both of these can be blocked.

Left anterior hemiblock is characterized by a mean QRS axis of $-45°$ or more. (When the mean QRS axis is $-45°$, left axis deviation is present and the height of the R wave in lead I [R_I] is equal to the depth of the S wave in lead aV_F [S_{aV_F}]. When the mean QRS axis is more negative than $-45°$, S_{aV_F} becomes larger than R_I.)

Left posterior hemiblock is characterized by right axis deviation. However, in making the diagnosis of left posterior hemiblock you must first exclude the other more common causes of right axis deviation (e.g., right ventricular hypertrophy, lateral wall infarction, chronic lung disease, or normal variants).

Questions

1. Draw the shape of the QRS complexes in leads V_1 and V_6 that would be expected with RBBB and LBBB.
2. Examine the following set of chest leads:
   a. What is the approximate QRS width?
   b. What conduction disturbance is present?
   c. Why are the T waves in leads V_1 to V_3 inverted?

3. Answer these questions about the following ECG:
   a. What is the QRS width?
   b. What type of axis deviation is present?
   c. What ventricular conduction disturbance is present?
   d. What evidence is there of left ventricular hypertrophy?

4. Examine the following 12-lead ECG and lead II rhythm strip carefully. Can you identify two conduction abnormalities?

5. Define the terms *"primary"* and *"secondary"* T wave abnormality.

True or false (6 to 8):

6. Left anterior hemiblock does not markedly widen the QRS complex.
7. LBBB is generally seen in patients with organic heart disease.
8. Bundle branch blocks may occur transiently.

Answers

1. See page 78.
2. a. 0.12 second.
   b. RBBB.
   c. Secondary T wave inversions may be seen in the right chest leads with RBBB. (See page 74 and answer 5 on the next page.)
3. a. 0.08 second (normal).
   b. Left axis deviation.
   c. Left anterior hemiblock.
   d. Tall R wave in lead aV_L (18 mm) with "strain" pattern in that lead. (See page 70.)

4. First-degree AV block (PR interval 0.24 sec) and LBBB.
5. *Primary* T wave abnormalities are due to actual changes in ventricular repolarization caused, for example, by drugs, ischemia, or electrolyte abnormalities. These abnormalities are independent of changes in the QRS complex. *Secondary* T wave changes, by contrast, are related entirely to alterations in the timing of ventricular depolarization and are seen in conditions in which the QRS is wide. For example, with bundle branch block a change in the sequence of depolarization also alters the sequence of repolarization, causing the T wave to point in a direction opposite the last deflection of the QRS complex. Thus, with RBBB the T waves will be secondarily inverted in leads with an rSR' configuration (e.g., V_1, V_2, and sometimes V_3). With LBBB the secondary T wave inversions will be seen in leads with tall wide R waves (V_5 and V_6). Secondary T wave inversions are also seen with ventricular paced beats (Fig. 7-8) and the Wolff-Parkinson-White preexcitation pattern (Fig. 10-20). Sometimes primary and secondary T wave changes are seen on the same ECG, as when ischemia develops in a patient with a bundle branch block (Fig. 8-21).
6. True.
7. True.
8. True.

8

Myocardial Ischemia and Infarction—I

TRANSMURAL ISCHEMIA AND Q WAVE INFARCT PATTERNS

In this chapter and the next we will be looking at one of the most important topics of clinical electrocardiography—the diagnosis of myocardial ischemia and infarction (ischemic heart disease). We begin with a discussion of basic terms.

MYOCARDIAL ISCHEMIA

Myocardial cells require oxygen and other nutrients to function. Oxygenated blood is supplied by the coronary arteries. If severe narrowing or complete blockage of a coronary artery causes the flow to become inadequate, ischemia of the heart muscle will develop. *Ischemia* means literally "to hold back blood." Myocardial ischemia may occur transiently. For example, patients who experience angina pectoris with exercise are having transient myocardial ischemia. If the ischemia is more severe, actual necrosis of a portion of heart muscle may occur. *Myocardial infarction* (MI) refers to myocardial necrosis ("heart attack"), which is usually caused by severe ischemia.

In this discussion we will be considering primarily ischemia and infarction of the left ventricle, the predominant chamber of the heart. Right ventricular infarction will be discussed briefly.

TRANSMURAL AND SUBENDOCARDIAL ISCHEMIA

Figure 8-1 diagrams a cross section of the left ventricle. Notice that it consists of an outer layer,

the *epicardium,* and an inner layer, the *subendocardium.* This distinction is important because myocardial ischemia may be limited to just the inner layer or may affect virtually the entire thickness of the ventricular wall (transmural ischemia).

MYOCARDIAL BLOOD SUPPLY

It is also important to understand certain basic facts about the blood supply to the left ventricle. The cardiac blood supply is delivered by the three main coronary arteries (Fig. 8-2). The right coronary artery supplies the inferior (diaphragmatic) portion of the heart as well as the right ventricle. The left anterior descending coronary artery generally supplies the ventricular septum and a large part of the left ventricular free wall. The left circumflex coronary artery supplies the lateral wall of the left ventricle. This circulation pattern may be variable. For example, in some cases the circumflex artery also supplies the inferior portion of the left ventricle. MIs tend to be *localized* to the portion (anterior or inferior) of the left ventricle supplied by one of these arteries.

TRANSMURAL ISCHEMIA WITH MI

We will begin by considering the effect of a transmural MI on the ECG. In the next chapter we will consider the ECG patterns of subendocardial ischemia and infarction.

Transmural infarction is characterized by ischemia and, ultimately, by necrosis of a portion of the entire thickness of the left ventricular wall. Not surprisingly, it generally produces changes in both myocardial depolarization (QRS complex) and myocardial repolarization (ST-T complex).

The earliest changes seen with an acute transmural infarction usually occur in the ST-T complex. There are two sequential phases of these ST-T changes: the *acute* and the *evolving*. The acute phase is marked by the appearance of ST segment elevations and sometimes tall positive (hyperacute) T waves in certain leads. The evolving phase (occurring after hours or days) is characterized by deep T wave inversions in those leads that previously showed ST elevations.

Transmural MI can also be described in terms of the location of the infarct: *anterior* means involving the anterior and/or lateral wall of the left ventricle; *inferior* means involving the inferior (diaphragmatic) wall of the left ventricle (Fig. 8-3). The anatomic location of the infarct determines the leads in which the typical ECG patterns appear. For example, with an acute anterior wall MI the ST segment elevations and tall hyperacute T waves

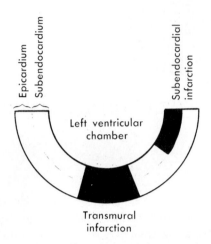

Fig. 8-1. Cross section of the left ventricle showing the difference between a *subendocardial* infarct, which involves the inner half of the ventricular wall, and a *transmural* infarct, which involves the full thickness (or almost the full thickness) of the wall.

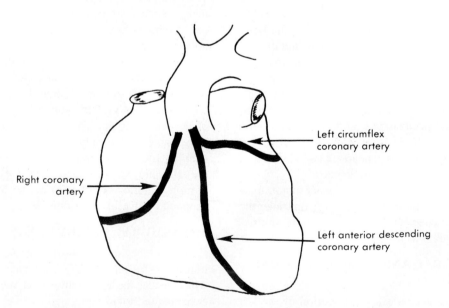

Fig. 8-2. Three major coronary arteries that supply blood to the heart.

appear in one or more of the anterior leads (chest leads V_1 to V_6, limb leads I and aV_L) (Fig. 8-4). With an inferior wall MI the ST segment elevations and tall hyperacute T waves are seen in inferior leads II, III, and aV_F (Fig. 8-5).

One of the most important characteristics of the ST-T changes seen with MI is their *reciprocity*. The anterior and inferior leads tend to show inverse patterns. Thus, with an anterior infarction with ST segment elevations in leads V_1 to V_6, I, and aV_L, leads II, III, and aV_F will often show

ST segment depression. Conversely, with an acute inferior wall infarction, leads II, III, and aV_F will show ST segment elevation, with reciprocal ST depressions often seen in one or more of leads V_1 to V_3, I, and aV_L. (These reciprocal changes are illustrated in Figures 8-4 and 8-5.)

The ST segment elevation seen with acute MI is called a "current of injury" and indicates that damage has occurred to the epicardial layer of the heart with a transmural infarction. The exact reasons why acute MI produces ST segment eleva-

Fig. 8-3. Myocardial infarcts are generally localized to either the anterior, **A,** or the inferior (diaphragmatic), **B,** portions of the left ventricle.

ECG SEQUENCE WITH ANTERIOR WALL INFARCTION

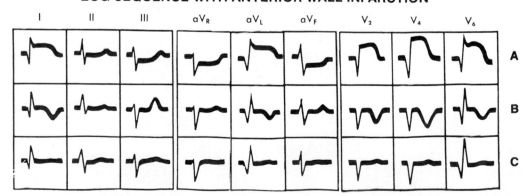

Fig. 8-4. **A,** Acute phase: ST elevations and new Q waves. **B,** Evolving phase: deep T wave inversions. **C,** Resolving phase: partial or complete regression of ST-T changes (and sometimes of Q waves). Notice in **A** and **B** the reciprocal ST-T changes in the inferior leads (II, III, and aV_F).

ECG SEQUENCE WITH INFERIOR WALL INFARCTION

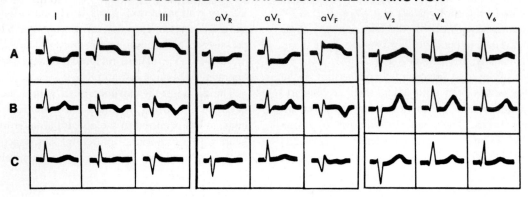

Fig. 8-5. **A,** Acute phase: ST elevations and new Q waves. **B,** Evolving phase: deep T wave inversions. **C,** Resolving phase: partial or complete regression of ST-T changes (and sometimes of Q waves). Notice in **A** and **B** the reciprocal ST-T changes in the anterior leads (I, aV_L, V_2, V_4).

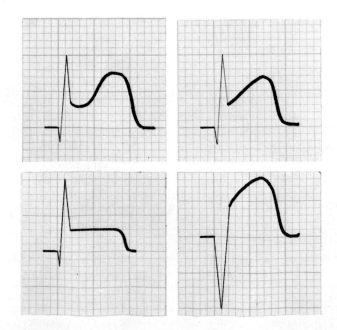

Fig. 8-6. ST segment elevations seen with acute infarction may have variable shapes.

tion are complex and not fully understood. Normally the ST segment is isoelectric (neither positive nor negative) because there is no net current flow at this time. Myocardial infarction alters the electrical charge on the myocardial cell membranes. As a result there is an abnormal current flow (current of injury) that produces the ST segment deviations.

The ST segment elevation seen with acute MI may have a variable appearance. The different shapes and appearances are shown in Figure 8-6). In some cases, notice that the ST segment is plateau shaped and in others dome shaped; sometimes it is obliquely elevated.

The ST segment elevations (and reciprocal ST depressions) are the *earliest* ECG signs of infarction and are generally seen within minutes of the infarct. Tall positive (hyperacute) T waves may also be seen at this time (Figs. 8-7 and 8-8) and have the same significance as the ST elevations. In some cases hyperacute T waves actually precede the ST elevations.

After a variable time lag (hours to days) the elevated ST segments start to return to the baseline. At the same time the T waves become inverted in leads that previously showed ST segment elevations. This phase of T wave inversions is called the evolving phase of the infarct. Thus, with an anterior wall infarction the T waves become inverted in one or more of the anterior leads (V_1 to V_6, I, aV_L). With an inferior wall infarction the T waves become inverted in one or more of the inferior leads (II, III, aV_F). These T wave inversions are illustrated in Figures 8-4 and 8-5.

QRS Changes: Q Waves of Infarction

Myocardial infarction, particularly when transmural, often produces distinctive changes in the QRS (depolarization) complex. The characteristic depolarization sign is the appearance of new Q waves.

Why do certain MIs lead to Q waves? Recall that a Q wave is simply an initial negative deflection of the QRS complex. If the entire QRS complex is negative $\left(\bigvee \right)$, we call it a *QS complex*.

Fig. 8-7. Chest leads from a patient with acute anterior wall infarction. **A,** Notice the tall positive (hyperacute) T waves in V_2 to V_5 in the earliest phase of the infarction. **B,** Recorded several hours later. There is marked ST segment elevation in the same leads (current of injury pattern) with abnormal Q waves in V_1 and V_2.

Fig. 8-8. Hyperacute T waves with anterior wall infarction. This patient was complaining of severe chest pain. Notice the very tall (hyperacute) T waves in the chest leads. There are also slight ST segment elevations in aV_L with reciprocal ST depressions in II, III, and aV_F. In V_4, note the atrial premature beat *(APB)*.

Λ Q wave (negative deflection) in any lead indicates that the electrical voltages are directed away from that particular lead. When transmural* infarction occurs, there is necrosis of heart muscle in a localized area of the ventricle; therefore the electrical voltages produced by this portion of the myocardium will disappear. Instead of positive (R) waves over the infarcted area, Q waves will be recorded (either a QR or a QS complex).

To summarize: Abnormal Q waves are characteristic markers of infarction. They signify the loss of positive electrical voltages caused by the death of heart muscle.

The new Q waves of an MI generally appear within the first day or so of the infarct. With an anterior wall infarction, they will be seen in one or more of leads V_1 to V_6, I, and aV_L (Fig. 8-4). With an inferior wall MI, they will appear in leads II, III, and aV_F (Fig. 8-5).

LOCALIZATION OF INFARCTIONS

As mentioned, MIs are generally localized to a specific portion of the left ventricle, affecting either the anterior or the inferior wall. Anterior infarcts (Figs. 8-9 to 8-11) are sometimes designated as anteroseptal, "strictly" anterior, or anterolateral/apical depending on the leads that show signs of the infarct.

Anterior Wall Infarctions

The characteristic feature of an anterior wall infarct is the *loss of normal R wave progression in the chest leads*. Recall that normally there is a progressive increase in the height of the R wave as you move from lead V_1 to lead V_6. An anterior infarct interrupts this progression, and the result is pathologic Q waves in one or more of the chest leads.

---

*As discussed in the next chapter, the equation of pathologic Q waves with transmural necrosis is an oversimplification. Not all transmural infarcts lead to Q waves, and not all Q wave infarcts correlate with transmural necrosis.

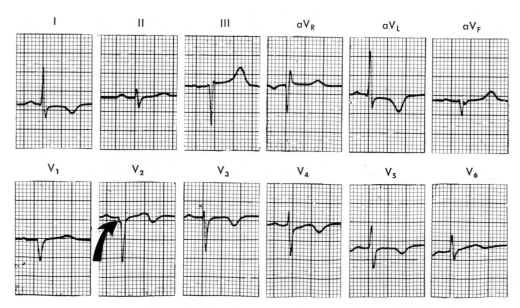

Fig. 8-9. Anterior wall infarction. Notice the QS complexes in leads V_1 and V_2, indicating anteroseptal infarction. There is also a characteristic notching (*arrow*, V_2) of the QS complex, often seen with infarcts. In addition, note the diffuse ischemic T wave inversions in leads I, aV_L, and V_2 to V_5, indicating generalized anterior wall ischemia.

Anteroseptal infarcts. Remember (from Chapter 4) that the ventricular septum is depolarized from left to right and that leads V_1 and V_2 show small positive (r) waves (septal r waves). Now consider the effect of damaging the septum. Obviously, there will be a loss of septal depolarization voltages; thus in leads V_1 and V_2 the r waves will be lost and an entirely negative (QS) complex will appear.

The septum is supplied with blood by the left anterior descending coronary artery, and septal in-farction generally suggests that there has been an occlusion of this artery or one of its branches.

"Strictly" anterior infarcts. Normally leads V_3 and V_4 show RS- or Rs-type complexes. If the anterior wall of the left ventricle is infarcted, the positive R waves that reflect the voltages produced by this muscle area will be lost. Instead, Q waves (as part of QS or QR complexes) will be seen in leads V_3 and V_4. A strictly anterior infarct generally results from occlusion of the left anterior descending coronary artery.

Fig. 8-10. Evolving anterior wall infarction. The patient sustained the infarct 1 week earlier. Notice the abnormal Q waves (I, aV_L, and V_2 to V_5) with slight ST segment elevations and deep T wave inversions. Left axis deviation resulting from left anterior hemiblock is present as well. (See Chapter 7.)

Anterolateral/anteroapical infarcts. An infarction of the lateral or apical wall of the left ventricle produces changes in the more laterally situated chest leads (V_5 and V_6). With these infarcts abnormal Q waves, as part of QS or QR complexes, appear in leads V_5 and V_6 (Fig. 7-7). The infarcts are often caused by occlusion of the left circumflex coronary artery, but they may also result from occlusion of the left anterior descending coronary artery or even a branch of the right coronary artery.

Differentiating anterior wall infarcts. The foregoing classification of anterior infarctions is not absolute. Often there is overlap. You can de-

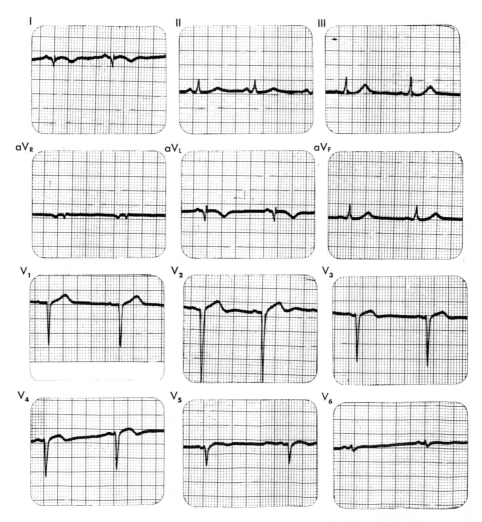

Fig. 8-11. Evolving anterior wall infarction. The infarct occurred 1 week earlier. Notice the poor R wave progression in leads V_1 to V_5 with Q waves in I and aV_L. T waves are slightly inverted in these leads. Right axis deviation in this case is the result of loss of lateral wall forces, with Q waves in I and aV_L.

Fig. 8-12. Acute inferior wall infarction. Notice the ST elevations in leads II, III, and aV$_F$ with reciprocal ST depressions in I and aV$_L$. Abnormal Q waves are also present in II, III, and aV$_F$.

Fig. 8-13. Inferior wall infarct. This patient sustained a myocardial infarction 1 month previously. Notice the abnormal Q waves and symmetric T wave inversions in leads II, III, and aV$_F$. There is also T wave flattening in V$_6$. Q waves and ST-T changes after infarction may persist indefinitely or may resolve partially or completely.

scribe Q wave MIs by simply referring to any infarct that shows ECG changes in one or more of leads I, aV_L, and V_1 to V_6 as "anterior" and then specifying which leads show Q waves and ST-T changes. Anterior infarctions associated with large Q waves in leads V_1 to V_5 or V_6 usually represent extensive damage and substantially reduced left ventricular function (ejection fraction) (Fig. 8-11).

Inferior Wall Infarctions

Infarction of the inferior (diaphragmatic) portion of the left ventricle is indicated by changes in leads II, III, and aV_F (Figs. 8-12 to 8-14). These three leads, as shown in the frontal plane axis diagram, are oriented downward or inferiorly (Fig. 5-1). Thus they will record voltages from the inferior portion of the ventricle. An inferior wall infarct may produce abnormal Q waves in leads II, III, and aV_F. It is generally caused by occlusion of the right coronary artery, less commonly by a left circumflex coronary obstruction.

"Posterior" Infarctions

The posterior (back) surface of the left ventricle can also be infarcted. This may be difficult to diagnose because characteristic abnormal ST elevations may not appear in any of the 12 conventional leads. Instead, tall R waves and ST depressions may occur in leads V_1 and V_2 (reciprocal to the Q waves and ST segment elevations that would be recorded at the back of the heart). During the evolving phase of such infarcts, when deep T wave inversions appear in the posterior leads, the anterior chest leads will show reciprocally tall positive T waves (Fig. 8-15).

In most cases of posterior MI the infarct extends either to the lateral wall of the left ventricle, producing characteristic changes in lead V_6, or to the inferior wall of that ventricle, producing characteristic changes in leads II, III, and aV_F (Fig. 8-15). Because of the overlap between *inferior* and *posterior* infarcts the more general term *"inferoposterior"* can be used when the ECG shows

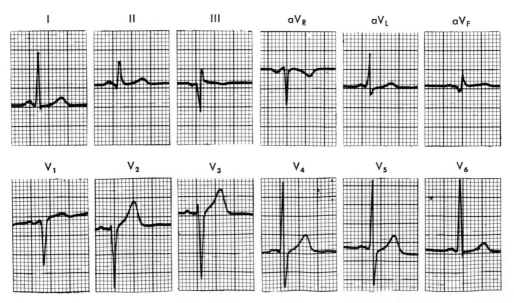

Fig. 8-14. Old inferior wall infarct. Notice the prominent Q waves in II, III, and aV_F from a patient who sustained an MI 1 year previously. The ST-T changes have essentially reverted to normal.

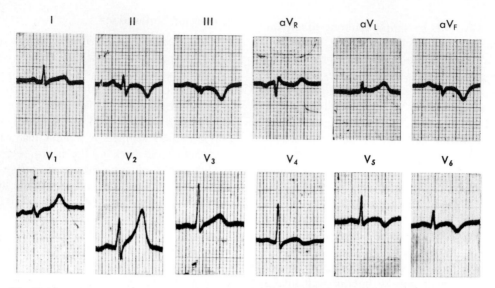

Fig. 8-15. Posterior infarction. Notice the tall R waves in V_1 and V_2. In addition, there is evidence of a prior inferior infarction (Q waves in II, III, aV_F) and probably a lateral infarction as well (T wave inversions in V_4 to V_6) Note also the reciprocally tall positive T waves in anterior precordial leads V_1 and V_2. (From Goldberger AL: *Myocardial infarction: electrocardiographic differential diagnosis,* ed 4, St Louis, 1991, Mosby.)

changes consistent with either inferior or posterior infarction.

Right Ventricular Infarctions

A related topic is right ventricular (RV) infarction. Clinical and autopsy studies have shown that patients with an inferoposterior infarct not uncommonly have associated RV involvement. In one postmortem study, RV infarction was found in about one of four cases of inferoposterior MI but not in cases of anterior MI. Clinically patients with an RV infarct may have elevated central venous pressure (distended neck veins) because of the abnormally high diastolic filling pressures in the right side of the heart. If the RV damage is severe, hypotension and even cardiogenic shock may result. AV conduction disturbances are not uncommon in this setting. The presence of jugular venous distension in a patient with an acute inferoposterior wall MI should always suggest this diagnosis. In addition, many of these patients will have ST ele-

vations in leads reflecting the right ventricle, such as V_1 and V_{3R} to V_{5R} (p. 26, footnote), as shown in Figure 8-16.

Recognition of RV infarction is of major clinical importance. Volume expansion may be critical in improving cardiac output in patients who are hypotensive and have a low or normal pulmonary capillary wedge pressure despite elevated central venous pressure.

SEQUENCE OF Q WAVES AND ST-T CHANGES WITH TRANSMURAL INFARCTIONS

Up to now we have discussed separately the ventricular depolarization (QRS) and repolarization (ST-T) changes produced by an acute MI. As shown in the examples in Figures 8-4 and 8-5, these changes occur sequentially.

Ordinarily the earliest sign of transmural ischemia is ST segment elevations (with reciprocal ST depressions). The ST elevations (current of injury

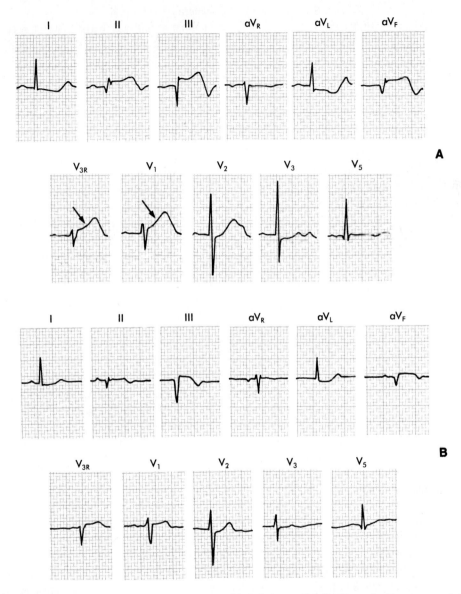

Fig. 8-16. Acute right ventricular infarction with inferior wall infarction. **A,** Q waves and ST segment elevations in leads II, III, and aV$_F$ are accompanied by ST elevations *(arrows)* in the right precordial leads (V$_{3R}$ and V$_1$). ST-T changes in V$_6$ are consistent with lateral wall ischemia. ST depressions in I and aV$_L$ are probably reciprocal to inferior lead ST elevations. **B,** Follow-up tracing obtained the next day showing diminution of the ST changes. (See also Question 129, page 283.) (From Goldberger AL: *Myocardial infarction: electrocardiographic differential diagnosis,* ed 4, St Louis, 1991, Mosby.)

pattern) usually persist for hours to days. During this same period Q waves will begin to appear in leads showing ST elevations. Following these changes, the ST segments start to return to the baseline; and the T waves become inverted during the evolving phase.

In the weeks or months following an infarct, what should you expect to happen to the Q waves and the ST-T changes just described? The answer is that you cannot make any certain predictions. In most cases the abnormal Q waves will persist for months, and even years, after the acute infarction. However, occasionally they will diminish in size and even disappear entirely. In some cases abnormal T wave inversions will persist indefinitely. In others there will be improvement but minor nonspecific ST-T abnormalities (such as slight T wave flattening) may persist (Figs. 8-4 and 8-5).

NORMAL AND ABNORMAL Q WAVES

One diagnostic problem frequently faced is deciding whether Q waves are abnormal. Not all Q waves are indicators of MI. For example, we normally expect to see a Q wave in lead aV_R. Furthermore, small "septal" q waves are normally seen in the left chest leads (V_4 to V_6) and in one or more of leads I, aV_L, II, III, and aV_F. Recall from Chapter 4 the significance of these septal q waves. The ventricular septum depolarizes from left to right. Left chest leads record this spread of voltages toward the right as a small negative deflection (q wave) as part of a qR complex, where the R wave represents the spread of left ventricular voltages toward the lead. When the electrical axis is horizontal, such qR complexes will be seen in leads I and aV_L. When the electrical axis is vertical, qR complexes will appear in leads II, III, and aV_F.

These normal septal q waves must be differentiated from the pathologic Q waves of infarction. Normal septal q waves are characteristically narrow and of low amplitude. As a rule septal q waves are less than 0.04 second in duration. A Q wave of 0.04 second or more in lead I, in all three infe-

rior leads (II, III, aV_F), or in leads V_3 to V_6 is generally abnormal.

What about a Q wave of 0.04 second or more width in leads V_1 and V_2? A large QS complex can be seen as a normal variant in lead V_1 and rarely in leads V_1 and V_2. However, QS waves in these leads may be the only evidence of an anterior septal MI. An abnormal QS complex resulting from infarction will sometimes show a notch as it descends or it may be slurred instead of descending and rising abruptly (Fig. 8-9). Further criteria for differentiating normal from abnormal Q waves in these leads lie beyond the scope of this book.

What about a wide Q wave in lead aV_L or Q waves in leads III and aV_F, which can also occur normally? Again, the precise criteria to differentiate normal from abnormal Q waves in these leads lie beyond the scope of this book. However, the following can be taken as general rules:

1. An inferior wall MI should be diagnosed with certainty only when abnormal Q waves are seen in leads II, III, and aV_F. If prominent Q waves appear just in leads III and aV_F, then the likelihood of MI is increased by the presence of abnormal ST-T changes in all three inferior limb leads.

2. An anterior wall MI should not be diagnosed from lead aV_L alone. Look for abnormal Q waves and ST-T changes in the other anterior leads (I and V_1 to V_6).

Furthermore, just as not all Q waves are abnormal, so not all abnormal Q waves are a result of MI. For example, poor R wave progression in the chest leads, sometimes with actual QS complexes in the right to middle chest leads (e.g., V_1 to V_3), may occur with left bundle branch block, left ventricular hypertrophy, and chronic lung disease in the absence of MI. Prominent noninfarctional Q waves are often a characteristic feature of hypertrophic cardiomyopathy (HCM), including the subset of patients with classic idiopathic hypertrophic subaortic stenosis (IHSS) (Fig. 8-17). Noninfarctional Q waves also occur with dilated cardiomyopathy (Fig. 10-18). As mentioned be-

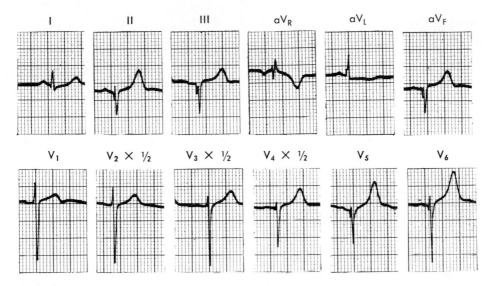

Fig. 8-17. Idiopathic hypertrophic subaortic stenosis (IHSS). Notice the prominent pseudoinfarctional Q waves, which are the result of septal hypertrophy. (From Goldberger AL: *Myocardial infarction: electrocardiographic differential diagnosis,* ed 4, St Louis, 1991, Mosby.)

fore, normal people may sometimes have a QS wave in lead V_1 and rarely in leads V_1 and V_2. Prominent Q waves in the absence of MI are sometimes referred to as a *pseudoinfarct pattern.**

VENTRICULAR ANEURYSM

After a large MI, in some patients a ventricular aneurysm will develop. An aneurysm is a severely scarred portion of infarcted ventricular myocardium that does not contract normally. Instead, during ventricular systole the aneurysmic portion bulges outward while the rest of the ventricle is contracting. Ventricular aneurysms may occur on the anterior or inferior surface of the heart. The ECG may be helpful in making the diagnosis of ventricular aneurysm following an MI. Patients with ventricular aneurysms frequently have persistent ST segment elevations following the infarct. As mentioned earlier, the ST segment elevations

seen with acute infarction generally resolve within several days. The persistence of ST segment elevations for several weeks or more is suggestive of a ventricular aneurysm (Fig. 8-18). However, the absence of persisting ST segment elevations does not rule out the possibility of an aneurysm.

Ventricular aneurysms are of clinical importance for several major reasons. They may lead to congestive heart failure. They may be associated with serious ventricular arrhythmias. A thrombus may form in an aneurysm and break off, resulting in stroke or some other embolic complication.

MULTIPLE INFARCTIONS

To this point we have discussed localized single infarcts. Not infrequently, however, patients may have two or more MIs at different times. For example, a new anterior wall infarct may develop in a patient with a previous inferior wall infarction. In such cases the ECG will initially show abnormal Q waves in leads II, III, and aV_F. During the anterior infarct new Q waves and ST-T changes will appear in the anterior leads. Figure 8-19 is the

---

*See Goldberger AL: *Myocardial infarction: electrocardiographic differential diagnosis,* ed 4, St Louis, 1991, Mosby.

Fig. 8-18. Anterior wall aneurysm. The patient sustained an infarct several months prior to this ECG. Notice the prominent Q waves in V_1 to V_3 and aV_L with persistent ST elevations in these leads and with reciprocal ST depressions in the inferior leads (II, III, and aV_F). Persistent ST elevations more than 2 to 3 weeks after an infarct suggest ventricular aneurysm.

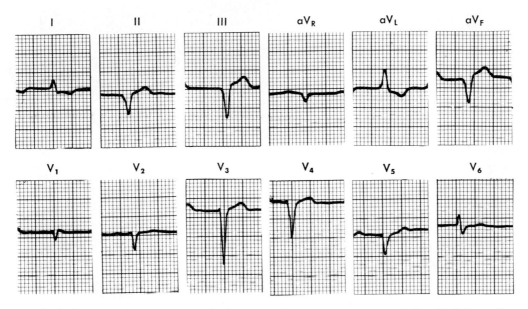

Fig. 8-19. Multiple infarcts. This ECG shows evidence of previous anterior wall and inferior wall MIs. Notice the poor R wave progression and QS complexes in chest leads V_1 to V_5, as well as the QS waves in II, III, and aV_F.

ECG of a patient with multiple infarcts (anterior and inferior).

SILENT MI

Most patients with acute MI have symptoms. They may experience the classic syndrome of crushing substernal chest pain. In other cases the pain may be atypical (feeling like indigestion or upper back or jaw pain). However, in some cases the patient may experience few if any symptoms ("silent" MI). Therefore it is not unusual to see abnormal Q waves on a patient's ECG that indicate a previous infarct, without any clinical history of a definite MI.

DIAGNOSIS OF MI IN THE PRESENCE OF BUNDLE BRANCH BLOCK

In some cases the diagnosis of infarction is made more difficult because the patient's baseline ECG will show a bundle branch block pattern or a bundle branch block may develop as a complication

of the infarct. Then the ECG picture becomes more complex.

Right Bundle Branch Block with MI

The diagnosis of an MI can be made relatively easily in the presence of RBBB. Remember that RBBB affects primarily the terminal phase of ventricular depolarization, producing a wide R′ wave in the right chest leads and a wide S wave in the left chest leads. MI affects the initial phase of ventricular depolarization, producing abnormal Q waves. When RBBB and an infarct occur together, there will be a combination of these patterns: the QRS complex will be abnormally wide (0.12 sec or more) as a result of the bundle branch block, lead V_1 will show a terminal positive deflection, and lead V_6 will show a terminal positive deflection, and lead V_6 will show a wide S wave; if the infarction is anterior, there will be a loss of R wave progression with abnormal Q waves in the anterior leads and characteristic ST-T changes; if it is

Fig. 8-20. Acute anterior wall infarction and the RBBB pattern. Notice the wide QRS complexes with an rSR′ wave in lead V_1 and a qRS pattern in V_5, indicating RBBB. There is, furthermore, a pattern of acute anterior wall infarction (Q waves and ST elevations in I and aV_L plus marked reciprocal ST depressions in II, III, and aV_F). Finally, notice the left axis deviations caused by the left anterior hemiblock. This combination (left anterior hemiblock and RBBB) is an example of bifascicular block and may herald complete (trifascicular) heart block in patients with an acute anterior wall infarction.

inferior, pathologic Q waves and ST-T changes will be seen in leads II, III, and aV$_F$. Figure 8-20 shows RBBB and acute MI. (See also Question 172, page 304.)

Left Bundle Branch Block with MI

The diagnosis of LBBB in the presence of MI is considerably more complicated and confusing than that of RBBB. The reason is that LBBB interrupts both the early and the late phases of ventricular stimulation (Chapter 7). It also produces secondary ST-T changes. As a general rule LBBB will hide the diagnosis of an infarct. *Thus a patient with a chronic LBBB pattern in whom an acute MI develops may not show the characteristic changes of infarction described in this chapter.* Occasionally patients with LBBB will manifest primary ST-T changes indicative of ischemia or actual infarction. The secondary T wave inversions of uncomplicated LBBB are seen in leads V$_4$ to V$_6$ (with prominent R waves). The appearance of T wave inversions in leads V$_1$ to V$_3$ (with prominent S waves) is a primary abnormality that cannot be ascribed to the bundle branch block itself (Fig. 8-21).

The problem of diagnosing infarction with LBBB is further complicated by the fact that the LBBB pattern has several features that resemble those seen with infarction. An LBBB pattern can therefore mimic an infarct pattern. Recall (from Chapter 7) that LBBB typically shows poor R wave progression in the chest leads because of the reversed way the ventricular septum is activated: from right to left, the opposite of what happens normally. Consequently, with LBBB, there is a loss of the normal septal R waves in the right chest leads. This loss of normal R wave progression simulates the pattern seen with an anterior wall infarct.

Figure 7-5 shows an example of LBBB with poor R wave progression. Anterior wall infarction was not present. Notice that the ST segments in the right chest leads are elevated, resembling the

Fig. 8-21. A, Typical left bundle branch block pattern. Notice the poor R wave progression in the right precordial leads and the discordance of QRS and ST-T vectors reflected by ST elevations in the right precordial leads and ST depressions with T wave inversions in the left precordial leads. **B,** Subsequently the ECG from this patient showed development of primary T wave inversions in V$_1$ to V$_3$ caused by anterior ischemia and probable infarction. (From Goldberger AL: *Myocardial infarction: electrocardiographic differential diagnosis,* ed 4, St Louis, 1991, Mosby.)

pattern seen during the hyperacute or acute phase of an infarction. ST segment elevation in the right chest leads is also commonly seen with LBBB in the absence of infarction.

As a general rule a patient with an LBBB pattern should not be diagnosed as having suffered a myocardial infarction simply on the basis of poor R wave progression in the right chest leads or ST elevations in those leads. However, the presence of Q waves as part of QR complexes in the left chest leads (V_5 and V_6) with LBBB generally indicates an underlying MI (Fig. 8-22). In addition, the appearance of ST elevations in the left chest leads or in other leads with prominent R waves suggests ischemia (Fig. 8-22, lead V_5).

In the next chapter this discussion of the ECG with ischemia and infarction will continue, focusing on *subendocardial* ischemia patterns.

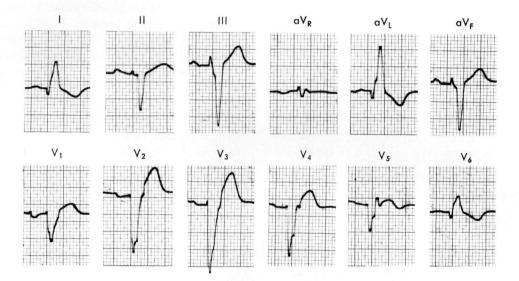

Fig. 8-22. Anterior wall infarction with LBBB. Notice the prominent Q waves in the left chest leads as part of QR complexes. See text. (From Goldberger AL: *Myocardial infarction: electrocardiographic differential diagnosis,* ed 4, St Louis, 1991, Mosby.)

REVIEW

Myocardial ischemia occurs when the blood supply to the myocardium is not adequate. *Myocardial infarction* (MI) refers to necrosis of the myocardium caused by severe ischemia.

Myocardial ischemia or infarction can affect the entire thickness of the ventricular muscle (*transmural* injury) or may be localized to just the inner layer of the ventricle (*subendocardial* ischemia or infarction). Transmural MI often (but not always) produces a typical sequence of ST-T changes and abnormal Q waves. The ST-T changes can be divided into two phases: (1) acute, marked by ST segment elevations (current of injury pattern) and sometimes tall positive T waves (hyperacute T waves), and (2) evolving, characterized by the appearance of deeply inverted T waves in leads that showed the hyperacute T waves and ST elevations. These ST-T changes occur during a period of hours or days and usually resolve over a period of weeks or months. During the first day or so after an infarction, new abnormal Q waves may appear in one or more leads.

When ST segment elevations persist for more than 2 or 3 weeks after an acute MI, this may signify that a ventricular aneurysm has developed. The abnormal Q waves tend to persist but may become smaller with time and, rarely, may even disappear.

Q wave MI can also be described in terms of its location. With an *anterior* infarction, ST segment elevations and abnormal Q waves occur in one or more of leads V_1 to V_6, I, and aV_L. (Reciprocal ST depressions may be seen in II, III, and aV_F.) With an *inferior* infarction, ST elevations and Q waves will appear in leads II, III, and aV_F and there may be reciprocal ST depressions in one or more of the anterior leads.

Right ventricular MI is a common complication of inferoposterior infarcts. In acute cases the ECG may also show elevated ST segments in the right chest leads.

The pathologic Q waves of infarction must be distinguished from normal Q waves. For example, small normal "septal" q waves as part of qR complexes may be seen in the left chest leads (V_4 to V_6), in leads II, III, and aV_F (with a vertical electrical axis), and in leads I and aV_L (with a horizontal axis). These septal q waves are normally less than 0.04 second in width.

A QS wave may be seen normally in lead V_1 and occasionally in leads V_1 and V_2. Q waves may also be seen as normal variants in leads aV_F, III, and aV_L.

Multiple MIs can occur, and the ECG will show old Q waves from the preceding infarct as well as new Q waves with ST-T changes from the current infarct.

When *right bundle branch block* complicates an acute MI, the diagnosis of both conditions is possible. The RBBB prolongs the QRS width, and lead V_1 shows a tall positive final deflection. In addition, abnormal Q waves and ST segment elevations resulting from the acute MI will be present in the chest leads (with an anterior MI) and in leads II, III, and aV_F (in inferior MI).

When *left bundle branch block* complicates an acute MI, it is often difficult to diagnose the MI because the LBBB may mask both the abnormal Q waves of the infarction and the ST segment elevations and T wave inversions of the ischemia. In addition, LBBB may produce QS waves in the right chest leads with ST segment elevations and poor R wave progression across the chest *without* MI. The presence of QR complexes in the left chest leads with LBBB is suggestive of underlying MI. T wave inversions in the right chest leads or ST segment elevations in the left chest leads or in leads with prominent R waves suggest ischemia with underlying LBBB.

Questions

See the end of Chapter 9.

9

Myocardial Ischemia and Infarction—II

SUBENDOCARDIAL ISCHEMIA AND NON–Q WAVE INFARCT PATTERNS

Transmural myocardial infarction (MI) may be associated with abnormal Q waves and the typical progression of ST-T changes described in Chapter 8. In other cases (described in this chapter), however, myocardial ischemia with or without actual infarction may be limited to the *subendocardial* layer (inner half) of the ventricle.

SUBENDOCARDIAL ISCHEMIA

How can subendocardial ischemia occur without transmural ischemia or infarction? The subendocardium is most distant from the coronary blood supply and closest to the high pressure of the ventricular cavity and therefore is particularly vulnerable to ischemia. It can become ischemic while the outer layer of the ventricle (epicardium) remains normally perfused with blood.

The most common ECG change with subendocardial ischemia is ST segment depression (Fig. 9-1). It may be limited to the anterior leads (I, aV_L, and V_1 to V_6) or to the inferior leads (II, III, and aV_F), or it may be seen more diffusely in both groups of leads. As shown in Figure 9-1, the ST depression with subendocardial ischemia has a characteristic squared-off shape. (ST segment elevation is usually seen in lead aV_R.)

Recall from the previous chapter that acute transmural infarction produces ST segment elevation, a current of injury pattern. This results from epicardial injury. With pure subendocardial isch-

emia just the opposite occurs—ST segment depression (except in lead aV_R, which often shows ST elevation).

To summarize: Myocardial ischemia involving primarily the subendocardium usually produces ST segment depression whereas acute ischemia involving the epicardium usually produces ST elevation. This difference in the direction of the injury current vector is depicted in Fig. 9-2.

ECG Changes with Angina Pectoris

The term *"angina pectoris"* refers to transient attacks of chest discomfort caused by myocardial ischemia. Angina is a symptom of coronary artery disease. The classic attack of angina is experienced as a dull, burning, or boring substernal pressure or heaviness. It is typically precipitated by exertion, stress, exposure to cold, and so on, and is relieved by rest and nitroglycerin.

Many (but not all) patients with classic angina will have an ECG pattern of subendocardial ischemia (with ST depressions) during an attack. When the pain disappears, the ST segments generally return to the baseline.

Figure 9-3 shows ST depressions during a spontaneous episode of angina. As just stated, not all patients with angina will have ST depressions during chest pain. The presence of a normal ECG does not rule out underlying coronary artery disease. However, the appearance of transient ST depres-

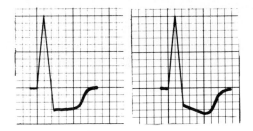

Fig. 9-1. Subendocardial ischemia may produce ST depressions.

SUBENDOCARDIAL INJURY:
ST Depression

TRANSMURAL (EPICARDIAL) INJURY:
ST Elevation

 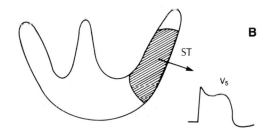

Fig. 9-2. Subendocardial versus epicardial injury currents. **A,** Acute subendocardial ischemia. The electrical forces *(arrow)* responsible for the ST segment are deviated toward the inner layer of the heart, causing ST depressions in lead V_5, which faces the outer surface of the heart. **B,** Acute epicardial ischemia as seen in a case of transmural MI. Electrical forces *(arrow)* responsible for the ST segment are deviated toward the outer layer of the heart, causing ST elevations in the overlying lead.

Fig. 9-3. This patient complained of chest pain while being examined. **A,** Notice the marked ST depressions in lead V_4. **B,** Five minutes later, after nitroglycerin, the ST segments have reverted to normal, with relief of the angina.

Fig. 9-4. Positive exercise test. **A,** Baseline rhythm strip from a patient with coronary artery disease. **B,** Notice the marked ST depressions with increased heart rate. (From Goldberger AL: *Myocardial infarction: electrocardiographic differential diagnosis,* ed 4, St Louis, 1991, Mosby.)

Fig. 9-5. Physiologic ST segment depression with exercise. Notice the J junction depression *(arrow)* with sharply upsloping ST segments. (From Goldberger AL: *Myocardial infarction: electrocardiographic differential diagnosis,* ed 4, St Louis, 1991, Mosby.)

sions with chest pain is a very strong indicator of myocardial ischemia.

Exercise Testing

Many patients with coronary artery disease will have a normal ECG while at rest; however, during exercise, ischemic changes may appear because of the extra oxygen requirements imposed on their heart by exertion. To assist in diagnosing coronary artery disease, the ECG can be recorded while the patient is being exercised under controlled conditions. Such *stress electrocardiography* is usually performed while the patient walks on a treadmill or pedals a bicycle. The test is stopped when the patient develops angina, fatigue, or diagnostic ST changes or when the heart rate reaches 85% to 90% of a maximum predetermined rate, predicted from the patient's age. (This is known as *submaximal testing.*)

Figure 9-4, *A,* is the normal resting ECG of a patient whereas 9-4, *B,* shows marked ST depressions recorded while the patient was exercising. The appearance of ST segment depressions constitutes a positive (abnormal) result. Most cardiologists accept horizontal or downward ST depressions of at least 1 mm or more, lasting at least 0.08 second, as a positive (abnormal) test result (Fig. 9-4, *B*). ST depressions of less than 1 mm, or depressions of only the J point, with a rapid upward sloping of the ST segment, are considered a negative (normal) test response (Fig. 9-5).

Exercise electrocardiography is often helpful in diagnosing coronary artery disease. However, like all tests, it may give both false-positive and false-negative results. For example, up to 10% of normal men and an even higher percentage of normal women will have false-positive exercise tests. False-positive tests (ST depressions without obstructive coronary disease) also can be seen in patients taking digitalis and in those with hypokalemia, left ventricular hypertrophy, ventricular conduction disturbances, or Wolff-Parkinson-White syndrome (p. 136). Furthermore, false-negative tests can occur despite the presence of significant underlying coronary artery disease. *Therefore, a normal exercise test does not exclude coronary artery disease.* *

To summarize: Subendocardial ischemia, such as occurs with typical angina pectoris (and as may sometimes be elicited with stress testing), often produces ST segment depressions in multiple leads.

Silent Myocardial Ischemia

A patient with coronary artery disease may have episodes of myocardial ischemia *without* angina; hence the term *"silent ischemia."* Silent ischemia is sometimes detected during exercise testing. The most useful way of assessing it is by ambulatory ECG (Holter) monitoring (Chapter 3). A 24-hour ECG monitoring of patients with coronary artery disease reveals a surprisingly high frequency of ST depressions *not* associated with angina. For further discussion of this important topic, refer to the Bibliography. (See also page 103.)

SUBENDOCARDIAL INFARCTION

If ischemia to the subendocardial region is severe enough, actual subendocardial infarction may occur. In such cases the ECG often shows persistent ST depressions instead of the transient depressions seen with reversible subendocardial ischemia.

Figure 9-6 shows an example of a non–Q wave infarction, with persistent ST depressions. Is it possible for Q waves to appear with pure subendocardial infarction? The answer is that if only the inner half of the myocardium is infarcted abnormal Q waves usually do not appear. Subendocardial infarction generally affects ventricular repolarization (ST-T complex) and not depolarization (QRS complex); but important exceptions may occur (pp. 117-118).

Another pattern sometimes seen in cases of non–Q wave infarction is T wave inversions with or without ST segment depressions. Figure 9-7 shows an infarction pattern with deep T wave in-

---

*Consult the Bibliography for a discussion of nuclear medicine imaging techniques with stress testing.

Fig. 9-6. Non–Q wave infarction. This patient complained of severe chest pain. Subsequently cardiac enzymes were elevated. Notice the marked ST depressions, best seen in chest leads V_2 to V_5, consistent with subendocardial ischemia. There is also a ventricular premature beat *(VPB)* in lead I. Slight ST elevations are seen in III and aV_R.

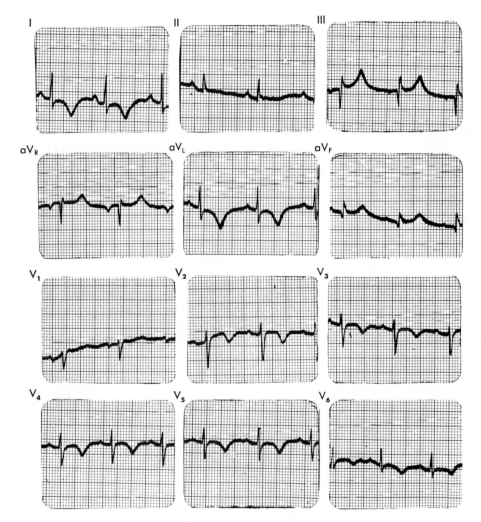

Fig. 9-7. Non–Q wave infarction. This patient complaining of chest pain had cardiac enzyme elevations. Notice the deep T wave inversions in leads I, aV$_L$, and V$_2$ to V$_6$. (Prominent Q waves in III and aV$_F$ represent an old inferior wall infarction.) Patients with acute infarcts may have deep ST segment depressions or T wave inversions without Q waves.

versions. (T wave inversions may also be seen in some cases of noninfarctional ischemia.)

To summarize: Non–Q wave infarction can be associated with either (1) persistent ST depressions or (2) T wave inversions.

VARIETY OF ECG CHANGES SEEN WITH MYOCARDIAL ISCHEMIA

It should be apparent by now that myocardial ischemia can produce a wide variety of ECG changes. For example, transmural infarction (discussed earlier) causes abnormal Q waves as well as ST segment elevations followed by T wave inversions. Ventricular aneurysm may be associated with persistent ST segment elevations. Subendocardial ischemia (seen, for example, during an anginal attack or during a stress test) may produce transient ST depressions. Actual subendocardial infarction may lead to persistent ST depressions or to T wave inversions without Q waves.

ECG Changes Associated with Noninfarctional Ischemia

The foregoing paragraph does not mention all the possible ECG patterns seen with myocardial ischemia. We will briefly consider several others that may occur.

Myocardial ischemia does not always cause diagnostic ST-T changes. In some patients the ECG may remain entirely normal during episodes of ischemia. In others there may be only subtle changes in the ST-T complex. For example, you may see just a slight T wave flattening or minimal T wave inversions. These are *nonspecific ST-T changes*. (See also Chapter 10.)

Nonspecific ST-T changes may be abnormal, but they are not definite indicators of ischemia. They may be a sign of ischemic heart disease. However, they may also be caused by many other conditions, such as drug effects, hyperventilation, or electrolyte abnormalities. Therefore you should *not* make a definite diagnosis of myocardial ischemia solely on the basis of nonspecific ST-T changes.

To complete our discussion of noninfarctional ischemia, we will consider one other condition,

Prinzmetal's angina. Recall that the ECG with classic or typical angina often shows the pattern of subendocardial ischemia with ST segment depressions. However, a small but important group of patients will have an atypical form of angina (first reported by Dr. Myron Prinzmetal). Their angina is atypical because during episodes of chest pain they have ST segment elevations, a pattern described previously with acute transmural infarction. In these patients with Prinzmetal's angina the ST segment elevations are transient. Following the episode of chest pain the ST segments usually return to the baseline, without the characteristic evolving pattern of Q waves and T wave inversions seen with acute transmural MI. Thus Prinzmetal's angina is atypical because the ECG shows ST elevations rather than the ST depressions seen with typical angina.

Patients with Prinzmetal's angina are also atypical because their chest pain often occurs at rest or at night (in contrast to classic angina pectoris, which usually occurs with exertion or emotional stress). Prinzmetal's angina pattern is significant because it is a marker of coronary artery *spasm*, causing transient transmural ischemia. These episodes of spasm may occur in patients with otherwise normal coronary arteries. In most cases, spasm is associated with high-grade coronary obstruction (Fig. 9-8). Increasing evidence implicates cocaine as another cause of coronary spasm.

At this point we can summarize the diversity of ECG changes seen with ischemic heart disease— including Q waves, ST segment elevations or depressions, tall positive T waves or deep T wave inversions, nonspecific ST-T changes, and even a normal ECG (Fig. 9-9).

DIFFERENTIAL DIAGNOSIS OF ST ELEVATIONS AND ST DEPRESSIONS

ST elevations (current of injury pattern) are the earliest sign of acute transmural ischemia with infarction. Transient elevations, as mentioned, are also seen with Prinzmetal's angina. ST elevations persisting for several weeks after an acute MI may be a sign of a ventricular aneurysm.

However, not all ST segment elevations are in-

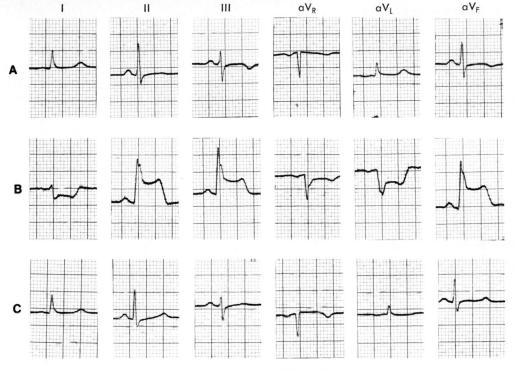

Fig. 9-8. Prinzmetal's (variant) angina with transient ST elevations. This patient, a 30-year-old man, had a history of exertional as well as rest angina. **A,** The baseline resting ECG shows nonspecific inferior lead ST-T changes. **B,** With chest pain, marked ST segment elevations occur in leads II, III, and aV_F and there are reciprocal ST depressions in I and aV_L. The rightward axis shift and slight widening of the QRS are consistent with left posterior hemiblock. **C,** Return of the ST segments to baseline after nitroglycerin administration. Cardiac catheterization in this case showed a severe right coronary obstruction with intermittent spasm producing total occlusion and transient ST elevations. (From Goldberger AL: *Myocardial infarction: electrocardiographic differential diagnosis,* ed 4, St Louis, 1991, Mosby.)

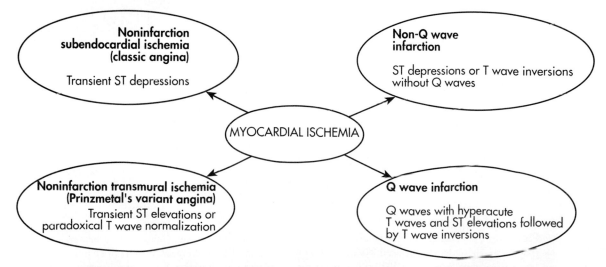

Fig. 9-9. Diversity of ECG changes with myocardial ischemia. T wave inversions may also occur with noninfarctional ischemia, and the ECG either be normal or show only nonspecific ST-T changes. (Adapted from Goldberger AL: *Myocardial infarction: electrocardiographic differential diagnosis,* ed 4, St Louis, 1991, Mosby.)

dicators of ischemia. For example, *acute pericarditis* (p. 131) is associated with ST elevations. (The ECG changes with acute pericarditis are described in Chapter 10.) In other cases ST elevation may occur as a *normal variant* (Fig. 10-15). Many young adults have them, usually most prominent in the chest leads. This pattern of benign ST segment elevation is called the "early repolarization variant" (also described in Chapter 10). Finally, chronic ST elevations are often seen in leads V_1 and V_2 associated with the patterns of *left ventricular hypertrophy* or *left bundle branch block*.

Subendocardial ischemia is usually characterized by ST segment depression. However, not all the ST depressions you will see are indicative of subendocardial ischemia. For example, in Chapter 6 we discussed the ST-T changes associated with *left ventricular hypertrophy* (strain pattern). As shown in Figure 6-12, the ST segment may be slightly depressed with left ventricular hypertrophy. Another cause is *acute transmural ischemia*. Remember that acute anterior wall ischemia may be associated with reciprocal ST depressions in one or more of leads II, III, and aV_F. Conversely, acute inferior wall ischemia may be associated with reciprocal ST depressions in one or more of the anterior leads (I, aV_L, V_1 to V_3). Therefore, whenever you see ST depressions, it is important to look at all the leads and to evaluate these changes in context.

The ST segment may also be depressed by two other important factors (both described in Chapter 10). The first is *digitalis effect*. As shown in Figure 10-1, digitalis may produce scooping of the ST-T complex with slight ST depression. The second factor is *hypokalemia*. As shown in Figure 10-9, with a low serum potassium the ST segment may be slightly depressed. Prominent U waves may also appear. In some cases it may be difficult to sort out which factors are responsible for the ST depressions you are seeing. For example, a patient with left ventricular hypertrophy may be taking digitalis and may also be having acute subendocardial ischemia.

DIFFERENTIAL DIAGNOSIS OF DEEP T WAVE INVERSIONS

Deep T wave inversions, as described previously, are usually seen during the evolving phase of a Q-wave MI (Fig. 8-4, *B*) and also sometimes

Fig. 9-10. Acute subarachnoid hemorrhage with giant T wave inversions. Subarachnoid hemorrhage may cause deeply inverted T waves, usually with markedly prolonged QT intervals, simulating the pattern seen in MI. (From Goldberger AL: *Myocardial infarction: electrocardiographic differential diagnosis,* ed 4, St Louis, 1991, Mosby.)

with a non–Q wave MI (Fig 9-7). They are the result of a delay in regional repolarization produced by the ischemic injury.

However, just as not all ST segment elevations reflect ischemia, so not all deep T wave inversions are abnormal. For example, T wave inversions may be seen normally in leads with a *negative QRS complex* (e.g., aV_R). The T wave may be normally inverted in lead V_1 and sometimes in lead V_2 in adults. Furthermore, as mentioned earlier (p. 43, footnote), some adults have a persistent *juvenile T wave inversion pattern* with inverted T waves in the right and middle chest leads (typically V_1 to V_3).

In addition, not all abnormal T wave inversions are caused by myocardial infarction. T wave inversions in the right chest leads may be caused by right ventricular strain (Fig. 10-16) and in the left chest leads by left ventricular strain (Fig. 6-10). Diffusely inverted T waves are seen during the evolving phase of pericarditis. Very deep widely splayed T wave inversions (with a long QT interval and sometimes prominent U waves) have been described in some patients with cerebrovascular accident, particularly subarachnoid hemorrhage *(CVA T wave pattern)* (Fig. 9-10). The cause of these marked repolarization changes with some types of cerebrovascular injury is not certain, but it probably reflects changes in the autonomic nervous system. As described in Chapter 7, secondary T wave inversions (resulting from abnormal depolarization) are seen in the right chest leads with RBBB and in the left chest leads with LBBB. Deep T wave inversions have also been reported following bouts of tachycardia (post-tachycardia T wave syndrome) and after electronic ventricular pacing (post-pacemaker T wave pattern). Patients with the mitral valve prolapse syndrome may have slightly inverted T waves in the inferolateral leads (II, III, aV_F, V_5, and V_6).

This list of noninfarctional factors causing T wave inversions is by no means complete, but it should convey the point that *T wave inversions are not always indicative of myocardial ischemia.* For a more complete discussion of the differential diagnosis of the ST-T changes of myocardial infarction, readers are referred to the Bibliography.

COMPLICATIONS OF MI

Up to now we have considered just the diagnosis of MI from the ECG and also the differential diagnosis of these patterns. We will conclude with a brief review of the major complications of MI.

The complications can be divided into two groups: (1) mechanical and (2) electrical. The *mechanical* complications include heart failure, cardiogenic shock, left ventricular aneurysm, rupture of the heart, pericarditis, papillary muscle dysfunction, infarct extension and expansion, and embolism. (Diagnosis of these problems lies outside the scope of this book.) The *electrical* complications include the arrhythmias and conduction disturbances seen as a consequence of myocardial ischemia. MI can cause virtually any arrhythmia, including sustained ventricular tachycardia or ventricular fibrillation leading to cardiac arrest. (The general subject of arrhythmias is discussed in Part II of this book.) The conduction disturbances include AV block (heart block) and intraventricular block (bundle branch block). (The conduction disturbances are discussed in Chapters 7 and 15.)

THE ECG IN MI: A CLINICAL PERSPECTIVE

One final note of caution should be made. The ECG is a reasonably sensitive, but hardly perfect, indicator of acute MI. Most patients with an acute MI will show the ECG changes described in Chapters 8 and 9. However, particularly during the early minutes or hours after an infarct, the ECG may be relatively nondiagnostic or even normal. Furthermore, as mentioned, an LBBB pattern may completely mask the changes of an acute infarct. Therefore the ECG must always be considered in clinical perspective and the diagnosis of myocardial ischemia or infarction not be dismissed simply because the ECG does not show the classic changes.

It should also be emphasized that the traditional distinction between transmural and subendocardial (nontransmural) MIs on the basis of the ECG findings is an oversimplification. In some cases extensive infarction may occur without Q waves while in others nontransmural injury may occur with Q waves. Furthermore, current evidence suggests that "subendocardial" infarction may have as ominous a long-term prognosis as "transmural" infarction. For these reasons electrocardiographers have largely abandoned the terms "transmural" and "subendocardial" and instead use *"Q wave"* and *"non−Q wave"* when describing an infarction.

REVIEW

Subendocardial ischemia generally produces ST segment depressions, which may appear only in the anterior leads (I, aV_L, and V_1 to V_6) or only in the inferior leads (II, III, and aV_F) or may appear diffusely in both groups of leads. (Lead aV_R usually shows ST segment elevations.)

These ischemic ST segment depressions may be seen during attacks of typical angina pectoris. Similar ST segment depressions may develop during exercise (with or without chest pain) in people with ischemic heart disease. Recording the ECG during exercise (stress electrocardiography) is a method of determining the presence of ischemic heart disease. ST segment depression of 1 mm or more, lasting 0.08 second or more, is generally considered a *positive* (abnormal) response. However, *false-negative* (normal) results can occur in patients with ischemic heart disease and *false-positive* results can occur in normal people.

Ischemic ST segment changes may also be detected during ambulatory ECG (Holter) monitoring. Analysis of these records has shown that many episodes of myocardial ischemia are not associated with angina pectoris ("silent ischemia").

With *non−Q wave infarction* the ECG may show persistent ST segment depressions or T wave inversions. Abnormal Q waves do not usually occur with subendocardial infarction limited to the inner half of the ventricular wall.

Prinzmental's angina occurs in patients with transient ST segment elevations, suggestive of epicardial or transmural ischemia, during attacks of angina. These patients often have atypical chest pain, which occurs at rest or at night, in contrast to classic angina, which is typically exertional and is associated with ST segment depressions. Prinzmetal's (variant) angina pattern is generally a marker of coronary artery spasm with or without underlying coronary obstructions.

The ST segment elevations of acute transmural MI can be simulated by the ST elevations of Prinzmetal's angina as well as by the normal variant ST elevations seen in some healthy people ("early repolarization pattern") and by the ST elevations of acute pericarditis.

The abnormal ST depressions of subendocardial ischemia may be simulated by the repolarization abnormalities of left ventricular hypertrophy, digitalis effect (Chapter 10), or hypokalemia (Chapter 10).

T wave inversions can be a sign of ischemia or infarction but may also occur in a variety of other settings (including normal variants, ventricular hypertrophy, pericarditis, subarachnoid hemorrhage, and secondary ST-T changes from bundle branch block).

Questions—Chapters 8 and 9

1. Answer these questions about the ECG below:
   a. What is the approximate heart rate?
   b. Are there any ST segment elevations?
   c. Are there any abnormal Q waves?
   d. What is the diagnosis?

2. Answer these questions about the following ECG:
   a. What is the approximate mean QRS axis?
   b. Is the R wave progression in the chest leads normal?
   c. Are the T waves normal?
   d. What is the diagnosis?

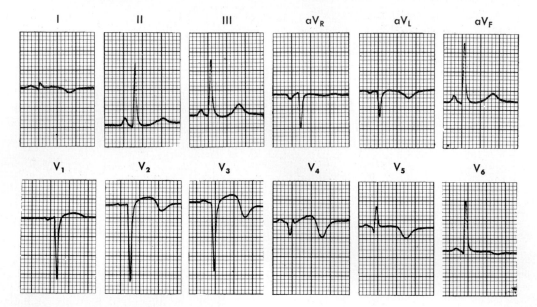

3. With acute *transmural anterior* wall ischemia, the ST segments in leads II, III, and aV_F are likely to be _____.

4. Persistent ST elevations several weeks or more after an infarct may be a sign of _____.

5. A patient with severe chest pain has persistent diffuse ST segment depressions with abnormal elevations of cardiac enzymes. The most likely diagnosis is
   a. Prinzmetal's angina
   b. Non–Q wave infarction
   c. Hyperacute infarction
   d. Angina pectoris

6. What ECG abnormality is shown and of what symptom might this patient have been complaining?

7. Does this ECG tracing show evidence of previous MI?

Answers

1. a. 100 beats/min.
   b. Yes. Leads II, III, and aV_F (with reciprocal ST depressions in leads V_2 to V_4, I, and aV_L).
   c. Yes. Best seen in leads III and aV_F.
   d. Acute inferior wall infarction.
2. a. About $+90°$. (Between $80°$ and $90°$ is acceptable.)
   b. No.
   c. No. Notice the inverted T waves in leads V_2 to V_6, I, and aV_L.
   d. Anterior wall infarction, possibly recent or evolving.
3. Reciprocally depressed.
4. Ventricular aneurysm.
5. b.
6. Marked ST segment depressions. This patient had severe ischemic chest pain with a non–Q wave infarct.
7. Yes. There is evidence of anterior wall infarction, with loss of R wave progression in the chest leads. There is also evidence of inferior wall infarction, with large Q waves in leads III and aV_F. In addition, notice the tall R wave in lead aV_L (14 mm) with repolarization abnormalities in leads I and aV_L. This patient had a history of hypertension, producing left ventricular hypertrophy.

10

Miscellaneous ECG Patterns

This chapter presents an electrocardiographic potpourri—a discussion of a number of ECG patterns that have not been covered in detail to this point. We will briefly discuss drug effects, electrolyte disturbances, pericardial disease and myocarditis, "early repolarization," pulmonary embolism, Wolff-Parkinson-White preexcitation, and several other miscellaneous ECG patterns.

DRUG EFFECTS

Numerous drugs can affect the ECG. Generally the changes produced are slight and nonspecific. However, several commonly used drugs produce distinctive ECG changes. We will briefly consider the patterns seen with digitalis, quinidine and related agents, and the psychotropics.

Digitalis is used to treat heart failure and certain arrhythmias. One of its effects is to shorten repolarization time in the ventricles. This shortens the QT interval and is associated with a characteristic scooping of the ST-T complex, as shown in Figures 10-1 and 10-2 *(digitalis effect)*. Notice that when digitalis effect occurs the ST segment and T wave are fused together and it is impossible to tell where one ends and the other begins. Digitalis effect can be seen in a patient taking therapeutic or toxic doses of any digitalis preparation (such as digoxin). Digitalis *effect* must be distinguished from digitalis *toxicity* (Chapter 16); the latter refers to arrhythmias, conduction disturbances, and systemic side effects produced by excessive amounts of digitalis.

Quinidine, procainamide, and disopyramide are antiarrhythmic drugs with similar properties. In contrast to digitalis, they prolong ventricular repolarization. Therefore they may prolong the QT interval and flatten the T wave. In toxic doses they may also prolong ventricular depolarization, leading to a widening of the QRS complexes* Occasionally these agents will produce prominent U waves resembling those seen with hypokalemia (p. 126).

Quinidine, a drug used to treat atrial or ventricular arrhythmias, may in selected cases actually cause fainting or even sudden death due to a torsade de pointes type of ventricular tachycardia (quinidine syncope), as described in Chapter 14. This *proarrhythmic* effect is most likely to occur with very long QT intervals and prominent U waves (Fig. 10-3).

Prolongation of the QT interval can occur with other cardiac antiarrhythmic drugs, including sotalol and amiodarone. Psychotropic drugs (e.g., the phenothiazines and tricyclic antidepressants) can markedly alter the ECG and, in toxic doses, induce a fatal ventricular tachyarrhythmia or asystole. They may also prolong the QRS, causing a bundle branch block-like pattern, or lengthen repolarization (long Q-T-U intervals), predisposing to torsade de pointes (p. 188). Figure 10-4 presents the typical findings, in this case from a young adult

---

*QRS prolongation may also occur with other antiarrhythmic drugs (e.g., propafenone, flecainide).

DIGITALIS EFFECT

Fig. 10-1. Notice the characteristic scooping of the ST-T complex produced by digitalis. Not all patients taking digitalis exhibit these changes, however.

DIGITALIS EFFECT

Fig. 10-2. Notice the characteristic scooping of the ST-T complex, best seen in leads V_5 and V_6. Low voltage is also present, with a total QRS amplitude of 5 mm or less in all six extremity leads.

QUINIDINE EFFECTS AND EARLY TOXICITY

Fig. 10-3. Lead V_6. Quinidine blood level 2.9 µg/ml (therapeutic range). Notice the prolonged repolarization with prominent U waves, similar to the pattern of hypokalemia. Patients in whom quinidine causes marked repolarization prolongation (often with large U waves) may be at increased risk of ventricular tachycardia (torsade de pointes, Chapter 14). This patient did, in fact, subsequently develop torsade de pointes.

Fig. 10-4. A, The ECG from a patient with tricyclic antidepressant overdose shows three major findings: sinus tachycardia (from anticholinergic and adrenergic effects), prolongation of the QRS (from slowed ventricular conduction), and prolongation of the QT (from delayed repolarization). **B,** A repeat ECG 4 days later shows persistent sinus tachycardia but normalization of the QRS and QT.

who took an overdose of tricyclic antidepressant. Notice the prolonged QRS and QT intervals, along with a sinus tachycardia.

ELECTROLYTE DISTURBANCES

Abnormal serum concentrations of potassium and calcium can produce marked effects on the ECG. Hyperkalemia can, in fact, be lethal because of its cardiac toxicity.

Hyperkalemia

Progressive hyperkalemia produces a distinctive sequence of ECG changes affecting both depolarization (QRS) and repolarization (ST-T). The normal serum potassium concentration is between 3.5 and 5.0 mEq/L. The first change seen with abnormal elevation of the serum potassium concentration is narrowing and peaking of the T waves. As shown in Figures 10-5 and 10-6 the T waves with hyperkalemia have a characteristic "tented" shape and may become quite tall. With further elevation of the serum potassium, the PR intervals become prolonged and the P waves are smaller and may disappear entirely. Continued elevations produce an intraventricular conduction delay, with widening of the QRS complexes (Figs. 10-5 to 10-7). As the concentration rises further, the QRS com-

plexes continue to widen, leading to a large undulating ("sine-wave") pattern (Fig. 10-5) and eventual asystole. The sequence of changes seen on the ECG with progressive hyperkalemia is outlined in Figure 10-5. Because hyperkalemia may be fatal, recognition of the earliest signs of T wave peaking may prove lifesaving. Hyperkalemia can be seen in several clinical settings. The most common is kidney failure, in which there is reduced excretion of potassium.

Hypokalemia

Hypokalemia also produces distinctive changes in the ST-T complex. The most common pattern seen is ST depressions with prominent U waves and prolonged repolarization* (Figs. 10-8 and 10-9). With hypokalemia the U waves typically become enlarged and may even exceed the height of the T waves. Hypokalemia can be caused by several factors. The most common are (1) urinary potassium losses resulting from diuretic therapy and

---

*Technically the QT interval with hypokalemia may remain normal while repolarization is prolonged (as shown by the prominent U waves). However, the T waves and U waves often merge, so QT intervals cannot always be accurately measured.

Fig. 10-5. The earliest change with hyperkalemia is peaking ("tenting") of the T waves. With progressive increases in serum potassium, the QRS complexes widen, the P waves decrease in amplitude and may disappear (Fig. 10-6), and, finally, a sine-wave pattern leads to asystole.

HYPERKALEMIA

Fig. 10-6. Notice the peaked T waves, widened QRS complexes, and prolonged PR intervals. Intermittently a junctional rhythm is present with no P waves.

(2) potassium losses associated with metabolic alkalosis from vomiting or gastric suction.

Hypercalcemia and Hypocalcemia

Hypercalcemia shortens, and hypocalcemia lengthens, ventricular repolarization (Fig. 10-10).

Hypercalcemia causes shortening of the QT interval. It may be life threatening at high levels and lead to coma and death. A short QT interval in a comatose patient is sometimes the first clue to the diagnosis of hypercalcemia. Hypercalcemia may be caused by numerous factors, including malignant tumors (especially breast and lung), multiple myeloma, hyperparathyroidism, and excessive amounts of vitamin D.

Hypocalcemia lengthens or prolongs the QT interval. Common causes include intestinal malabsorption, pancreatitis, kidney failure, and hypoparathyroidism.

It should be noted that patients may have clinically significant hypocalcemia or hypercalcemia without diagnostic ECG changes.

Fig. 10-7. In this patient the K^+ concentration was 8.5 mEq/L. Notice the absence of P waves and the bizarre wide QRS complexes.

HYPOKALEMIA

Fig. 10-8. Variable ECG patterns may be seen with hypokalemia, ranging from slight T wave flattening to the appearance of prominent U waves, sometimes with ST depressions or T wave inversions. These patterns are not directly related to the specific level of serum potassium.

HYPOKALEMIA

Fig. 10-9. The serum K^+ was 2.2 mEq/L. Notice the prominent U waves.

HYPOCALCEMIA   NORMAL   HYPERCALCEMIA

QT 0.48 sec
QT$_C$ 0.52

QT 0.36 sec
QT$_C$ 0.41

QT 0.26 sec
QT$_C$ 0.36

Fig. 10-10. Hypocalcemia prolongs the QT interval by stretching out the ST segment. Hypercalcemia decreases the QT by shortening the ST segment.

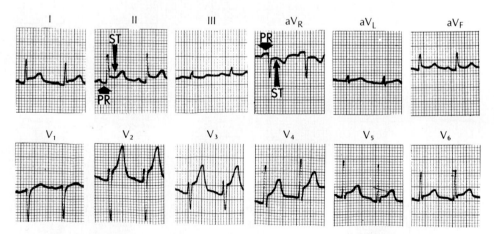

Fig. 10-11. Acute pericarditis causing diffuse ST segment elevations in I, II, aV$_F$, and V$_2$ to V$_6$, with reciprocal ST depressions in aV$_R$. By contrast, a concomitant atrial current of injury causes PR segment elevations in aV$_R$ with reciprocal PR depressions in the left chest leads and lead II. (From Goldberger AL: *Myocardial infarction: electrocardiographic differential diagnosis*, ed 4, St Louis, 1991, Mosby.)

PERICARDITIS AND PERICARDIAL EFFUSION

Pericarditis (inflammation of the pericardium) may be caused by a number of factors—including viral or bacterial infection, metastatic tumors, collagen vascular diseases, myocardial infarction, cardiac surgery, and uremia.

As mentioned in Chapter 8, the ECG patterns of pericarditis resemble those seen with acute myocardial infarction. The early phase of acute pericarditis is usually characterized by ST segment elevations. This is a current of injury pattern resulting from the inflammation of the heart's surface (epicardium) that often accompanies pericardial inflammation. Figure 10-11 shows an example of the ST segment elevations with acute pericarditis. A major difference between these and the ones occurring with myocardial infarction is their distribution. The ST segment elevations with acute myocardial infarction are characteristically limited to either the anterior leads because of the localized area of the infarct. The pericardium envelops the heart, and the ST-T changes occurring with pericarditis are therefore more generalized. ST elevations are typically seen in both anterior and inferior leads. For example, in Figure 10-11 notice the elevations in leads I, II, aV_L, aV_F, and V_2 to V_6.

Not only does acute pericarditis affect ventricular repolarization (the ST segment), it also affects repolarization of the atria, which starts during the PR segment (end of the P wave to beginning of the QRS). In particular, pericardial inflammation often causes an atrial current of injury, reflected by elevation of the PR in lead aV_R and depression of the PR in other limb leads and the left chest leads (V_5 and V_6). Thus with acute pericarditis the PR and ST segments typically point in opposite directions—the PR being elevated (often by only 1 mm or so) in aV_R, the ST being usually slightly depressed in that lead. Other leads may show PR depression and ST elevation.*

---

*This constitutes an exception to the earlier statement (p. 16) that repolarization of the atria generally is not recorded on the ECG.

Figure 10-11 illustrates these subtle but often helpful repolarization changes seen with acute pericarditis. The presence of PR changes may be a useful clue in the differential diagnosis of ST segment elevation, suggesting acute pericarditis as the cause.

The ST elevations seen with acute pericarditis are sometimes followed (after a variable time) by T wave inversions (Fig. 10-12). This sequence of elevations and inversions is the same as that described with myocardial infarction. In some cases the T wave inversions caused by pericarditis will resolve completely with time and the ECG will return to normal. In other cases they may persist for long periods.

We have concentrated on the similarity between the ECG patterns of acute pericarditis and acute myocardial infarction because both may produce ST segment elevations followed by T wave inversions. However, the ST-T changes with pericarditis, as noted, tend to be more diffuse than the localized changes of myocardial infarction. Another major difference is that pericarditis does not produce abnormal Q waves, such as those seen with certain infarcts. With MI, abnormal Q waves occur because of the death of heart muscle and the consequent loss of positive depolarization voltages. (See Chapter 8.) Pericarditis, on the other hand, generally causes only a superficial inflammation and does not produce actual myocardial necrosis. Thus abnormal Q waves never result from pericarditis alone.

Pericardial effusion refers to an abnormal accumulation of fluid in the pericardial sac. In most cases this fluid accumulates as the result of pericarditis. In some cases, however, such as myxedema (hypothyroidism) or rupture of the heart, pericardial effusion may occur in the absence of pericarditis. The major clinical significance of pericardial effusion is the danger of cardiac tamponade, in which the fluid actually "chokes off" the heart, leading to a drop in blood pressure and sometimes to cardiac arrest. (See Chapter 17.)

The most common ECG sign of pericardial effusion (with or without actual tamponade) is low voltage of the QRS complexes. In such cases the

PERICARDITIS, EVOLVING PATTERN

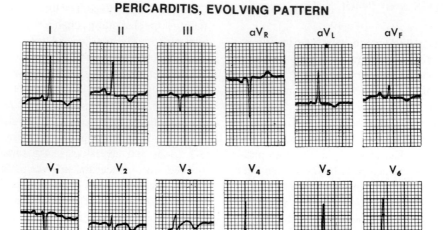

Fig. 10-12. Notice the diffuse T wave inversions in leads I, II, III, aV_L, aV_F, and V_2 to V_6.

ELECTRICAL ALTERNANS IN PERICARDIAL TAMPONADE

Fig. 10-13. In patients with pericardial effusion and cardiac tamponade, electrical alternans may develop. Notice the beat-to-beat alternation in the P-QRS-T axis caused by swinging of the heart in a large pericardial effusion. Relatively low QRS voltage and sinus tachycardia are also present.

low voltage is probably due to short-circuiting of cardiac voltages by the fluid surrounding the heart.

In our discussion of hypertrophy patterns (Chapter 6), the criteria for high voltage were mentioned. *Low voltage* is said to be present when the total amplitude of the QRS complexes in each of the six limb leads is 5 mm (0.5 mV) or less.* Figure 10-2 shows an example of low voltage.

Following is a list of the major factors that can lead to low voltage complexes:

1. Obesity
2. Emphysema
3. Pericardial effusion
4. Hypothyroidism
5. Diffuse myocardial injury (e.g., extensive myocardial infarction or myocardial fibrosis)
6. Infiltration of the heart muscle (e.g., amyloidosis)
7. Normal variant

Obesity can cause low voltage because of the fat tissue that lies between the heart and the chest wall. In patients with emphysema there is increased inflation of the lungs. This extra air acts to insulate the heart. Of the causes of low voltage listed, obesity and emphysema are among the most common. However, when you see low voltage (particularly with sinus tachycardia), pericardial effusion should always be high on your list because it can lead to fatal tamponade (p. 213).

Myxedema (hypothyroidism), as noted, may cause a pericardial effusion without actual pericarditis. Hypothyroidism also generally causes sinus bradycardia (Chapter 11). Therefore the combination of low voltage and sinus bradycardia should suggest the possible diagnosis of myxedema.

Electrical alternans is another pattern that can occur with pericardial effusion and tamponade (Fig. 10-13). It is characterized by a beat-to-beat shift in the QRS axis associated with mechanical swinging of the heart to-and-fro in a large accumulation of fluid. It is virtually pathognomonic of cardiac tamponade, although *not* every patient with tamponade will manifest this pattern.

To summarize: Pericarditis causes a diffuse current of injury pattern with ST segment elevations in the anterior and inferior leads, followed by T wave inversions in those leads. Abnormal Q waves, however, are not seen with pericarditis alone. Pericardial effusion is one of the causes of low voltage on the ECG.

MYOCARDITIS

A variety of conditions, for example, certain viral infections, may be associated with inflammation of the heart muscle (myocarditis). The ECG findings with myocarditis are quite variable, ranging from nonspecific ST-T changes to the repolarization changes that occur with acute pericarditis. In some cases the ECG of focal myocarditis may exactly simulate that of acute myocardial infarction, even with Q waves. Atrial or ventricular arrhythmias can occur with myocarditis, as can AV or ventricular conduction disturbances.

EARLY REPOLARIZATION VARIANT

Recall, from Chapter 4, that the normal ST segment is isoelectric, riding along the baseline and gradually rising into the T wave. (See Figure 2-10.) Although slight deviations (generally less than 1 mm) may be seen in normal people, more marked ST elevations may signify an abnormal condition (e.g., myocardial infarction, Prinzmetal's angina, ventricular aneurysm, or pericarditis).

In Figure 10-14, from a *normal* young adult, notice the marked elevation of the ST segments. This is a benign variant known as the *early repolarization pattern*. With early repolarization the ST segments in the chest leads may rise to 3 mm above the baseline. Although most common in young people, such elevations can also occur in older persons, simulating the pattern seen with acute pericarditis or MI. However, they are stable and do not undergo the evolutionary sequence seen with acute pericarditis; and they are not associated with reciprocal ST depressions (except in lead aV_R), contrary to what is observed with acute MI.

PULMONARY EMBOLISM

The ECG is not a sensitive test for pulmonary embolism. In some cases the obstruction produced

---

*Low voltage in the limb leads may or may not be accompanied by low voltage in the chest leads (defined as a total QRS amplitude of 10 mm or less in V_1 to V_6).

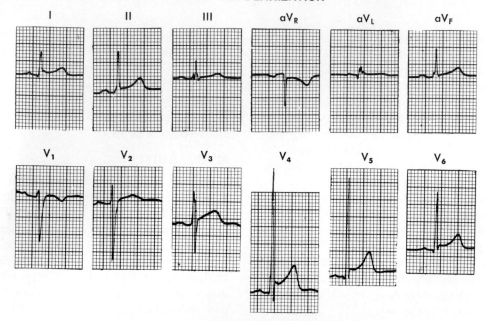

Fig. 10-14. ST segment elevation, usually most marked in the chest leads, is sometimes seen as a normal variant. This "early repolarization" pattern may be confused with ST segment elevations of acute myocardial infarction or pericarditis.

ACUTE PULMONARY EMBOLISM

Fig. 10-15. Several features occasionally seen with pulmonary embolism are sinus tachycardia, S waves in lead I with Q waves and T wave inversions in lead III ($S_I Q_{III} T_{III}$ pattern), and poor R wave progression with T wave inversions (right ventricular "strain") in chest leads V_1 to V_4 resulting from acute right ventricular overload.

by an embolus in the pulmonary artery system can lead to ECG changes, but generally there is no single pattern that is always diagnostic. The following may all be seen (Fig. 10-15):

1. Sinus tachycardia (Other arrhythmias also occur, such as ventricular ectopy and atrial fibrillation.)
2. A right ventricular "strain" pattern (inverted T waves in leads V_1 to V_4)
3. The so-called $S_1Q_{III}T_{III}$ pattern (an S wave in lead I and a new Q wave in lead III with T wave inversion in that lead) (This pattern, which may simulate that produced by acute inferior wall MI, is probably due to acute right ventricular dilation.)
4. Shifting of the QRS axis to the right
5. ST segment depressions indicative of subendocardial ischemia
6. An incomplete or complete RBBB pattern (wide rSR' in lead V_1)

The appearance of these changes, particularly in combination, is suggestive but not diagnostic of pulmonary embolism. Many patients with massive pulmonary emboli will have only minor, relatively nonspecific, changes on their ECG. Thus both the diagnostic sensitivity and the specificity of the ECG with pulmonary embolism are limited. Figure 10-15 shows a classic example of the changes seen with pulmonary embolism.

CHRONIC LUNG DISEASE (EMPHYSEMA)

Patients with chronic lung disease from emphysema often have a relatively characteristic combination of ECG findings (Fig. 10-16)—including (1) low voltage, (2) poor R wave progression in the chest leads, and (3) a vertical or rightward QRS axis in the frontal plane. Excessive pulmonary air trapping causes the low voltage. The poor R wave progression results, in part, from the downward displacement of the diaphragm; thus the chest

CHRONIC LUNG DISEASE

Fig. 10-16. Notice the characteristic relatively low voltages in the limb leads, right axis deviation, P pulmonale, and poor R wave progression. T wave inversions (V_1 to V_5) are due to right ventricular "strain."

leads are actually placed *relatively* higher than usual. In addition, right ventricular dilation may contribute to the delayed chest lead transition zone. Finally, the anatomically vertical position of the heart in the chest of a patient with emphysema, and sometimes right ventricular enlargement, causes the mean QRS axis to be vertical or even rightward (greater than +100°). Tall, relatively narrow, P waves due to right atrial overload (Fig. 10-16) may also be present.

CONGESTIVE HEART FAILURE

Congestive heart failure (CHF) is a complex syndrome that may result from multiple causes—including ischemic heart disease, systemic hypertension, valvular heart disease, and cardiomyopathy. The ECG may provide helpful clues to a specific diagnosis in some of these patients. For example, prominent Q waves and typical ST-T changes suggest underlying ischemic heart disease. Left ventricular hypertrophy patterns (Chapter 6) may be seen with hypertensive heart disease, aortic valve disease (stenosis or regurgitation), or mitral regurgitation. The combination of left atrial enlargement (or atrial fibrillation) and signs of right ventricular hypertrophy should suggest mitral stenosis (Fig. 19-1). Left bundle branch block (Chapter 7) may be seen with congestive heart failure caused by ischemic heart disease, valvular abnormalities, hypertension, or cardiomyopathy.

In some patients marked enlargement and decreased function of the left (and often the right) ventricle occur without coronary artery disease, hypertension, or significant valvular lesions. The term *"dilated (congestive) cardiomyopathy"* is applied in such cases. Dilated cardiomyopathy can be idiopathic or associated with chronic excessive alcohol ingestion (alcoholic cardiomyopathy), viral infection, or some other etiology.

Patients with dilated cardiomyopathy from any cause may have a distinctive ECG pattern (the *ECG-CHF* triad) characterized by

1. Relatively low limb lead voltages (such that the QRS in each of the six limb leads ≤ 8 mm in amplitude)
2. Relatively prominent precordial lead QRS voltages (such that the sum of the S wave in either lead V_1 or lead V_2 plus the R wave in V_5 or V_6 ≥ 35 mm)
3. Poor R wave progression defined by a QS- or rS-type complex in leads V_1 to V_4

When this triad is present (Fig. 10-17), it strongly suggests underlying cardiomyopathy but does not indicate a specific etiology. It may occur not only with primary dilated cardiomyopathy but also with severe heart disease due to previous infarcts or significant valvular dysfunction. Furthermore, it is of only modest sensitivity; that is, its absence does not exclude underlying cardiomyopathy.

WOLFF-PARKINSON-WHITE SYNDROME

The Wolff-Parkinson-White (WPW) syndrome is an unusual and distinctive ECG abnormality caused by *preexcitation* of the ventricles. Normally the electrical stimulus passes to the ventricles from the atria via the AV junction. The physiologic lag of conduction through the AV junction results in the normal PR interval of 0.12 to 0.2 second. Imagine the consequences of having an extra pathway between the atria and ventricles that would *bypass* the AV junction and *preexcite* the ventricles. This is exactly what occurs with the WPW syndrome: an atrioventricular (AV) bypass tract* connects the atria and ventricles, circumventing the AV junction (Fig. 10-18).

Preexcitation of the ventricles with the WPW syndrome produces the following three characteristic changes on the ECG (Figs. 10-19 and 10-20):

1. The QRS is widened, giving the superficial appearance of a bundle branch block pattern. However, the wide QRS is caused not by a delay in ventricular depolarization but by early stimulation of the ventricles. (The QRS will be widened to the degree that the PR is shortened.)
2. The PR is shortened (often but not always <0.12 sec) because of ventricular preexcitation.
3. There is slurring, or notching, of the upstroke of the QRS complex. This is called a *delta* wave.

---

*Formerly called the bundle of Kent.

ECG-CHF TRIAD

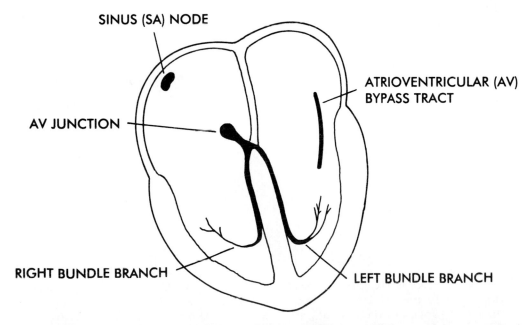

Fig. 10-17. Severe idiopathic dilated cardiomyopathy in a 29-year-old man. Poor precordial R wave progression simulates anterior wall infarction. The triad of relatively low limb lead QRS voltages, prominent precordial QRS voltages, and poor R wave progression in the chest leads is highly suggestive of dilated cardiomyopathy. (From Goldberger AL: *Myocardial infarction: electrocardiographic differential diagnosis,* ed 4, St Louis, 1991, Mosby.)

Fig. 10-18. Anatomy of the preexcitation syndrome (Wolff-Parkinson-White) pattern. In a small percentage of the population an accessory fiber (atrioventricular bypass tract) connects the atria and ventricles. The consequences of this extra conduction path are discussed in the text.

WPW PREEXCITATION

- • Short PR
- • Wide QRS
- • Delta Wave (arrow)

Fig. 10-19. Preexcitation via the bypass tract in Wolff-Parkinson-White is associated with the triad of findings shown here.

Figures 10-19 and 10-20 show the WPW pattern, with its classic triad of a widened QRS, a short PR interval, and a delta wave. Notice that it superficially resembles a bundle branch block pattern because of the widened QRS complexes. Depending on which area of the ventricles is preexcited first, the ECG may show a pattern simulating that of either a right bundle branch block with tall R waves in the right chest leads or a left bundle branch block with a predominantly negative QS in lead V_1.

The significance of the WPW syndrome is twofold: First, patients with this pattern are prone to arrhythmias, especially paroxysmal supraventricular tachycardia (PSVT) (Fig. 10-21). Second, the ECG of these patients is often mistaken as indicating a bundle branch block or myocardial infarction (Fig. 10-20).

Fig. 10-20. Notice the characteristic triad of the Wolff-Parkinson-White pattern: wide QRS complexes, short PR intervals, and delta waves *(arrows)* that are negative in some leads here (e.g., II, III, and aV_F) and positive in others (aV_L and V_4 to V_6). The Q waves in leads II, III, and aV_F are the result of abnormal ventricular conduction (negative delta waves) rather than an inferior myocardial infarction.

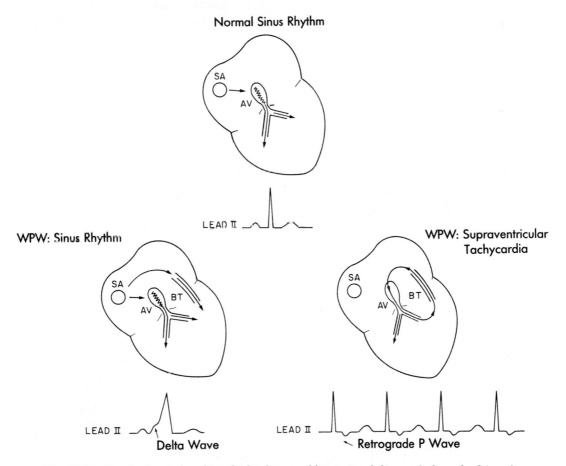

Fig. 10-21. Conduction during sinus rhythm in normal hearts *(top left)* spreads from the SA node to the AV node and then down the bundle branches. The *jagged line* in the AV node indicates physiologic slowing of conduction there. With Wolff-Parkinson-White *(top right)* an abnormal accessory conduction pathway called a bypass tract *(BT)* connects the atria and ventricles. With WPW during sinus rhythm the electrical impulse is conducted quickly down the bypass tract, preexciting the ventricles before the impulse arrives via the AV node. Consequently, the PR is short and the QRS is wide, with slurring at its onset (delta wave) representing the preexcitation. WPW also predisposes to a reentrant-type supraventricular tachycardia *(bottom)* in which a premature atrial beat may spread down the normal pathway to the ventricles, travel back up the bypass tract, and recirculate down the AV node again. This "circus movement" can then repeat itself over and over, resulting in a tachycardia. Notice the normal QRS and retrograde (negative) P wave in lead II during this type of bypass tract tachycardia. (See Chapter 12.)

The WPW syndrome predisposes to PSVT because of the presence of an extra conduction pathway. For example, a premature impulse traveling down the AV junction may recycle up the accessory pathway and then back down the AV junction, and so on.* This type of recirculating impulse is an example of *reentry*.

Another type of preexcitation variant, the Lown-Ganong-Levine (LGL) pattern, is caused by a bypass tract that connects the atria and AV junction. Bypassing the AV node results in a short PR interval (less than 0.12 sec). However, the QRS width is not prolonged, because ventricular activation occurs normally. Therefore the LGL pattern consists of a normal-width QRS with a short PR and no delta wave; the WPW consists of a wide QRS with a short PR and a delta wave (Fig. 10-19). Patients with the LGL pattern may also have reentrant-type PSVT or paroxysmal atrial fibrillation or flutter.†

DIFFERENTIAL DIAGNOSIS OF WIDE QRS COMPLEXES

Discussion of the WPW syndrome allows us now to review all the major ECG patterns that produce a widened QRS complex. This list includes four major categories:

1. Bundle branch blocks, including the classic RBBB or LBBB patterns
2. "Toxic" conduction delays caused by some extrinsic factor, such as hyperkalemia or drugs (quinidine, propafenone and related antiarrhythmics, phenothiazines, tricyclic antidepressants)
3. Beats arising in the ventricles, which may be ventricular premature beats (p. 177), ventricular escape beats (Fig. 17-14), or pacemaker beats (p. 80)
4. Wolff-Parkinson-White type preexcitation

Differentiation among these possibilities is usually easy. Right and left bundle branch blocks have been described (Chapter 7). Hyperkalemia produces widening of the QRS complex, often with loss of P waves. Widening of the QRS in any patient taking an antiarrhythmic or psychotropic should always suggest possible drug toxicity. Pacemakers generally produce an LBBB pattern with a pacemaker spike before each QRS. The WPW syndrome is recognized by the combination of a short PR interval and a wide QRS, usually with a delta wave.

ST-T CHANGES: SPECIFIC AND NONSPECIFIC

The concluding topic of Part I of this book is a review of the major factors causing ST-T (repolarization) changes. The term *"nonspecific ST-T change,"* defined earlier (Chapter 9), is commonly used in clinical electrocardiography. Many factors (e.g., drugs, ischemia, electrolyte imbalances, infections, and pulmonary disease) can affect the ECG. As mentioned above, the repolarization phase (ST-T complex) is particularly sensitive to such effects and can show a variety of nonspecific changes as a result of multiple factors (Figs. 10-22 and 10-23). These changes include slight ST depressions, T wave flattening, and slight T wave inversions (Fig. 10-22).

In contrast to these nonspecific ST-T changes, there are certain fairly specific changes associated with particular conditions (e.g., the tall tented T waves of hyperkalemia). Some of these relatively specific ST-T changes are shown in Figure 10-24. However, even such apparently specific changes can be misleading. For example, ST elevation is characteristic of acute transmural myocardial in-

---

*When PSVT develops in a patient with the WPW syndrome, the QRS complex generally becomes narrow. The widened QRS seen with WPW during normal sinus rhythm occurs because the stimulus travels concomitantly down the bypass tract and down the AV junction, resulting in a *fusion* beat. When PSVT occurs, the impulse usually travels down the AV junction and back up the bypass tract in a retrograde fashion, resulting in a loss of the delta wave. (The role of bypass tracts in paroxysmal supraventricular tachycardia is discussed further in Chapters 12 and 18.)

†Most persons with a short PR interval and normal QRS do not have LGL preexcitation, however. A relatively short PR may be seen as a normal variant without a bypass tract due to accelerated AV conduction. Therefore do not "over-read" an ECG on which the only noteworthy finding is a short PR.

Normal T wave

Nonspecific ST-T changes

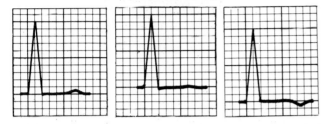

Fig. 10-22. Flattening of the T wave (*left* and *middle*) or slight T wave inversion *(right)* is an abnormal but relatively nonspecific change that may be caused by numerous factors.

Fig. 10-23. Nonspecific ST-T changes. Notice the diffuse T wave flattening.

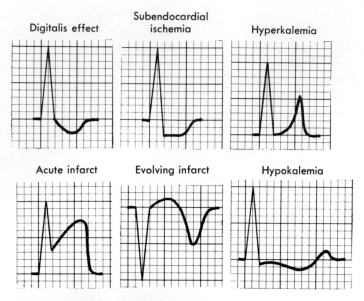

Fig. 10-24. Relatively specific ST-T changes. Note, however, that they are not absolutely specific for the abnormalities shown.

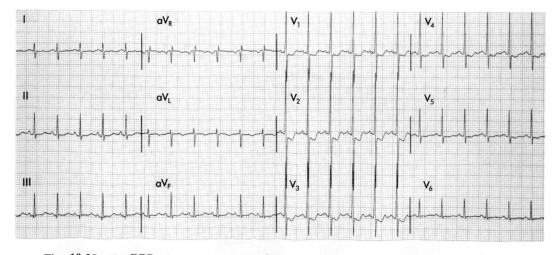

Fig. 10-25. The ECG of healthy neonates shows a pattern resembling that of right ventricular hypertrophy, with tall right precordial R waves and right axis deviation, which reflects the physiologic predominance of the right ventricle during fetal development. Note also the sinus tachycardia and the relatively narrow QRS complexes.

farction, yet ST elevations are also seen in Prinz-metal's angina and ventricular aneurysms as well as in pericarditis and benign (normal) early repolarization. Similarly, deep T wave inversions are most characteristic of ischemia but may occur in other conditions as well (pp. 116-117).

To summarize: Repolarization abnormalities (ST-T changes) can be grouped into two general categories: First are the nonspecific ST-T changes, which include slight ST segment deviation and flattening or inversion of the T wave. These are not diagnostic of any particular condition but must always be interpreted in clinical context. Second are the relatively specific ST-T changes that are more strongly, but not always definitively, diagnostic of some particular underlying cause (for example, hyperkalemia or myocardial ischemia).

PEDIATRIC ELECTROCARDIOGRAPHY

The normal ECG patterns seen in children differ considerably from those seen in adults (Chapter 4). The topic of pediatric electrocardiography falls outside the scope of this book, but a few critical points of difference between pediatric and adult ECGs will be mentioned briefly. The normal ECG of a neonate resembles the pattern seen in right ventricular hypertrophy, with tall R waves in the right chest leads and right axis deviation (Fig. 10-25). During the first decade of life the T waves in the right to middle chest leads are normally inverted. This pattern sometimes persists into adolescence and adulthood and is called the *juvenile* T wave variant. Children and young adults may also have high voltage in the chest leads as a normal variant. (See Chapter 6.)

REVIEW

The ECG can be influenced by numerous factors.

Many *drugs* affect it. *Digitalis effect* refers to the characteristic scooped-out depression of the ST segment produced by therapeutic doses of digitalis. (*Digitalis toxicity* refers to the arrhythmias and conduction disturbances produced by excessive doses of digitalis.) *Quinidine, procainamide,* and *disopyramide* as well as certain *psychotropic* drugs can prolong the QT interval and, in toxic doses, markedly widen the QRS complex. These drugs may also cause a potentially lethal type of ventricular tachycardia called *torsade de pointes* (Chapter 14). Patients likely to develop this complication often show prolonged QT intervals and/or large U waves.

Electrolyte disturbances can also affect the ECG. *Hyperkalemia* typically produces a sequence of changes. First, there is narrowing and peaking (tenting) of the T wave. Further elevation of the serum potassium concentration leads to PR prolongation and then to loss of P waves and to QRS widening, followed by a "sine-wave" pattern and asystole. *Hypokalemia* may produce ST depressions and prominent U waves. The QT interval becomes prolonged. (In some cases you are actually measuring the QU and not the QT interval, because it may be impossible to tell where the T wave ends and the U wave begins.) *Hypercalcemia* may shorten the QT interval, and *hypocalcemia* may prolong it.

Pericarditis produces diffuse ST segment elevations, usually in one or more of the chest leads and also in leads I, aV_L, II, and aV_F. PR segment elevation in lead aV_R with PR depression in other leads may be caused by an atrial current of injury. Abnormal Q waves do not develop. The ST segment elevations may be followed by T wave inversions after a variable period.

Pericardial effusion often produces *low voltage* of the QRS complex (QRS amplitude of 5 mm or less in all six extremity leads). Low voltage is not specific for pericardial effusion but may also occur with obesity, emphysema, and diffuse myocardial injury or infiltration or as a normal variant.

Pericardial effusion complicated by *cardiac tamponade* is usually associated with sinus tachycardia and low voltage complexes. Some of these patients will also have *electrical alternans,* a pattern characterized by a beat-to-beat shift in the QRS axis.

Myocarditis can produce ST-T changes that are nonspecific or that resemble the changes of pericarditis or myocardial infarction. It may also be associated with arrhythmias.

Normally the ST segment is isoelectric. However, in some healthy people, young adult males in particular, there will be normal ST segment elevations *(early repolarization variant),* usually best seen in the chest leads (up to 3 mm of elevation). The pattern may simulate that of acute MI or pericarditis but does not show the successive changes usually occurring with those pathologies.

Pulmonary embolism may produce any of the following patterns: (1) sinus tachycardia and various arrhythmias, (2) right ventricular "strain" T wave inversions, (3) $S_IQ_{III}T_{III}$, (4) right axis shift, (5) ST depressions resulting from subendocardial ischemia, and (6) acute RBBB.

The *WPW pattern* shows (1) a short PR interval (usually but not always <0.12 sec), (2) a wide QRS complex, and (3) slurring or notching of the initial part of the QRS complex. This slurring is called a *delta* wave. Patients with the WPW pattern are particularly prone to attacks of reentrant-type paroxysmal supraventricular tachycardias (PSVT). Another form of preexcitation, the Lown-Ganong-Levine pattern, is characterized by a short PR interval and a normal QRS.

The differential diagnosis of ECG patterns with a wide QRS complex includes four major possibilities: (1) right or left bundle branch block, (2) toxic conduction delays caused by hyperkalemia or certain drugs, (3) beats arising in the ventricles, such as VPBs or pacemaker beats, and (4) WPW preexcitation.

Questions

1. The following factors may all affect ventricular repolarization (ST-T complex). Put an "L" next to those that may prolong ventricular repolarization (lengthen the QT interval). Put an "S" next to those that may shorten the QT interval.

   Digitalis   Hypokalemia

   Quinidine   Hypocalcemia

   Procainamide   Hypercalcemia

2. Put an "X" next to those factors that can widen the QRS complex.

   Hypokalemia

   Hyperkalemia

   Wolff-Parkinson-White syndrome

   Digitalis effect

   Quinidine toxicity

   Right bundle branch block

3. Which of the following factors can produce ST segment elevations?

Hypokalemia
Early repolarization pattern
Digitalis effect
Ventricular aneurysm
Hypocalcemia
Right bundle branch block
Pericarditis

4. Match ECGs *A, B,* and *C* with the following causes:

Digitalis effect
Hyperkalemia
Hypokalemia

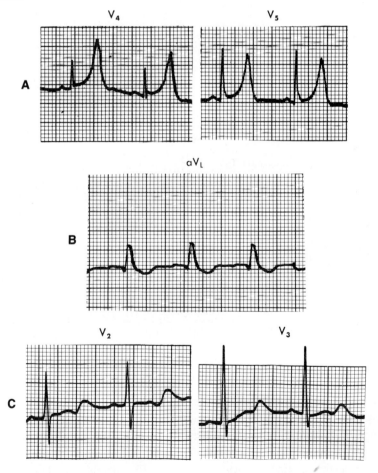

5. What caused the wide QRS in the following ECG?
   a. Right bundle branch block
   b. Quinidine toxicity
   c. Posterolateral infarction
   d. Wolff-Parkinson-White pattern
   e. Hyperkalemia

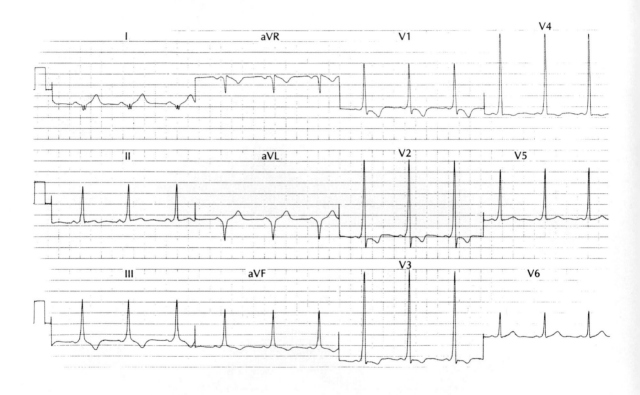

Answers

1. Digitalis (S); quinidine (L); procainamide (L); hypokalemia (L); hypocalcemia (L); hypercalcemia (S).

2. Hyperkalemia (X); Wolff-Parkinson-White syndrome (X); quinidine toxicity (X); right bundle branch block (X).

3. Early repolarization variant; ventricular aneurysm; pericarditis.

4. Digitalis effect, *B;* hyperkalemia, *A;* hypokalemia, *C*.

5. d.   Notice the diagnostic triad of a wide QRS, short PR interval, and delta wave (slurred initial portion of the QRS). Compare this with Figure 10-20, which also shows the Wolff-Parkinson-White pattern. WPW patterns are at times mistaken for hypertrophy (tall R waves) or infarction (*pseudoinfarction* Q waves).

II

CARDIAC RHYTHM DISTURBANCES

Sinus Rhythms

NORMAL SINUS RHYTHM

The diagnosis of normal sinus rhythm (NSR) was described in Chapter 3. When the sinus (SA) node is pacing the heart, atrial depolarization spreads from right to left and downward toward the AV junction. An arrow representing this depolarization wave will point downward and toward the left. Therefore, with normal sinus rhythm, the P wave is negative in lead aV_R and positive in lead II (Figs. 4-3 and 11-1).

By convention, *normal sinus rhythm* is usually defined as sinus rhythm with a heart rate between 60 and 100 beats/min. Sinus rhythm with a heart rate of less than 60 beats/min is called *sinus bradycardia;* one with a heart rate greater than 100 beats/min is *sinus tachycardia.*

REGULATION OF THE HEART RATE

The heart, like the other organs of the body, has a special nerve supply from the autonomic nervous system that controls involuntary muscle action. The autonomic nerve supply to the heart (and, in particular, the SA and AV nodes) consists of two opposing groups of fibers: the sympathetic nerves and the parasympathetic nerves. Sympathetic stimulation produces an increased heart rate and also increases the strength of myocardial contraction. Parasympathetic stimulation (from the vagus nerve) produces a slowing of the heart rate as well as a slowing of conduction through the AV nodal area. In this way the autonomic nervous system exerts a counterbalancing control of the heart rate.

The sympathetic nervous system acts as a cardiac accelerator while the parasympathetic (vagal) system produces a braking effect. For example, when you become excited or upset, increased sympathetic stimuli (and diminished parasympathetic tone) result in an increased heart rate and increased contractility, producing the familiar sensation of a pounding heart (palpitations).*

SINUS TACHYCARDIA

Sinus tachycardia *is simply sinus rhythm with a heart rate exceeding 100 beats/min.* Generally in adults the heart rate with sinus tachycardia is between 100 and 180 beats/min.

Figure 11-2 shows an example of sinus tachycardia. Each QRS complex is preceded by a P wave. Notice that the P waves are positive in lead II. With sinus tachycardia at very fast rates, the P wave may merge with the preceding T wave and become difficult to distinguish.

Sinus tachycardia is an "arrhythmia," but not necessarily an abnormal rhythm. Indeed, most normal persons develop a sinus tachycardia during exercise or excitement. In general, a sinus tachycardia will be seen with any condition that produces

---

*Palpitations may be associated with a normal heartbeat, with isolated premature beats (atrial or ventricular), or with an actual run of extra heartbeats (due, for example, to atrial fibrillation, paroxysmal supraventricular tachycardia, or ventricular tachycardia).

NORMAL SINUS RHYTHM

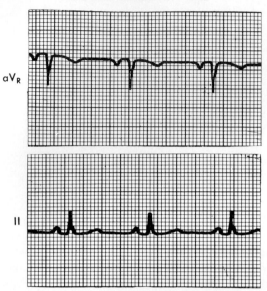

Fig. 11-1. Each QRS complex is preceded by a P wave that is negative in aV$_R$ and positive in II.

an *increase* in sympathetic tone or a *decrease* in vagal tone.

The following conditions are commonly associated with sinus tachycardia:

1. Anxiety, excitement, and exertion
2. Drugs that increase sympathetic tone (e.g., epinephrine, dopamine, tricyclic antidepressants, isoproterenol, and cocaine)
3. Drugs that block vagal tone (e.g., atropine)
4. Fever, many infections, septic shock
5. Congestive heart failure (Sinus tachycardia caused by increased sympathetic tone is generally seen with pulmonary edema.)
6. Pulmonary embolism (Sinus tachycardia is the most common arrhythmia seen with acute pulmonary embolism [Chapter 10].)
7. Acute myocardial infarction, which may produce virtually any arrhythmia (Sinus tachycardia persisting after an acute infarct is generally a bad prognostic sign and implies extensive heart damage.)
8. Hyperthyroidism (Sinus tachycardia occurring at rest may be an important diagnostic clue.)
9. Intravascular volume loss due to bleeding, vomiting, diarrhea, pancreatitis, dehydration, and related conditions
10. Alcohol intoxication or withdrawal

Treatment of sinus tachycardia must be directed at the underlying cause (e.g., infection, hyperthyroidism, congestive heart failure).

Fig. 11-2. Sinus tachycardia.

SINUS BRADYCARDIA

With sinus bradycardia, sinus rhythm is present and the heart rate is less than 60 beats/min (Fig. 11-3). It commonly occurs in the following conditions:

1. As a normal variant (Many people have a resting pulse rate of less than 60 beats/min, and trained athletes may have a resting or sleeping pulse rate as low as 35 beats/min.)
2. Drugs that increase vagal tone (e.g., digitalis or edrophonium) or that decrease sympathetic tone (e.g., the beta blockers) (In addition, calcium channel–blocking drugs such as diltiazem hydrochloride and verapamil may cause marked sinus bradycardia.)
3. Hypothyroidism
4. Hyperkalemia
5. "Sick sinus syndrome" (Some patients, particularly elderly ones, will have marked sinus bradycardia without obvious cause, probably from degenerative disease of the sinus node or surrounding tissue. The "sick sinus syndrome" is discussed further at the end of this chapter and in Chapter 18. See also Figure 11-6.)
6. Sleep apnea syndrome
7. Carotid sinus hypersensitivity syndrome
8. Vasovagal reactions

Most people with moderate sinus bradycardia have no symptoms. If the heart rate is very slow (in the 40s), light-headedness and even syncope may occur. Treatment requires decreasing the dose of or discontinuing medications (e.g., beta blockers or calcium-channel blockers). In cases of chronic sinus bradycardia causing symptoms (as in the *sick sinus syndrome*) an electronic pacemaker may be needed. (See Chapter 20.)

SINUS ARRHYTHMIA

Even in healthy persons the sinus (or SA) node does not pace the heart at a perfectly regular rate. There is normally a slight beat-to-beat variation. Sometimes (Figs. 11-4 and 11-5), when this variability is more accentuated, the term "*sinus arrhythmia*" is used.

The most common cause of sinus arrhythmia is respiration. Respiratory sinus arrhythmia is a normal finding, particularly in children and young adults. With inspiration the heart rate normally increases slightly, and with expiration it decreases slightly, because of changes in vagal tone occurring during the different phases of respiration (Fig. 11-4). A *nonphasic sinus arrhythmia* at rest, though not strictly abnormal, has no specific pathologic or therapeutic significance. In this situation the heart rate varies from beat to beat without relation to the respiratory cycle (Fig. 11-5).

SINUS PAUSES, SINUS ARREST, AND ESCAPE BEATS

Up to this point we have considered normal sinus rhythm, sinus tachycardia, sinus bradycardia,

Fig. 11-3. Sinus bradycardia. Notice the negative P waves, because this is lead aV$_R$.

Fig. 11-4. Phasic sinus arrhythmia. Normally there is a slight increase in the heart rate with inspiration and a slight decrease with expiration.

MONITOR LEAD

Fig. 11-5. Nonphasic sinus arrhythmia. The monitor lead shows a markedly irregular rhythm. Each QRS complex is preceded by a P wave, with a constant PR interval. This arrhythmia was associated with acute myocarditis. (Notice that the T waves are biphasic.)

Fig. 11-6. Sinus pause in a patient with sick sinus syndrome. The monitor lead shows sinus bradycardia with a long pause (about 2.4 sec).

Fig. 11-7. Junctional escape beat *(JE)*. The monitor strip shows a sinus pause with each escape beat. The wide QRS is due to an underlying bundle branch block.

and sinus arrhythmia. Suppose the sinus node fails to stimulate the atria for one or more beats. Such dysfunction may occur intermittently, with simply a missed beat (no P wave or QRS complex) at occasional intervals, or it may be more extreme.* An example of the latter is *sinus pause* or *arrest* (Fig. 11-6), in which the SA node fails to stimulate the atria for a prolonged period. This leads to cardiac arrest with asystole unless the sinus node regains function or some other pacemaker (escape pacemaker) takes over. Fortunately, other parts of the cardiac conduction system are capable of producing electrical stimuli and functioning as an escape pacemaker in these circumstances. Escape beats may come from the atria, the AV node, or the ventricles. Figure 11-7 shows a junctional escape beat. (The characteristics of escape beats are described in Chapter 12.)

Sinus block or sinus arrest can be caused by numerous factors, including hypoxia, myocardial ischemia or infarction, hyperkalemia, digitalis toxicity, and toxic reactions to other drugs such as the beta blockers and calcium-channel blockers (diltiazem, verapamil). The sinus node region, particularly in elderly persons, may undergo degenerative changes with periods of SA dysfunction and even arrest leading at times to light-headedness and syncope. The term *"sick sinus syndrome"* refers to this type of SA node dysfunction (Figs. 11-6 and 18-13).

To summarize: The term *"arrhythmia"* refers to any heart rhythm other than strictly normal sinus rhythm. Sinus bradycardia, sinus tachycardia, sinus arrhythmia, and SA block are all arrhythmias. However, sinus bradycardia in a resting person, sinus tachycardia with exercise, and respiratory sinus arrhythmia are all normal findings. In other settings, such as with hypothyroidism or pulmonary emboli, sinus bradycardia or sinus tachycardia, respectively, may be an important diagnostic clue.

The next few chapters describe important arrhythmias in which the cardiac pacemaker is located *outside* the sinus node—in the atria, AV junction, or ventricles.

---

*There are two distinct mechanisms for sinus node dysfunction: sinus pacemaker failure and sinoatrial (SA) block. The former is due to actual failure of the SA node to electrically fire (depolarize) for one or more beats. The latter results when the SA node fires but the impulse is apparently blocked from exiting the node and stimulating the atria. From a clinical viewpoint, distinguishing between SA pacemaker dysfunction and SA (exit) block is usually not essential.

REVIEW

With *normal sinus rhythm* (NSR) each heartbeat originates in the sinus node. The P wave is always negative in lead aV_R and positive in lead II. The rate is between 60 and 100 beats/min.

With *sinus tachycardia* the heart rate is greater than 100 beats/min while with *sinus bradycardia* it is less than 60 beats/min. There are multiple causes of sinus bradycardia and sinus tachycardia, and both arrhythmias may occur normally.

With *sinus arrhythmia* there is variability of the sinus rate from beat to beat, and it may be either phasic with respiration or nonphasic. *SA* dysfunction (due to pacemaker cell failure or "exit" block) may lead to sinus pauses or, in extreme cases, *SA arrest*. Prolonged sinus arrest will cause fatal asystole unless NSR resumes or unless *escape beats* from other foci in the atria, AV junction, or ventricles take over. SA dysfunction may be seen particularly in elderly people as a consequence of the *sick sinus syndrome*. Digitalis toxicity or toxic reactions to other drugs (beta blockers, calcium blockers) must always be excluded in anyone with marked sinus bradycardia, SA pauses or sinus arrest.

Questions

1. Is normal sinus rhythm present?

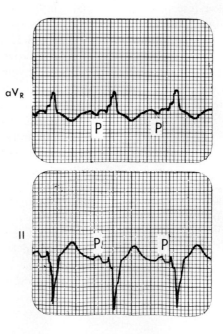

2. Is normal sinus rhythm present?

Answers

1. Yes. The P waves are negative in lead aV_R and positive in lead II. Don't be confused by the unusual QRS complexes (positive in lead aV_R and negative in lead II) produced by the abnormal axis deviation. Diagnosis of normal sinus rhythm depends only on the P waves.
2. No. Each QRS complex is preceded by a P wave. However, notice that the P waves are *negative* in lead II. These retrograde P waves indicate an ectopic pacemaker, probably located in a low atrial site near the AV junction.

12

Supraventricular Arrhythmias—I

PREMATURE ATRIAL AND AV JUNCTIONAL BEATS, PAROXYSMAL SUPRAVENTRICULAR TACHYCARDIAS, AV JUNCTIONAL RHYTHMS

The intrinsic pacemaker of the heart is the sinus (SA) node, and normally it initiates each heartbeat. However, pacemaker stimuli can arise from other parts of the heart—the atria, the AV junction, or the ventricles. The terms *"ectopy," "ectopic pacemaker,"* and *"ectopic beat"* are used to describe these non-sinus beats. Ectopic beats are often premature; that is, they come before the next sinus beat is due. Thus we may find atrial premature beats (APBs), AV junctional premature beats (JPBs), and ventricular premature beats (VPBs). Ectopic beats can also come after a pause in the normal rhythm, as in the case of AV junctional or ventricular *escape* beats. Ectopic beats originating in the AV junction (node) or atria are referred to as *supraventricular* (i.e., coming from *above* the ventricles).

In this chapter and the next, ectopic atrial and AV junctional (supraventricular) rhythms are described. Chapter 14 deals with ventricular ectopy.

ATRIAL AND AV JUNCTIONAL (NODAL) PREMATURE BEATS

Atrial premature beats (APBs)* result from ectopic stimuli; that is, they arise from somewhere

in either the left or the right atrium but not in the sinus node. The atria therefore are depolarized from an ectopic site. Following an atrial or junctional depolarization, the stimulus may spread normally through the His-Purkinje system into the ventricles. For this reason, ventricular depolarization (the QRS) is generally not affected by APBs or JPBs.

APBs have the following major features (Figs. 12-1 to 12-3):

1. The atrial depolarization is premature, occurring before the next normal P wave is due.
2. The QRS complex of the APB is often preceded by a visible P wave that usually has a slightly different shape and/or different PR interval from the P wave seen with normal sinus beats. The PR interval of the APB may be either longer or shorter than the PR interval of the normal beats. In some of these cases the P wave may be "buried" in the T wave of the preceding beat.
3. Following the APB there is generally a slight pause before the normal sinus beat resumes.*
4. The QRS complex of the APB is usually identical or very similar to the QRS complex of the preceding beats. Remember that with APBs the atrial pacemaker is in an ectopic

---

*The terms *"atrial premature contractions," "atrial premature beats," "atrial premature depolarizations,"* and *"atrial extrasystoles"* are used synonymously. The designation "premature beat" or "depolarization" is preferred by most cardiologists because not every premature stimulus is associated with an actual mechanical contraction of the atria or ventricles.

---

*This pause is due to "resetting" of the SA node pacemaker by the premature atrial stimulus.

Fig. 12-1. Atrial premature beats (*arrows*). Notice, in **A,** the APB after the fourth sinus beat and, in **B,** the blocked APB also after the fourth sinus beat. The premature P wave falls on the T wave of the preceding beat and is not followed by a QRS complex because the AV node is still in a refractory state.

Fig. 12-2. Atrial bigeminy. Each sinus beat is followed by an atrial premature beat (or premature atrial complex).

Fig. 12-3. This rhythm strip shows sinus rhythm with three atrial premature beats (APBs). The first two (marked ●) are conducted with right bundle branch block aberrancy (rSR′ in V_1). The third (○) is conducted with normal ventricular activation. Notice how the first two premature P waves come so early in the cardiac cycle that they fall on the T waves of the preceding sinus beats, making these T waves slightly taller.

location but the ventricles are usually depolarized in a normal way. This contrasts with ventricular premature beats (VPBs), discussed in Chapter 14, in which the QRS complex is usually very wide because of abnormal depolarization of the ventricles.

5. Occasionally APBs will result in aberrant ventricular conduction so the QRS is wider than normal. Figure 12-3 shows an example of such beats causing delayed depolarization of the right ventricle. Thus these APBs are associated with right bundle branch block *aberrancy*.

6. Sometimes when an APB is very premature, the stimulus will reach the AV junction just after it has been stimulated by the preceding normal beat. Because the AV junction, as all other conductive tissues, requires time to recover its capacity to conduct impulses, this premature atrial stimulus may reach the junction when it is still *refractory*. In such cases the APB may not be conducted to the ventricles and no QRS complex will appear. This situation results in a *blocked* APB. The ECG will show a premature P wave *not* followed by a QRS complex (Fig. 12-1, *B*). After the blocked P wave, there is a brief pause before the next normal beat resumes. The blocked APB therefore produces a slight irregularity of the heartbeat. If you do not search carefully for these blocked APBs, you will overlook them.

Atrial premature beats may occur frequently (e.g., five or more times per minute) or sporadically. Two occurring consecutively are referred to as an *atrial couplet*. Sometimes, as shown in Figure 12-2, each sinus beat will be followed by an APB. This pattern is referred to as *atrial bigeminy*.

Clinical Significance

Atrial premature beats are very common. They may occur both in persons with a normal heart and in persons with virtually any type of organic heart disease. Finding APBs does not imply that an individual has cardiac disease. In normal subjects they may be seen with emotional stress, hyperthyroidism, excessive intake of caffeine, or the administration of sympathomimetic agents (epinephrine, isoproterenol, theophylline). APBs may produce palpitations—the patient may complain of feeling a skipped beat or an irregular pulse. APBs may also be seen with various types of structural heart disease. Frequent APBs are sometimes the forerunner of atrial fibrillation (Chapter 13) or other atrial tachyarrhythmias.

PAROXYSMAL SUPRAVENTRICULAR TACHYCARDIAS (PSVTs)

Premature supraventricular beats may occur singly or repetitively. A sudden run of three or more constitutes a paroxysmal supraventricular tachycardia (PSVT). Episodes of PSVT may be brief and nonsustained (e.g., lasting from three beats up to 30 seconds). Sustained episodes (greater than 30 seconds) may last for minutes, hours, or longer. The topic of PSVTs is actually quite involved. Therefore the following brief discussion is intended to give an introduction and overview. Students and clinicians wishing to pursue this important area of cardiology in more detail should refer to the Bibliography.

There are three major types of PSVT: (1) paroxysmal atrial tachycardia (PAT and related rhythms), (2) AV nodal reentrant tachycardia (AVNRT), and (3) tachycardias involving a bypass tract of the type seen in the Wolff-Parkinson-White syndrome (discussed in Chapter 10). We will briefly consider these three types of arrhythmias, which are depicted schematically in Figure 12-4.

Paroxysmal atrial tachycardia (PAT). This rhythm is defined simply as three or more consecutive APBs (Fig. 12-5). Most episodes appear to be due to an ectopic (non-sinus) pacemaker located in either the left or the right atrium that fires off "automatically" in a rapid way. A sustained episode lasting 30 seconds or longer, particularly at a rapid rate, may cause light-headedness or even syncope (fainting) and in susceptible individuals can induce angina or congestive heart failure. The atrial rate with PAT may be as high as 200 or so beats per minute (range 100 to 250). PAT has been observed in patients without apparent structural cardiac abnormality as well as in those with virtu-

Fig. 12-4. Major types of paroxysmal supraventricular tachycardia (PSVT). **A,** The reference rhythm is normal sinus. **B,** With atrial tachycardia, a focus *(X)* outside the sinus node fires off automatically at a rapid rate. **C,** With AV nodal reentrant tachycardia (AVNRT) the cardiac stimulus originates as a wave of excitation that spins around the AV nodal (junctional) area. As a result retrograde P waves may be buried in the QRS or appear immediately before or just after the QRS *(arrows)* due to nearly simultaneous activation of the atria and ventricles. **D,** A similar type of reentrant (circus movement) mechanism may occur with a bypass tract of the type found in Wolff-Parkinson-White syndrome (Fig. 10-21). Note the retrograde P wave *(arrow)* in lead II, somewhat after the QRS. (See Josephson and Wellens [1990] for further details.)

Fig. 12-5. Paroxysmal atrial tachycardia (a type of PSVT) terminating spontaneously with the abrupt resumption of sinus rhythm. The P waves of the tachycardia (rate, about 150/min) are superimposed on the preceding T waves.

PAROXYSMAL SUPRAVENTRICULAR TACHYCARDIA (PSVT)

Fig. 12-6. Notice the marked regularity of rhythm in this PSVT, with a rate of about 170 beats/min. It is probably due to a rapidly circulating impulse in the AV node (junction) and thus is referred to as an AV nodal reentrant tachycardia (AVNRT). No P waves are visible.

Fig. 12-7. Paroxysmal supraventricular tachycardia (PSVT) treated with carotid sinus massage. The first 14 beats in this rhythm strip show the tachyarrhythmia with a rate of about 140 beats/min and no visible P waves. Carotid sinus massage resulted in its abrupt termination, with the appearance of normal sinus rhythm. (The PSVT here is probably an AVNRT; see Figure 12-6.)

ally any type of heart disease.* Short episodes may require no special therapy, but longer runs causing symptoms are usually treated initially with antiarrhythmic drugs.

AV nodal reentrant tachycardia (AVNRT). This rhythm, which was formerly considered a variant of PAT, is actually a distinct arrhythmia due to a rapidly circulating impulse in the AV node area. The term reentry (introduced in Chapter 10) describes situations in which a cardiac impulse literally spins around and around and appears to "chase its own tail." These rhythms are therefore sometimes referred to as "circus-movement" tachycardias. Reentry can occur in virtually any part of the heart. (For example, in the ventricles it will lead to premature ventricular beats and sometimes to ventricular tachycardia.)

AVNRT produces a very rapid and regular supraventricular rhythm with rates typically between 140 and 250 beats per minute (Fig. 12-6). It may occur in subjects with otherwise normal hearts or in persons with underlying heart disease. Runs of AVNRT are generally initiated by an atrial premature beat.

With AVNRT, as indicated by the name, the reentrant rhythm originates in the AV nodal area and spreads simultaneously or nearly simultaneously up the atria and down the ventricles. (See Figure 12-4.) As a consequence the P waves are usually hidden in the QRS complex since the atria and ventricles are activated simultaneously. In other cases the P waves may appear just before or just after the QRS and be difficult to see. They will be negative in lead II because of this retrograde (bottom-to-top) activation of the atria. Episodes of AVNRT may cease spontaneously or may require treatment. The initial therapy usually involves attempts to increase vagal tone, since the vagus nerve slows conduction in the AV node. This "braking effect" may interrupt the reentrant mechanism (Fig. 12-7). Increasing vagal tone can be accomplished with the Valsalva maneuver (instruct the patient to strain against a closed glottis by bearing down as for a bowel movement) or with carotid sinus massage.

A variety of drugs are used to interrupt the reentrant mechanism in AVNRT. Clinically the two most often enlisted in the acute setting are adenosine and verapamil. Digoxin and beta blockers also are useful in selected cases. Other drugs may be used and are discussed in references in the Bibliography.

Younger patients and individuals without significant underlying cardiovascular disease may tolerate heart rates up to 250 beats/min with complaints only of palpitations or light-headedness. However, in patients with limited cardiac reserve a heart rate above 160 beats/min (or even less) can have disastrous consequences. In these persons myocardial ischemia or even infarction may occur. The patient may also develop congestive heart failure or hypotension. In such emergency circumstances—when any PSVT is associated with angina, congestive heart failure, or severe hypotension and when initial therapy with vagal maneuvers and rapid-acting drugs fails—electrical cardioversion may be required.

Electrical cardioversion is the use of a direct current shock to treat certain tachyarrhythmias.* The shock is administered with special paddles placed on the chest wall. In treating some arrhythmias (e.g., ventricular flutter or ventricular fibrillation) an *unsynchronized* DC shock is given. In treating PSVT and other supraventricular arrhythmias (e.g., atrial fibrillation and atrial flutter) it is essential to give a *synchronized* DC shock. The shock is synchronized with the QRS so it does not occur during the *vulnerable period* of ventricular repolarization (simultaneous with the apex of the T wave). NOTE: DC shocks given to the heart during the vulnerable period may produce ventricular fibrillation. *Therefore, in treating PSVT, a **synchronized** DC shock must be given.* See the Bibliography for details.

For patients with recurrent episodes of AVNRT,

---

*See Chapter 16 for a brief discussion of PAT *with block* resulting from digitalis toxicity and Chapter 18 for a discussion of *multifocal atrial tachycardia* (MAT).

*The electrical shock depolarizes the heart, interrupting abnormal rhythms and allowing the sinus node to regain control of the cardiac electrical cycle.

a special form of therapy called *radiofrequency* (RF) *catheter ablation* may be curative. This mode of therapy, which is becoming increasingly widespread, involves delivering short pulses of RF current through an intracardiac catheter placed near the AV node during an electrophysiologic procedure. It produces a very small burn that effectively blocks the part of the circuit supporting the reentrant-type wave. Readers wishing more details about catheter ablation therapy for AVNRT as well as for other arrhythmias should consult the Bibliography.

PSVT due to a "concealed" bypass tract. A third common cause of PSVT has already been introduced in the discussion of preexcitation syndromes (p. 156). As you recall, the Wolff-Parkinson-White syndrome is related to the presence of a so-called bypass tract that connects the atria and ventricles, circumventing the AV node. Patients with this type of atrioventricular bypass tract may develop a tachycardia due to a reentrant mechanism in which the impulse travels down the normal conduction system (AV node and His bundle) into the ventricles, recycles rapidly up into the atria via the bypass tract, and then goes down the AV node again. Repetition of this large reentrant circuit leads to a type of PSVT.

Of interest is the fact that in some patients the bypass tract is concealed—that is, it never becomes evident during sinus rhythm but appears only when a tachycardia starts.* The ECG with a concealed bypass tract type of PSVT is very similar to that just described with AVNRT. One subtle difference is that many patients with tachycardia associated with a concealed bypass tract have distinctly seen retrograde P waves that are located between consecutive QRS complexes (Fig. 12-5).

The therapy of PSVT due to a concealed bypass tract is quite similar to that of AVNRT, with drugs (e.g., adenosine) for acute episodes and evaluation by electrophysiologic testing for the possibility of radiofrequency catheter ablation of the bypass tract. Indeed, the most successful applications of radiofrequency ablation technology to date have been in the therapy of tachycardias associated with bypass tracts.

Summary. You should suspect a PSVT particularly when you see a rhythm strip showing a rapid and typically very regular rate at around 200 beats per minute (range 100 to 250). The mechanism may be due to reentry in the AV node (AVNRT) or may involve a concealed bypass tract (a variant of the Wolff-Parkinson-White syndrome), or it may be due to a rapid automatically firing ectopic focus located in either atrium (PAT). The differential diagnosis of PSVT and other supraventricular tachycardias is discussed further in Chapter 18.

AV JUNCTIONAL RHYTHMS

With atrial premature beats the ectopic pacemaker is located somewhere in the atria outside the SA node. Under certain circumstances the AV junction may also function as an ectopic pacemaker, producing an AV junctional rhythm. In some discussions the term "AV nodal" or "nodal" is used to refer to an AV junctional rhythm. The terms *"AV junctional," "junctional," "AV nodal,"* and *"nodal"* are all essentially synonymous.

In Chapter 4 the basic mechanism of AV junctional rhythms and the pattern seen with AV junctional escape beats were described. When the AV junction is the cardiac pacemaker, the atria are stimulated in a *retrograde* fashion, from bottom to top. An arrow representing the spread of atrial depolarization with junctional rhythm will point upward, just opposite the direction of atrial depolarization when normal sinus rhythm is present (Fig. 4-3). This retrograde stimulation of the atria will produce a positive P wave in lead aV_R and a negative P wave in lead II (Fig. 4-5). With AV junc-

---

*To be evident during sinus rhythm, the bypass tract must conduct impulses rapidly from atria to ventricles, bypassing the AV node. This produces a short PR, a wide QRS, and a delta wave, the classic triad of WPW (Fig. 10-20). In some patients with a bypass tract, the pathway does not conduct antegrade very effectively, but can still conduct retrograde under certain conditions, thereby allowing an impulse to reenter the atria from the ventricles. Bypass tracts that conduct only in a retrograde direction causing PSVT are said to be "concealed."

tional rhythm the ventricles will be depolarized normally (unless a bundle branch block is present), resulting in a narrow QRS complex.

In some cases of AV junctional rhythm the atria will be stimulated just before the ventricles. In other cases the stimulus may reach the ventricles first. Finally, in many cases the atria and the ventricles will be stimulated simultaneously. If the atria are stimulated first, the P wave will precede the QRS complex. (A retrograde P wave preceding the QRS also occurs with some ectopic atrial beats from the lower part of either atrium. However, the distinction between such "low" ectopic atrial and AV junctional beats is usually not of clinical importance.) If the ventricles are first to be stimulated, the QRS will precede the P wave. If atrial and ventricular depolarizations are simultaneous, the P wave will be "buried" in the QRS and not be seen.

To summarize: AV junctional beats can be recognized on the ECG by one of the following three patterns (Fig. 12-8):

1. Retrograde P waves (positive in lead aV$_R$, negative in lead II) immediately preceding the QRS complexes
2. Retrograde P waves immediately following the QRS complexes
3. Absent P waves (buried in the QRS), so the baseline between QRS complexes is flat

AV Junctional Escape Rhythms

AV junctional escape beats were mentioned in the section on sinus arrest (p. 153). An AV junctional escape beat (Fig. 12-9) is simply a beat that comes after a pause when the normal sinus pacemaker fails to function. The AV junctional escape beat therefore is a "safety beat." Following this escape beat, the normal sinus pacemaker may resume function. However, if it does not, a slow AV junctional escape rhythm may continue. An AV junctional escape rhythm is a consecutive run of AV junctional beats. The heart rate is usually slow, between 30 and 50 beats/min.

Figure 12-10 shows an example of an AV junctional escape rhythm. It is not surprising that the basic rate of the AV junction is slower than that

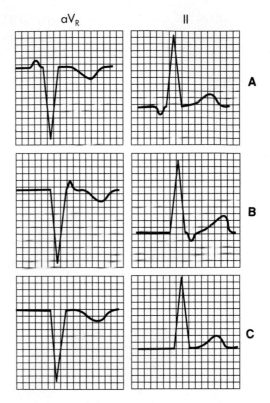

Fig. 12-8. AV junctional (nodal) beats produce P waves that point upward in lead aV$_R$ and downward in II— just the opposite of what is seen with sinus rhythm. The P wave may just precede the QRS complex, **A,** follow it, **B,** or occur simultaneously with it, **C.** In the last instance no P wave will be visible.

of the SA node. If the AV junction had a faster inherent rate, it would compete with the SA node for control of the heartbeat.

AV junctional escape rhythms can be seen in a number of clinical settings—digitalis toxicity (Chapter 16), toxic reactions to beta blockers or calcium-channel blockers (diltiazem, verapamil), acute myocardial infarction, hypoxemia, hyperkalemia. Treatment depends on the cause (for example, stopping the digitalis or oxygenating the patient). If the heart rate becomes excessively slow with an AV junctional rhythm, then drugs such as

Fig. 12-9. The junctional escape beat *(JEB)* comes after a pause and is followed by a junctional premature beat *(JPB)*. Notice the retrograde (inverted) P wave preceding the JPB in this lead II rhythm strip.

JUNCTIONAL ESCAPE RHYTHM

Fig. 12-10. This strip shows a slow junctional escape rhythm at about 40 beats/min with no visible P waves and a flat baseline between QRS complexes.

atropine (a vagal blocker) or isoproterenol (a sympathomimetic stimulant) may be used acutely to increase the heart rate.

As is true of AV junctional escape rhythms, the AV junctional tachycardias can arise in a number of settings. Probably the most common has already been discussed, AV nodal reentrant tachycardia (AVNRT, Fig. 12-4), which is due to a rapidly recirculating impulse in the nodal part of the AV junction. AV junctional tachycardias can also be due to abnormally enhanced automaticity. Interested readers should consult the Bibliography.

REVIEW

Stimuli that pace the heart can arise not only in the sinus (SA) node but in other cardiac tissues as well—the atria, AV junction, or ventricles.

The terms *"ectopy," "ectopic pacemaker,"* and *"ectopic contraction* or *beat"* are used to describe these stimuli. There are two major categories of ectopic beats:

1. *Premature* (extra beats that come before the next normal beat is expected; examples include APBs, JPBs, and VPBs, originating in the atria, AV junction, and ventricles, respectively)
2. *Escape* (usually AV junctional or ventricular beats that are *not* premature but come after a pause in the normal rhythm)

APBs show the following:

1. Usually there is a different-shaped P wave with a slightly longer or shorter PR interval than in the preceding complexes. Sometimes the P wave will be hidden in the T wave of the preceding normal beat.
2. Occasionally the atrial stimulus cannot penetrate the AV junction. In such cases of *blocked* APBs the premature P wave will *not* be followed by a QRS complex.

PSVTs are a sudden run of three or more supraventricular beats. There are three common types:

1. AV nodal reentrant tachycardia (AVNRT)
2. Reentrant tachycardia involving a bypass tract
3. Paroxysmal atrial tachycardia (PAT)

These rhythms are schematized in Figure 12-4.

AV junctional rhythms show the following features:

1. The P wave, when seen, is negative in lead II and positive in aV$_R$, just the reverse of the pattern seen with normal sinus rhythm. These are called *retrograde* P waves.
2. The retrograde P wave may immediately precede or follow the QRS complex.
3. In many cases the retrograde P wave will be buried within the QRS complex. When this occurs, the baseline between QRS complexes remains completely flat.

AV junctional rhythms are categorized as junctional escape rhythms and junctional tachycardias. An AV junctional escape rhythm is a run of AV junctional beats with a slow rate, generally between 30 and 50 beats/min. AV junctional tachycardia, by contrast, is a more rapid run of three or more consecutive beats originating in the AV junction. A common type is AV nodal reentrant tachycardia. Other types are due to increased automaticity of AV junctional pacemaker cells.

Questions

1. Why might the patient whose rhythm strip is shown below complain of occasional palpitations?

V$_1$

2. What is the beat marked X?

3. a. What is the approximate heart rate?
   b. What class of arrhythmia is present?
      (1) Sinus tachycardia
      (2) Paroxysmal supraventricular tachycardia (PSVT)
      (3) Atrial flutter
      (4) Atrial fibrillation
      (5) Multifocal atrial tachycardia (MAT)

Answers

1. The palpitations could be due to occasional APBs. Notice that the fifth complex here is an APB (or possibly a JPB, since the P wave is not seen).

2. Junctional escape beat. Notice that it comes after a pause in the normal rhythm and is not preceded by a P wave.

3. a. Approximately 210 beats/min. (Count the number of QRS complexes in 6 seconds and multiply by 10.)
   b. (2) PSVT. There may be a retrograde P wave just after the QRS, making AV nodal reentrant tachycardia the most likely mechanism for the PSVT. However, a concealed bypass tract cannot be excluded here.

13

Supraventricular Arrhythmias—II

ATRIAL FLUTTER AND ATRIAL FIBRILLATION

Atrial flutter and atrial fibrillation (Fig. 13-1) are two distinct but related tachyarrhythmias. Like paroxysmal supraventricular tachycardia (PSVT), they are *ectopic*. In other words, with all three types the atria are being stimulated *not* from the SA node but from an ectopic site or sites. With PSVT the atria are stimulated at a rate generally between 140 and 250 beats/min. With atrial flutter the atrial rate is even faster, generally between 250 and 350 beats/min. Finally, with atrial fibrillation the atrial depolarization rate is typically between 400 and 600 beats/min.*

With both atrial flutter and atrial fibrillation there are no discrete P waves on the ECG. Instead we see characteristic flutter (F) waves and fibrillation (f) waves representing continuous atrial electrical activity. Notice the pronounced *sawtooth* shape of the F waves and the rapid "tremulous" f waves in Figure 13-1.

ATRIAL FLUTTER

With atrial flutter the stimulation rate is about 300 per minute (Fig. 13-2). What happens to the ventricles during this rapid bombardment of the atria? The answer is that with atrial flutter (and atrial fibrillation) the ventricular (QRS) rate varies depending on the ability of the AV junction to transmit stimuli from the atria to the ventricles. If the ventricles respond to each flutter wave, then the ventricular rate will be around 300 beats per minute. Most commonly the ventricular rate with atrial flutter is about 150, 100, or 75 beats per minute. Atrial flutter with a ventricular response of 150 beats/min is called 2:1 flutter because the ratio of the atrial rate (300) to the ventricular rate (150) is 2 to 1. Atrial flutter with a ventricular rate of 100 beats/min is 3:1, and with 75 beats/min usually 4:1. As mentioned, atrial flutter with a ventricular rate equal to the atrial rate, 300 beats/min, or 1:1 flutter, is very rare. Characteristically patients with atrial flutter will increase or decrease their ventricular rate by stepwise fractions of the atrial rate (Fig. 13-1). Thus a patient may change abruptly from atrial flutter with a ventricular response of 75 to 100 beats/min, to 150 beats/min, or rarely even to 300 beats/min. In some patients the ventricular response with atrial flutter will be more variable.*

Clinical Significance

Atrial flutter is rarely seen in people with normal hearts. This is in contrast to atrial fibrillation (described later), which may occur transiently in

---

*The electrophysiologic mechanisms for the rapid-traveling waves that underlie atrial flutter and fibrillation are the subject of ongoing investigations. (See the Bibliography.)

*The QRS pattern of "group beating" (p. 193) is not uncommon with atrial flutter and represents a Wenckebach-type variant associated with bombardment of the AV node by frequent atrial depolarization waves (e.g., at 300/min).

Fig. 13-1. Atrial flutter and fibrillation. Notice the sawtooth waves with atrial flutter *(F)* and the irregular fibrillatory waves with atrial fibrillation *(f)*.

ATRIAL FLUTTER

Fig. 13-2. A, Notice the variable appearance of flutter waves in different leads. In I the waves are barely apparent while in II and III the classic "sawtooth" waves appear. The ventricular rate is about 160 beats/min, and the flutter rate is about 320 beats/min; thus 2:1 conduction is present. **B,** Carotid sinus massage produces marked slowing of the ventricular rate by increasing vagal tone.

normal individuals. Atrial flutter is not specific for any particular type of heart disease but occurs, for example, in patients with valvular heart disease, acute myocardial infarction, chronic ischemic heart disease, cardiomyopathy, hypertensive heart disease, lung disease, and pulmonary emboli as well as after cardiac surgery.

Treatment Considerations

Treatment of atrial flutter depends on the clinical condition. In some patients atrial flutter will revert spontaneously to normal sinus rhythm. In others who are hypoxic, treatment with oxygen may help restore normal sinus rhythm.

Patients in atrial flutter with a rapid ventricular response are usually treated initially with one or a combination of drugs (digitalis, beta blockers, calcium-channel blockers) to slow impulse conduction through the AV node. Occasionally they will convert to sinus rhythm spontaneously in the course of this initial therapy. In other cases a second drug (e.g., quinidine or procainamide) is added to help convert the flutter to normal sinus rhythm.

In many patients atrial flutter will persist despite pharmacologic therapy. Fortunately, it is one of the arrhythmias most easily treated with electrical cardioversion. As described in Chapter 12, a synchronized DC shock is given with the patient properly anesthetized.

Another way of attempting to convert atrial flutter is with very rapid pacing of the atria by means of a temporary pacing wire (known as *overdrive*

pacing). The details of this therapy, however, lie outside the scope of this book.*

To summarize: Atrial flutter is a tachyarrhythmia in which the atria are stimulated (depolarized) usually at a rate of 250 to 350 beats/min, with a ventricular response that is often some fraction of the atrial rate (½, ¼, etc.). Atrial flutter may be treated with special drugs, synchronized DC shock, or rapid atrial pacing.

ATRIAL FIBRILLATION

With atrial fibrillation, one of the most commonly seen arrhythmias, the atria are stimulated (depolarized) at a very rapid rate, up to 600 times/min. This fibrillatory activity produces a characteristically irregular wavy pattern in place of the normal P waves. The irregular waves, seen in Figure 13-3, are called *fibrillatory* or *f waves*. In some cases the f waves are relatively coarse (Fig. 13-4). In others a fine fibrillation is seen (Fig. 13-5). Atrial fibrillation therefore is characterized by rapid oscillatory depolarization of the atria, producing irregular undulations of the ECG baseline without discrete P waves.

Because of the rapid atrial depolarization rate, the AV junction in patients with atrial fibrillation is being bombarded by innumerable stimuli from the atria. If every stimulus (each f wave) penetrated the AV junction, the ventricles would beat

---

*Catheter ablation techniques (p. 162) have also been used with success in selected cases.

Fig. 13-3. Rapid undulation of the baseline due to fibrillatory (f) waves. There are no true P waves, and the ventricular rate is irregular.

Fig. 13-4. Coarse atrial fibrillatory waves with a rapid ventricular response. This patient has hyperthyroidism. (The commonly used term "rapid atrial fibrillation" is actually a misnomer since "rapid" is intended to refer to the ventricular rate rather than the atrial rate. The same is true for "slow atrial fibrillation.")

ATRIAL FIBRILLATION

Fig. 13-5. Fibrillatory waves may be hard to find. In this tachyarrhythmia no atrial waves are evident. The ventricular rate is about 140 beats/min and irregular. Although no clear fibrillatory waves are visible here, the rhythm is nevertheless atrial fibrillation.

ATRIAL FIBRILLATION

Fig. 13-6. Another example of atrial fibrillation. Here the relatively subtle fibrillation waves give the baseline between irregularly spaced R waves a wrinkly appearance.

at a rate of up to 600 times/min, with obvious consequences to the patient. Fortunately, the AV junction is refractory to most of these impulses and allows only a fraction to reach the ventricles. In patients with a normal AV junction in whom atrial fibrillation suddenly develops, the ventricular rate is generally between 110 and 180 beats/min.* Figure 13-5 shows an example of atrial fibrillation with a ventricular rate of about 140 beats/min. Characteristically, the ventricular rate with atrial fibrillation is haphazardly irregular because the AV junction is being stimulated in an apparently random fashion by the rapidly fibrillating atria.

To summarize: There are two ECG characteristics of atrial fibrillation. First, you will see the irregular wavy baseline produced by the rapid f waves. Second, the ventricular (QRS) rate is usually quite irregular. When the ventricular rate is very fast (Fig. 13-6), it may be difficult to distinguish the f waves. However, in such cases the diagnosis of atrial fibrillation can usually be made by finding a very irregular ventricular rate in the absence of distinct P waves.

General Clinical Aspects

In some patients atrial fibrillation occurs *paroxysmally* and may last for only minutes, hours, or days. Some individuals may experience only one or occasional episodes; others will have multiple recurrences. In other patients it is *chronic* and may persist indefinitely.

Atrial fibrillation can occur both in normal persons and in patients with a variety of cardiac diseases. Paroxysmal atrial fibrillation may be associated with emotional stress or excessive alcohol consumption in otherwise healthy people. In such cases it often spontaneously reverts to normal sinus rhythm or is converted easily with pharmacologic therapy alone.

Atrial fibrillation is also one of the most frequently observed arrhythmias in patients with or-

ganic heart disease. Common pathologic substrates include coronary artery disease, hypertensive heart disease, and valvular heart disease. Patients with coronary artery disease may go into atrial fibrillation for the first time during an acute myocardial infarction or as a consequence of chronic ischemic myocardial disease, presumably due to atrial dilation or fibrosis. Atrial fibrillation is also commonly caused by valvular heart disease, particularly when there is mitral valve involvement. For example, severe mitral stenosis or mitral regurgitation will produce atrial enlargement, predisposing to atrial arrhythmias.

Atrial fibrillation also occurs in other conditions. For example, patients with thyrotoxicosis (hyperthyroidism) may go into atrial fibrillation (Fig. 13-5). Atrial fibrillation (or flutter) is not uncommon following cardiac surgery. It may also occur with pericardial disease, myocarditis, pulmonary emboli, cardiomyopathies, and other forms of heart disease.

Clinical Consequences

What happens physiologically when atrial fibrillation develops? Normally, after the P wave, the atria contract and pump blood into the ventricles. With atrial fibrillation, normal atrial depolarization is lost and the atria fibrillate (quiver) instead of contracting synchronously. In these circumstances the normal atrial "kick" is lost, and the result is decreased cardiac output (since ventricular filling is decreased) and sometimes thromboembolization.

Decreased cardiac output. Hemodynamically the most significant effect of atrial fibrillation is decreased cardiac output, which will be especially marked in patients with underlying cardiac impairment and in elderly people, who appear to be more dependent on atrial contraction for filling of the ventricles. In addition, the amount of this decreased output will depend on the ventricular rate with atrial fibrillation. The faster the rate, the more decreased the cardiac output will be. Thus the patient in atrial fibrillation at a rate of 180 beats/min is more likely to be hypotensive or in congestive heart failure than would be the case with a rate of

---

*Always consider factors such as hypoxemia, severe anemia, fever, congestive heart failure, and hyperthyroidism, which can contribute to the rapid ventricular response and which, until corrected, may make rate control much more difficult.

100 beats/min. In patients with coronary artery disease this rapid ventricular rate can cause myocardial ischemia and even infarction (Chapter 8).

To summarize: Decreased cardiac output with atrial fibrillation reflects two major factors: (1) the loss of normal atrial contractility (atrial kick) and (2) the rapid ventricular rate. The drop in cardiac output with atrial fibrillation (as with any tachyarrhythmia) can produce one (or more) of the following three clinical problems: congestive heart failure, hypotension (rarely even shock), and myocardial ischemia. Initial clinical assessment of the patient in atrial fibrillation must focus on these three areas. Is the patient showing signs of severe congestive failure (difficulty breathing, rales in the chest)? Is the patient's blood pressure low? Is there evidence of myocardial ischemia with anginal chest pain and/or ECG signs of acute ischemia or actual infarction (ST segment depressions or elevations)? *Patients in atrial fibrillation associated with pulmonary edema, hypotension, or acute myocardial ischemia require emergency therapy.*

Atrial thrombi and embolization. The second problem, resulting from the stagnation of blood, is a tendency in some patients for atrial thrombi to develop and dislodge into the arterial circulation, causing peripheral embolism. The thrombi can produce a cerebrovascular accident, occlusion of the blood supply to the legs, and other complications.

The risk of thrombus formation and embolization is highest in patients with chronic atrial fibrillation due to rheumatic mitral valve disease. However, it also occurs in patients with atrial fibrillation due to other causes (so-called "nonrheumatic atrial fibrillation").

Treatment

We will not discuss the details of treating atrial fibrillation but instead will focus more broadly on the general clinical approach to patients with this arrhythmia. There are two principal ways of converting atrial fibrillation to sinus rhythm. The first is *pharmacologically*. The second is with *electrical cardioversion*, the same as that described for PSVT and atrial flutter.

Drug therapy, if successful, generally takes hours or days to convert atrial fibrillation to sinus rhythm. Electrical cardioversion has an immediate effect. However, patients in chronic atrial fibrillation (present for months or years) may not convert to normal sinus rhythm with any therapy. This is particularly true in cases of chronic heart disease with extremely dilated atria that are not capable of normal depolarization. Furthermore, the patient with a very large left atrium or with long-standing atrial fibrillation will often revert to atrial fibrillation eventually, even if electrical or pharmacologic cardioversion was initially successful.

There are at least four major clinical questions to ask in approaching patients with atrial fibrillation. First, is the arrhythmia causing a life-threatening decrease in cardiac function, as indicated by myocardial ischemia, hypotension, or congestive heart failure? As a general rule, patients in acute atrial fibrillation that is producing myocardial ischemia, shock, or pulmonary edema should be considered candidates for electrical cardioversion if they do not respond promptly to drug therapy. Second, is the atrial fibrillation acute or chronic? Third, does the patient require short- or long-term anticoagulation? Fourth, what is the cause of the arrhythmia?

In most cases acute paroxysmal atrial fibrillation does not require immediate electrical cardioversion. Drug therapy alone can be used initially to control the ventricular rate. Digitalis, beta blockers and calcium-channel blockers (verapamil, diltiazem) all act by slowing conduction of stimuli through the AV node.* In atrial fibrillation, as noted, the AV node is being bombarded by stimuli from the atria, which are fibrillating 400 to 600 times/min. A prime initial clinical concern in patients with atrial fibrillation is to slow the ventricular rate. In patients with atrial fibrillation and a rapid ventricular rate, digitalis given intravenously

---

*Digitalis acts primarily by increasing vagal tone. Beta blockers decrease sympathetic tone. Calcium-channel blockers directly interfere with conduction by impairing the cellular entry of calcium ions, which play a major role in electrical impulse transmission in the AV node.

(or even orally) can generally slow the ventricular rate below 100 beats/min in a matter of hours. Beta blockers and calcium-channel blockers may act more rapidly. Some patients with paroxysmal atrial fibrillation may actually convert to normal sinus rhythm spontaneously or after being given these drugs. In other cases it is necessary to add another type drug (e.g., quinidine, procainamide, propafenone, or amiodarone) to try to restore normal atrial depolarization.

The usual sequence in treating atrial fibrillation pharmacologically is to slow the ventricular response with the drugs described above. If sinus rhythm is not restored after rate slowing, then the addition of quinidine or a related drug* is often considered. Quinidine alone may sometimes increase conduction through the AV node (because of its vagolytic effect). Therefore it should never be given to a patient in atrial fibrillation unless the ventricular rate has first been slowed (usually to less than 100 beats/min). Elective DC cardioversion is generally reserved for patients who fail to respond to an initial trial of drug therapy.

Attempts to convert atrial fibrillation to sinus rhythm with either pharmacologic therapy or DC cardioversion should not be made unless the patient has been sufficiently anticoagulated or atrial thrombus formation has been convincingly excluded (e.g., by transesophageal echocardiography). The reason for this caveat is that restoration of normal atrial contractility during sinus rhythm may cause dislodgment of an atrial thrombus formed during the fibrillation. Thrombus formation becomes more likely the longer the duration of the fibrillation, but it may also occur with fibrillation of relatively short duration. Patients in

chronic or paroxysmal atrial fibrillation that cannot be converted to sinus rhythm are candidates for long-term anticoagulation with warfarin or aspirin. Current guidelines for specific anticoagulation regimens before and after attempted cardioversion in paroxysmal or chronic atrial fibrillation are given in the Bibliography.

Some patients in chronic atrial fibrillation who cannot be converted to sinus rhythm have an uncontrollably fast ventricular response despite intensive drug therapy. A relatively new approach to this problem is ablation of the AV node by radiofrequency current delivered by a special cardiac catheter (p. 162). Since this therapy often results in complete heart block, a permanent pacemaker must also be implanted.

At the same time that you are starting to treat any patient in atrial fibrillation, you should be thinking of possible causes of this arrhythmia. Search for evidence of coronary artery disease, alcohol excess, hypertensive heart disease, cardiomyopathy, valvular disease, or pericardial disease. A blood test for thyroid function should be obtained in any patient with unexplained atrial fibrillation, since thyrotoxicosis is a treatable cause of this arrhythmia. Remember: Some patients, including young adults, may go into paroxysmal atrial fibrillation without underlying heart disease. The term *"lone atrial fibrillation"* is sometimes used to describe the condition in which chronic atrial fibrillation develops in a patient without identifiable structural heart disease.

Patients with underlying AV nodal disease may develop atrial fibrillation with a slow ventricular response in the absence of drug therapy. If the ventricular rate becomes exceedingly slow, a permanent pacemaker may be required.

Atrial Fibrillation and Other Arrhythmias

Atrial fibrillation (or atrial flutter) may occur with other arrhythmias and conduction disturbances, just as you can have sinus rhythm with ventricular premature beats (VPBs), AV heart block, and so on. Figure 13-7 shows an example of atrial fibrillation with VPBs. Atrial fibrillation or flutter can also occur with complete heart block

---

*Procainamide and disopyramide have electrophysiologic actions similar to those of quinidine. The role of newer antiarrhythmic agents (e.g., amiodarone, sotalol, flecainide, and propafenone) is currently being evaluated in the therapy of atrial fibrillation. A number of cardiac surgical procedures designed to restore normal conduction are also under investigation for patients with refractory atrial fibrillation associated with incapacitating symptoms or hemodynamic instability despite medical therapy. (See the Bibliography for articles discussing these complicated therapeutic issues.)

Fig. 13-7. Atrial fibrillation with ventricular premature beats (VPBs).

Fig. 13-8. Atrial fibrillation with complete AV block. The ventricular rate is very slow and regular because of the block. (Notice the right bundle branch block morphology of the QRS complexes.)

(Fig. 13-8), and in such cases there is a very slow and regular ventricular response. In any patient with atrial fibrillation and a very slow ventricular rate, always think of possible digitalis toxicity (Chapter 16).

Atrial fibrillation with the Wolff-Parkinson-White syndrome is discussed on page 225.

Occasionally, it will be difficult to decide whether atrial fibrillation or atrial flutter is present (p. 236). The coarse atrial fibrillatory waves may resemble flutter waves (Fig. 19-3). In some of these cases the arrhythmia is referred to as flutter-fibrillation and has the same clinical significance and treatment as atrial fibrillation.

REVIEW

Atrial flutter shows the following:

1. Characteristic sawtooth flutter waves instead of discrete P waves
2. A constant or variable ventricular rate (e.g., one QRS complex with every fourth flutter wave, 4:1 flutter; one QRS with every two flutter waves, 2:1 flutter, and the ventricular rate half the atrial rate; or the rare 1:1 flutter, in which the ventricles contract about 300 times a minute)

Atrial flutter rarely occurs in normal hearts but is most often seen in patients with valvular heart disease, ischemic heart disease, lung disease, cardiomyopathy, or pulmonary emboli, and after cardiac surgery. It may be treated with a synchronized DC shock (cardioversion), with drug therapy, or with rapid atrial pacing.

Atrial fibrillation shows the following:
1. Rapid irregular undulations of the baseline (fibrillatory waves) instead of P waves
2. A ventricular rate that is usually grossly irregular

In some cases atrial fibrillation occurs chronically. In others it is paroxysmal. Occasionally it is seen in healthy people. Common causes are coronary artery disease, hypertensive heart disease, and mitral valve disease. It may also occur with hyperthyroidism, cardiomyopathy, excess alcohol, cardiac surgery, pulmonary emboli, and chronic pericarditis. It may be seen with other arrhythmias (e.g., ventricular ectopy or complete heart block). With an extremely slow ventricular rate (50 beats/min or less) it may signify digitalis toxicity.

Sustained atrial fibrillation sometimes can be converted to normal sinus rhythm with DC cardioversion or by means of drugs.

Questions

1. Answer the following questions about the rhythm strip below:
   a. What is the atrial rate?   b. What is the ventricular rate?
   c. What is this arrhythmia?

2. Answer the following questions about this rhythm strip:
   a. What is the *average* heart rate?
   b. What is the rhythm?

3. The atrial rate with atrial flutter is *(faster, slower)* than the atrial rate with atrial fibrillation.

4. The atrial rate with atrial flutter is *(faster, slower)* than that with atrial tachycardia.

5. The ventricular rate with atrial fibrillation is always greater than 100 beats/min (true or false).

Answers

1. a. About 300 beats/min.
   b. About 75 beats/min.
   c. Atrial flutter with 4:1 AV conduction.
2. a. About 70 beats/min. (Count the number of RR cycles in 6 seconds and multiply by 10.)
   b. Atrial fibrillation. (This is a subtle example, because the fibrillatory waves are of very low amplitude. The diagnosis of atrial fibrillation is suspected when an irregular ventricular response is found along with fine wavering of the baseline between QRS complexes.)
3. Slower.
4. Faster.
5. False.

14

Ventricular Arrhythmias

The three preceding chapters have focused on *supra*ventricular arrhythmias—rhythm disturbances arising in the sinus node, atrial, or AV junctional (node) areas with normal ventricular depolarization. Now we will consider another major ECG topic, the ventricular arrhythmias. Ectopic (non-sinus) beats frequently arise in the ventricles themselves, producing *premature ventricular complexes, ventricular tachycardia,* and sometimes *ventricular fibrillation*.

VENTRICULAR PREMATURE BEATS

Ventricular premature beats (VPBs)* are premature depolarizations arising in the ventricles, analogous to atrial premature beats (APBs) and junctional premature beats (JPBs), which are supraventricular. Recall that with APBs and JPBs the QRS complex is usually of normal width because the stimulus spreads normally through the bundle branches to the ventricles. With VPBs, however, the premature depolarizations arise in either the right or the left ventricle. Therefore the ventricles are not stimulated simultaneously, and the stimulus spreads through the ventricles in an aberrant direction. Thus the QRS complexes will be wide with VPBs, just as they are with the bundle branch block patterns. Figures 14-1 to 14-8 show some examples.

---

*In the ECG literature the terms *"ventricular premature beat"* (VPB), *"ventricular premature depolarization"* (VPD), *"ventricular extrasystole,"* and *"premature ventricular complex"* or *"contraction"* (PVC) are used interchangeably.

VPBs have two major characteristics*:
1. They are premature and occur before the next normal beat is expected.
2. They are aberrant in appearance. The QRS is abnormally wide (usually 0.12 sec or more), and the T wave and QRS usually point in opposite directions.

VPBs usually precede a sinus P wave. Occasionally they will appear just after a sinus P wave but before the normal QRS (Fig. 14-7). Sometimes they will be followed by a non-sinus P wave (negative in lead II) that has arisen due to retrograde stimulation of the atria by the premature ventricular beat.

Features

Clinicians tend to comment on a number of features of VPBs that may have clinical relevance.

Frequency. The frequency of VPBs refers to how many are seen per minute or other unit of time. It may range from one or an occasional isolated premature depolarization to many.

VPBs may occur in various combinations. Two in a row (Fig. 14-4) are referred to as a *pair* or *couplet*. Three or more in a row are, by definition,

---

*The basic electrophysiologic mechanisms responsible for VPBs are a subject of active investigation. VPBs may arise by at least three mechanisms—*reentrant waves*, increased *spontaneous depolarizations* of ventricular cells (enhanced automaticity), and *triggered activity* or *afterdepolarizations* (i.e., premature firing of ventricular cells triggered by the previous depolarization).

Fig. 14-1. A ventricular premature beat (VPB) is recognized because it comes before the next normal beat is expected and it has a wide aberrant shape. (Also notice the long PR interval in the normal sinus beats, indicating first-degree AV block.)

Fig. 14-2. Notice the wide aberrant shapes of ventricular premature beats compared to the QRS complexes of APBs, which generally resemble the sinus QRS complexes.

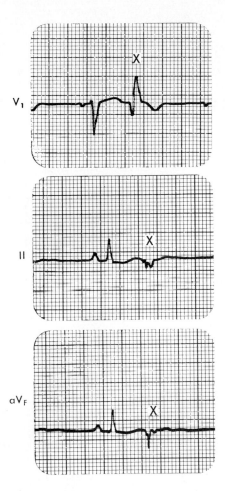

Fig. 14-3. Notice that the same ventricular premature beat (X) recorded simultaneously in three different leads has different shapes. Compare this with Figure 14-9, illustrating multiform VPBs that show different shapes in the same lead.

Monitor lead

Fig. 14-4. Two ventricular premature beats (V) are termed "paired VPBs" or a "couplet." These also show the R on T phenomenon. (See text and Figure 14-10.)

NONSUSTAINED VENTRICULAR TACHYCARDIA

Fig. 14-5. Notice the two short bursts of nonsustained ventricular tachycardia, defined as three or more consecutive VPBs.

Fig. 14-6. Ventricular premature beats. **A,** Ventricular bigeminy. Each normal sinus impulse is followed by a VPB (marked X). **B,** Ventricular trigeminy. After every two sinus impulses a VPB occurs.

ventricular tachycardia (Fig. 14-5). Sometimes, as shown in Figure 14-6, *A*, isolated VPBs occur so frequently that each normal beat is followed by a VPB. This produces a distinctive repetitive grouping of one normal beat–one VPB, called *ventricular bigeminy*. The sequence of two normal beats with a VPB is *ventricular trigeminy*.

Coupling interval. The term "coupling interval" is frequently used and refers to the interval between the VPB and the preceding normal beat. In many cases, when there are multiple VPBs, *fixed coupling* will occur, with the coupling interval approximately the same for each VPB (Fig. 14-6). At other times VPBs may show a *variable coupling interval*. Clinically, fixed and variably coupled VPBs are generally approached in the same fashion.

Compensatory pause. As you may have noticed, APBs and VPBs are usually followed by a pause before the next normal beat. The pause may be longer than that following an APB, but there are exceptions. A fully compensatory pause (Fig. 14-7) indicates that the interval between the normal QRS complexes immediately before and immediately after the VPB is exactly twice the basic RR interval. A fully compensatory pause is more characteristic of VPBs than of APBs. Sometimes a VPB will fall almost exactly between two normal beats, and in such cases it is said to be *interpolated* (Fig. 14-8).

Uniform and multiform VPBs. These terms are used to describe the appearance of VPBs in a lead. Uniform VPBs, as the name implies, have the same appearance in any lead and arise from the same anatomic site (focus) (Fig. 14-5). (They will, of course, have different shapes in different leads, just as normal beats will.) By contrast, multiform VPBs have different morphologies in the same lead (Fig. 14-9). Multiform VPBs often, though not always, arise from different foci. Uniform VPBs are uni*focal* but multi*form* VPBs are not necessarily multi*focal*. Uniform VPBs may occur in healthy people or in persons with underlying organic heart disease. Multiform VPBs usually indicate that organic heart disease is present.

R on T phenomenon. The *R on T* or "VPB on T" phenomenon refers to VPBs that are timed so they fall near the peak* of the T wave of the pre-

---

*Or at the nadir of a negative T wave.

FULLY COMPENSATORY PAUSE

$$R_1—R_2$$
520 msec

$$R_3—R_4$$
1040 msec

Fig. 14-7. Some ventricular premature beats cause a fully compensatory pause—the interval between the two sinus beats that surround the VPB (R_3 and R_4 in this case) being exactly two times the normal interval between sinus beats (R_1 and R_2). Notice that the P waves come on time, except that the third P wave is interrupted by the VPB and therefore is not conducted through the AV junction, which is still refractory. The next (fourth) P wave also comes on time. The fact that the sinus node is continuing to pace despite the VPB results in the fully compensatory pause.

INTERPOLATED VPB

Fig. 14-8. Sometimes a ventricular premature beat (marked X here) will fall between two normal beats, in which case it is *interpolated*.

MULTIFORM VPBs

Fig. 14-9. The multiform ventricular premature beats shown here have different shapes in the same lead. (Compare with Figure 14-3.)

Monitor lead

Fig. 14-10. A ventricular premature beat (marked X) falling near the peak of the T wave of the preceding beat may predispose to ventricular tachycardia or ventricular fibrillation, particularly when this "R on T" phenomenon occurs in the setting of acute myocardial ischemia or infarction.

ceding normal beat (Figs. 14-10 and 14-16). Those falling on the T wave are noteworthy in that they may precipitate ventricular tachycardia or fibrillation, particularly in the course of an acute MI or myocardial ischemia or with very long QT intervals (p. 188). Recall from the discussion of synchronized DC cardioversion (p. 161) that the peak of the T wave is a time during which an external stimulus is especially likely to produce ventricular tachycardia or fibrillation. However, ventricular tachycardia and ventricular fibrillation most commonly occur without a preceding "R on T" beat, and most "R on T" beats do not precipitate a sustained ventricular tachyarrhythmia.

Clinical Significance

VPBs are among the most commonly seen arrhythmias. They may occur both in normal hearts and in serious organic heart disease. Individuals with VPBs may be asymptomatic or may complain of palpitations (i.e., sensations of a "skipped" or "extra" beat). VPBs may be a stable and benign finding or the precursor of cardiac arrest and sudden death from ventricular fibrillation. Clearly, clinicians need certain ground rules to help decide when they are of concern. A few general principles will be discussed here.

As mentioned, VPBs are not uncommon in normal adults of all age groups, although they occur more frequently with advancing age. Young adults, for example, may have them because of anxiety or excessive caffeine intake. Certain drugs (e.g., epinephrine, isoproterenol, and aminophylline) used in asthmatics can provoke them in normal hearts. Nevertheless, finding frequent VPBs should always prompt a careful search for underlying cardiac disease (heart murmurs, abnormal echocardiographic findings, etc.) and a careful drug history. Occasional or even frequent isolated VPBs in an otherwise healthy person are not usually a source of concern. VPBs are also common in subjects with mitral valve prolapse and may be seen with virtually any type of heart disease. For example, a patient with valvular, hypertensive, or ischemic heart disease with or without myocardial infarction may have them. VPBs are the most com-

mon arrhythmia seen with acute myocardial infarction.

As noted, VPBs can be caused by the effects on the heart of numerous drugs (e.g., epinephrine, isoproterenol, and aminophylline, which are cardiac stimulants). Ventricular ectopy is also an important sign of digitalis toxicity (discussed in Chapter 16). VPBs may be seen with electrolyte disturbances, such as hypokalemia or hypomagnesemia, and in patients with lung disease or hypoxemia from any cause.

Treatment Considerations

Treatment of VPBs depends on several factors. In every case a search should be made for possibly reversible causes. Elimination of excessive caffeine intake and certain drugs as well as reduction of anxiety may be effective in patients with occasional to frequent VPBs. Judicious administration of oxygen to hypoxemic patients or treatment of hypokalemia or hypomagnesemia may be sufficient in appropriate cases. Withholding digitalis and checking the serum digoxin level are mandatory in any patient who develops VPBs while taking digitalis.

VPBs occurring during an *acute* MI are of particular concern because of the increased risk of ventricular tachycardia and ventricular fibrillation in this setting. Cardiologists often use intravenous lidocaine or procainamide to treat patients with an acute infarction who are having very frequent VPBs (greater than 5 per minute), paired VPBs (2 in a row), or VPBs showing the R on T phenomenon. However, enthusiasm for the use of prophylactic lidocaine in all patients with an acute MI has waned due to its lack of efficacy in improving mortality rates and its potential for toxicity.

Drug Therapy

The use of antiarrhythmic drugs in asymptomatic patients with frequent VPBs, including short runs of ventricular tachycardia, should be strongly discouraged. As noted, VPBs are common in healthy people. Even in patients with underlying heart disease there is no evidence that suppression of frequent isolated VPBs or short runs of ventricular tachycardia with drugs improves survival. Perhaps more important, the drugs used to treat ventricular ectopy (e.g., quinidine, procainamide, disopyramide, mexiletine, propafenone, encainide, and flecainide) all have grave and sometimes life-threatening side effects. Furthermore, they may actually make the situation worse by, paradoxically, increasing the severity of the ectopy *(proarrhythmic effect)*. Indeed, treating a patient with "antiarrhythmic" drugs may sometimes provoke a potentially fatal ventricular tachyarrhythmia.*

For more complete discussion of these complex and sometimes controversial therapeutic issues the reader is referred to the Bibliography. It should be emphasized again that whenever you are confronted by a patient with frequent VPBs it is always important to search for potentially reversible causes (in particular, hypokalemia, hypomagnesemia, and certain drugs). Correcting metabolic problems or drug effects may obviate the need to treat the patient with additional, potentially toxic, medications.

VENTRICULAR TACHYCARDIA

VPBs are important primarily because they may be a precursor of sustained ventricular tachycardia and ventricular fibrillation, which are life-threatening arrhythmias. *Ventricular tachycardia is, by definition, simply a run of three or more consecutive VPBs.* Examples are shown in Figures 14-5 and 14-11 to 14-13. It may occur as a single brief event, as multiple *nonsustained* episodes, or as a persistent run of rapid beats. The heart rate is generally between 100 and 200 beats/min but may be faster.

Sustained ventricular tachycardia (lasting more than 30 sec) is a life-threatening arrhythmia for two major reasons. First, most patients are not able to maintain an adequate blood pressure at very rapid ventricular rates and eventually become hypotensive. Second, the condition may degenerate

---

*Refer to the Bibliography for a discussion of the well-known Cardiac Arrhythmia Suppression Trial (CAST study), which demonstrated the life-threatening proarrhythmic effects of certain drugs in patients with prior MI.

into ventricular fibrillation (Fig. 14-14), causing immediate cardiac arrest.

Ventricular tachycardia can also be characterized as *monomorphic* (Fig. 14-12, *A*) or *polymorphic* (Fig. 14-18) depending on whether consecutive VPBs are the same or variable in a single lead.

Very rapid ventricular tachycardia with a sine-wave appearance is sometimes referred to as *ventricular flutter* and often leads to ventricular fibrillation (Fig. 14-15).

Occasionally you may be required to treat a patient who is having a sustained run of very rapid ventricular tachycardia while on a cardiac monitor and has become pulseless. In such cases you can try giving the patient a sharp punch to the midsternum with your clenched fist. This treatment, termed *"thump version"* (Fig. 14-13) (p. 210, footnote), may by itself restore a normal heart rhythm in a case of ventricular tachycardia. While it is being tried, the electrical cardioverter should be charged up; if the thump does not restore normal rhythm, the patient must be given a DC shock. Immediately preceding or following electrical cardioversion, the patient should be started on intravenous medication to suppress further ectopy and the cause of the ventricular tachycardia should be carefully sought.

Causes and Therapy of Recurrent Sustained Ventricular Tachycardia

Sustained ventricular tachycardia, which may lead to syncope or sudden death, rarely occurs in patients without underlying heart disease. Most patients with this type of high-grade ventricular ectopy (i.e., long runs of VT) have some basic structural cardiac abnormality, usually prior MI, myocarditis, or other cardiomyopathy associated with fibrosis (scarring) or hypertrophy. The most common cause of sustained monomorphic ventricular tachycardia in American adults is coronary artery disease, usually with prior myocardial infarction. Only some of these patients can be successfully managed with antiarrhythmic drug therapy. Others with refractory ventricular tachycardia will require one of the nonpharmacologic modalities mentioned on page 187. The important role of in-

PAROXYSMAL NONSUSTAINED VENTRICULAR TACHYCARDIA

Monitor - continuous strip

Fig. 14-11. The monitor lead shows short bursts of VT.

SUSTAINED VENTRICULAR TACHYCARDIA TERMINATED BY DC SHOCK

DC shock

Fig. 14-12. A, Long run of "monomorphic" VT. **B,** Normal sinus rhythm restored after direct current cardioversion.

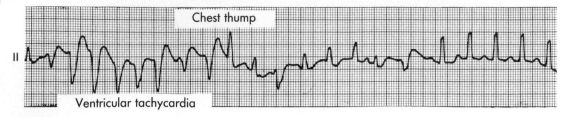

Fig. 14-13. VT terminated by a thump on the chest ("thump version").

VENTRICULAR FIBRILLATION

Fig. 14-14. VF may produce both coarse and fine waves. Immediate defibrillation should be performed.

Fig. 14-15. Ventricular tachycardia *(VT)* and ventricular fibrillation *(VF)* recorded during cardiac arrest. The rapid sine-wave type of ventricular tachycardia seen here is sometimes referred to as ventricular flutter.

vasive *electrophysiologic studies* in evaluating patients with sustained ventricular tachycardia is discussed in references within the Bibliography.

Some patients, usually those with severe organic heart disease, are at high risk for life-threatening recurrences of sustained ventricular tachycardia or ventricular fibrillation despite pharmacologic medical therapy. For these individuals a special device, called an *implantable cardioverter defibrillator* (ICD), has been developed to deliver an electric shock directly to the heart during a life-threatening tachycardia. Readers interested in the ICD as well as in other *nonpharmacologic modalities* for treating refractory ventricular arrhythmias (surgery,

anti-tachycardia pacemakers, catheter ablation techniques) should consult the Bibliography and other more specialized sources.

ACCELERATED IDIOVENTRICULAR RHYTHM

Figures 14-16 and 14-17 present a distinctive arrhythmia that has been called "accelerated idioventricular rhythm" (AIVR) or "slow ventricular tachycardia." Recall that with typical ventricular tachycardia the heart rate is faster than 100 beats/min. With AIVR it is usually between 50 and 100 beats/min, and the ECG shows wide QRS complexes without associated P waves.

ACCELERATED IDIOVENTRICULAR RHYTHM

Fig. 14-16. AIVR in a case of acute inferior wall infarction. The first four beats show the typical pattern, followed by a return of sinus rhythm, then the reappearance of AIVR. Notice that the fifth, sixth, twelfth, and thirteenth QRS complexes are "fusion beats" due to the near-simultaneous occurrence of a sinus beat and a ventricular beat.

Fig. 14-17. Accelerated idioventricular rhythm *(AIVR)* and nonsustained polymorphic ventricular tachycardia *(VT)* occurring together. Notice the "VPB on T" beats that initiate both the AIVR and the VT episodes.

AIVR is particularly common with acute myocardial infarction and may be a sign of reperfusion after the use of thrombolytic agents. It is generally short lived, lasting for minutes or less, and usually requires no specific therapy. Treatment (by the administration of intravenous lidocaine or procainamide) is indicated if it occurs with actual ventricular tachycardia (Fig. 14-17), particularly in the setting of acute MI.

In many cases (Fig. 14-16) AIVR appears to be a benign "escape" rhythm that competes with the underlying sinus mechanism. When the sinus rate slows, AIVR appears; and when the sinus rate speeds up, the arrhythmia disappears. In other cases (Fig. 14-17) AIVR is initiated by premature beats rather than by escape beats. This latter type is more likely to be associated with actual ventricular tachycardia.

VENTRICULAR FIBRILLATION

With ventricular fibrillation (Figs. 14-14 and 14-15) the ventricles do not beat in any coordinated fashion but instead fibrillate or quiver asynchronously and ineffectively. There is no cardiac output, and the patient becomes unconscious immediately. Ventricular fibrillation is one of the three major ECG patterns seen with cardiac arrest. The other two are *asystole* and *electromechanical dissociation* (Chapter 17).

The ECG in ventricular fibrillation shows characteristic fibrillatory waves with an irregular pattern that may be either coarse or fine (Fig. 14-14).

Ventricular fibrillation requires immediate defibrillation with an unsynchronized DC shock. Patients who have just been resuscitated from an episode of ventricular fibrillation are generally given an immediate dose of an intravenous antiarrhythmic drug in an attempt to suppress further ventricular ectopy.

This tachyarrhythmia can occur in patients with heart disease of any type. It may be preceded by a warning arrhythmia (e.g., VPBs or ventricular tachycardia) or may occur spontaneously. It is the most common cause of *sudden cardiac death* (p. 215) in patients with an acute myocardial infarction, although it may occur in normal hearts as well, sometimes because of drugs (e.g., epinephrine).

TORSADE DE POINTES: A SPECIAL FORM OF VENTRICULAR TACHYCARDIA

A special type of polymorphic ventricular tachycardia has been called "torsade de pointes," a French term meaning "twisting of the points." Figure 14-18 shows an example of this distinctive tachycardia. Notice how the direction of the QRS complexes appears to rotate cyclically, pointing downward for several beats and then twisting and pointing upward in the same lead.

Torsade de pointes is important because of its diagnostic and therapeutic implications. As shown in Figure 14-18, it classically occurs in the setting of delayed ventricular repolarization, evidenced by *prolongation of the QT intervals or the presence of prominent U waves*. It is often initiated by a VPB that occurs near or on the T or U wave of the preceding beat. Reported causes include

1. Drugs, particularly quinidine (quinidine syncope, p. 123) and related antiarrhythmic agents (disopyramide and procainamide) as well as psychotropic agents (phenothiazines and tricyclic antidepressants)
2. Electrolyte imbalance, including hypokalemia, hypomagnesemia, and hypocalcemia, which prolong repolarization
3. Miscellaneous factors (e.g., severe bradyarrhythmias, hereditary long-QT syndromes, and occasionally acute myocardial ischemia)

Recognition of torsade is critical because it is often caused by drugs conventionally recommended in treating ventricular tachycardia (i.e., quinidine or procainamide). Therapy of torsade therefore should include removing or correcting causative factors (drug toxicity, electrolyte imbalance). In emergency settings a temporary pacemaker may be inserted to accomplish "overdrive" suppression of the arrhythmia by increasing the underlying heart rate and thereby decreasing ventricular repolarization time. Intravenous magnesium sulfate has proved highly useful for this arrhythmia. Drug therapy with bretylium tosylate, isopro-

"Torsade de pointes"
ventricular tachycardia

Fig. 14-18. Notice the shifting polarity and amplitude of the QRS complexes during a bout of ventricular tachycardia. This is the hallmark of torsade de pointes. There is also QT prolongation (0.52 sec) in the normal sinus beats. (See Question 2, page 190.)

terenol, or lidocaine may be required in selected cases. Sustained episodes of torsade require attempted cardioversion. However, the arrhythmia will often recur unless causative factors (drug effect, electrolyte imbalance, underlying bradycardia) are corrected. For further discussion of this important topic, readers should consult the Bibliography.

REVIEW

Ventricular premature beats (VPBs) have the following characteristics:
1. They are premature, occurring before the next normal beat is expected.
2. They have an aberrant shape. The QRS is abnormally wide, usually 0.12 second or more in duration, and the T wave and QRS usually point in opposite directions.

VPBs may occur with varying *frequency*. Two in a row are called a *couplet*. Three or more in a row constitute *ventricular tachycardia*. When a VPB occurs regularly after each normal beat, this is called *ventricular bigeminy*. When the rhythm is two normal beats followed by a VPB, this is *ventricular trigeminy*.

A VPB is often followed by a compensatory pause before the next beat.

Uniform VPBs have the same shape in a single lead. *Multiform* VPBs have different shapes in the same lead.

When a VPB occurs simultaneously with the apex of the T wave of the preceding beat, this is called an *R on T phenomenon*. It may be the precursor of ventricular tachycardia or ventricular fibrillation, particularly in the setting of acute MI or long QT syndromes.

VPBs may occur both normally and with organic heart disease.

Ventricular tachycardia is a run of three or more VPBs. Short runs of ventricular tachycardia are called *nonsustained*. *Sustained* ventricular tachycardia refers to episodes lasting more than 30 seconds, which may lead to syncope or even cardiac arrest.

Ventricular fibrillation occurs when the ventricles stop beating and, instead, fibrillate or twitch in an ineffective fashion. It is one of the three major ECG patterns seen with cardiac arrest; the other two are *asystole* and *electromechanical dissociation* (Chapter 17).

Accelerated indioventricular rhythm (AIVR) is a ventricular arrhythmia that resembles a slow ventricular tachycardia with a rate between 50 and 100 beats/min. It is commonly seen with myocardial infarction and is usually self-limited.

Torsade de pointes is the name of a form of ventricular tachycardia in which the QRS complexes in the same lead appear to twist periodically and turn in the opposite direction. It is generally seen in the setting of delayed ventricular repolarization (increased QT interval or prominent U waves) due to drugs (quinidine), electrolyte abnormalities (hypokalemia, hypomagnesemia), or other factors.

Questions

1. What is the arrhythmia shown below?

2. Which arrhythmia does this rhythm strip show?

MONITOR
LEAD

3. Name three potentially treatable causes of VPBs.

4. What is the rhythm here?

Answers

1. Ventricular tachycardia (monomorphic)
2. Torsade de pointes. Notice the changing orientation and amplitude of the QRS complexes. Contrast this with the ECG in Question 1, where all QRS complexes are the same.
3. Hypoxemia, digitalis toxicity, hypokalemia, hypomagnesemia. (See page 183.)
4. Sinus rhythm with ventricular bigeminy.

15

AV Heart Block

Heart block is the general term for atrioventricular (AV) conduction disturbances. Normally the AV junction (node) acts like an apparent bridge between the atria and the ventricles. The PR interval, as mentioned earlier, is primarily a measure of the lag in AV conduction between initial stimulation of the atria and initial stimulation of the ventricles. The normal PR interval is between 0.12 and 0.2 second. Heart block occurs when there is impaired transmission through the AV junction, either transiently or permanently. The mildest form is called *first-degree heart block*.* With this pattern the PR interval is uniformly prolonged above 0.2 second. *Second-degree heart block* is an intermediate grade of AV conduction disturbance in which there is *intermittent* failure of impulse transmission between atria and ventricles. The most extreme form is *third-degree* or *complete heart block*. In this case the AV junction does not conduct any stimuli between the atria and ventricles. These three degrees of heart block are described in the present chapter, along with the related topic *AV dissociation*.

FIRST-DEGREE HEART BLOCK

With first-degree heart block the PR interval is prolonged above 0.2 second and is constant from beat to beat (Fig. 15-1).

---

*The term first-degree AV block is actually a misnomer since the impulse is not blocked but delayed. A preferable term, therefore, is simply *"prolonged PR interval."*

First-degree heart block does not produce any symptoms or any significant change in cardiac function. There are numerous causes, and most factors that produce first-degree AV block can also produce second- and third-degree block. For example, digitalis, which has a vagal effect on the AV junction, can produce any degree of heart block. Other drugs such as quinidine, any of the numerous beta blockers, and the calcium blockers (verapamil and diltiazem) can also cause severe depression of AV conduction.

Patients with ischemic heart disease may have heart block of any degree. This may occur with chronic myocardial ischemia over a long time or with an acute myocardial infarction. Varying degrees of heart block are particularly common with inferior wall infarction because the right coronary artery, which generally supplies the inferior wall, also usually supplies the AV junction. In addition, acute inferior MI is often associated with increased vagal tone. Heart block during inferior wall infarction tends to be transient.

Hyperkalemia may cause first-degree heart block. Other signs of hyperkalemia (as mentioned in Chapter 10) include peaking of the T waves and widening of the QRS complexes. First-degree AV block may occur with acute rheumatic fever. Occasionally, mild first-degree block is seen as a normal variant.

SECOND-DEGREE AV BLOCK

Second-degree AV block is somewhat more complicated because there are two types—Mobitz

FIRST DEGREE AV BLOCK

Fig. 15-1. With first-degree AV block the PR interval is uniformly prolonged above 0.2 second with each beat. **A** and **B** are from different patients.

I (also called Wenckebach block) and Mobitz II. Despite this imposing nomenclature, the two types of second-degree block are actually not too difficult to understand.

Mobitz Type I (Wenckebach) AV Block

With the Wenckebach pattern, each stimulus from the atria to the ventricles appears to have a more difficult time passing through the AV junction. Finally, a point is reached where the stimulus is not conducted at all. This *blocked beat* is followed by relative recovery of the AV junction, and the whole cycle starts again.

The characteristic ECG picture of Wenckebach block therefore is a progressive lengthening of the PR interval from beat to beat until finally a beat is "dropped." The dropped beat is a P wave that is not followed by a QRS complex, indicating failure of the AV junction to conduct the stimulus from the atria to the ventricles. Furthermore, the PR interval following the nonconducted P wave will be shorter than the PR interval of the beat just before the nonconducted P wave. Figure 15-2 di-

agrammatically depicts the Wenckebach phenomenon, and Figure 15-3 shows an actual example of this pattern. The number of P waves occurring before a QRS is dropped may vary. In many cases it will be just two or three. What characterizes the Wenckebach pattern is the general sequence of a progressive lengthening of the PR interval followed by a nonconducted P wave.

As you can see from the examples, the Wenckebach cycle also produces a distinct clustering of QRS complexes separated by a pause that results from the dropped beat. Any time you encounter an ECG with this type of *group beating,* suspect a Wenckebach block and look for the diagnostic pattern of lengthening PR intervals.

Clinically patients with the Wenckebach type of AV block are usually without symptoms unless the ventricular rate is very slow. The pulse rate is irregular.

Common causes of Wenckebach block include drugs (digitalis, beta blockers, calcium-channel blockers [diliazem and verapamil]) and ischemic heart disease. Wenckebach block is not uncommon

WENCKEBACH (MOBITZ TYPE I) SECOND-DEGREE AV BLOCK

Fig. 15-2. The PR interval lengthens progressively with successive beats until one P wave is not conducted at all. Then the cycle repeats itself. Notice that the PR interval following the nonconducted P wave is shorter than the PR of the beat just before it.

WENCKEBACH (MOBITZ TYPE I) SECOND-DEGREE AV BLOCK

Fig. 15-3. Notice the progressive increase in PR intervals, with the third P wave in each sequence not followed by a QRS. Wenckebach block produces a characteristically syncopated rhythm with grouping of the QRS complexes *(group beating)*.

Table 15-1. Mobitz I Versus Mobitz II AV Block

	Mobitz I	Mobitz II
	0.18 0.24 0.18	0.18 0.18 0.18
Pattern of block	Cycles of gradually increasing PR followed by nonconducted P	Abrupt nonconducted P without preceding PR changes
Usual location of block	AV node	His bundle or bundle branches
Occurrence with acute MI	Inferior	Anterior
Risk of progression to complete heart block	Low	High
Indication for permanent pacemaker	Not usually	Usually

with acute inferior wall infarction. In such cases it is usually transient and generally does not require any specific treatment except for observation, since these patients may progress into complete heart block. Of note, Wenckebach AV block may also occur in athletes at rest, due to a physiologic increase in vagal tone.

Mobitz Type II AV Block

Mobitz type II AV block is a rarer and more serious form of second-degree heart block. Its characteristic feature is the sudden appearance of a nonconducted sinus P wave without the progressive prolongation of PR intervals seen in Mobitz type I (AV Wenckebach) block.*

Mobitz type II block is generally a sign of severe conduction system disease involving regions below the AV node (i.e., the His-Purkinje system). Since patients with this form of block often progress into complete heart block, cardiologists generally consider this an indication for a pacemaker. Unlike Wenckebach (Mobitz type I) block, Mobitz type II is *not* usually seen with digitalis excess or with inferior wall infarction. However, Mobitz type II may be seen with anterior wall MI, and these patients often progress into complete heart block. Therefore cardiologists generally treat a patient with an anterior wall infarction and Mobitz type II AV block by inserting a pacemaker.

A comparison of Mobitz I and Mobitz II blocks is given in Table 15-1.

---

*A point of common confusion: It should be noted that 2:1 AV block per se does not always indicate a Mobitz type II block. Not uncommonly 2:1 AV block is due to a Wenckebach (Mobitz I) mechanism in which the block simply occurs after every other P wave. In such cases careful search of a long rhythm strip will often reveal 3:2, 4:3, etc. types of Wenckebach in addition to the 2:1 periods. Furthermore, in most (but not all) cases of AV Wenckebach the QRS complex is of normal duration. By contrast, when 2:1 is due to a Mobitz II mechanism the His-Purkinje system (not just the AV node) is involved and the QRS duration is often prolonged. Thus 2:1 block with a narrow QRS most likely represents AV Wenckebach. However, 2:1 block with a wide QRS may be due to either mechanism. Definitive assessment in any case of chronic 2:1 block requires an intracardiac electrophysiologic study.

THIRD-DEGREE (COMPLETE) HEART BLOCK

First- and second-degree heart blocks are examples of *incomplete* block because the AV junction does conduct at least some stimuli to the ventricles. With complete heart block, there is no transmission of stimuli from the atria to the ventricles. Instead, the atria and the ventricles are paced independently. The atria generally continue to be paced by the sinus node. The ventricles, however, are paced by an escape pacemaker located somewhere below the point of block in the AV junction. The resting ventricular rate with complete heart block may be lower than 30 or as high as 50 or 60 beats/min. The atrial rate is generally faster than the ventricular rate.

Examples of complete heart block are shown in Figures 15-4 and 15-5. The ECG with sinus rhythm and complete heart block has the following characteristics:

1. P waves are present, with a regular atrial rate faster than the ventricular rate.
2. QRS complexes are present, with a slow (usually fixed) ventricular rate.
3. The P waves bear no relation to the QRS complexes, and the PR intervals are completely variable since the atria and ventricles are electrically disconnected.
4. Complete heart block may also occur in a patient whose basic atrial rhythm is flutter or fibrillation. In these cases the ventricular rate is very slow and almost completely regular (Fig. 13-8).

With complete heart block the QRS complexes may be either of normal width (Fig. 15-4) or abnormally wide (Fig. 15-5) with the appearance of a bundle branch block pattern. The width of the QRS complexes depends in part on the location of the blockage in the AV junction. If the block is in the first part (the AV node), the ventricles will be stimulated normally by a junctional pacemaker and the QRS complexes will be narrow (Fig. 15-4) unless the patient has an underlying bundle branch block. If the block is within, or particularly below, the His bundle, the ventricles will be paced

THIRD-DEGREE (COMPLETE) AV BLOCK

Fig. 15-4. Complete heart block is characterized by independent atrial *(P)* and ventricular (QRS) activity. The atrial rate is always faster than the ventricular rate. The PR intervals are completely variable. Some P waves fall on the T wave, distorting its shape. Others may fall in the QRS complex and be "lost." Notice that the QRS complexes are of normal width, indicating that the ventricles are being paced from the AV junction. Compare this with Figure 15-5, which shows complete heart block with wide very slow QRS complexes because the ventricles are likely being paced from below the AV junction (idioventricular pacemaker).

Fig. 15-5. Another example of complete heart block, showing a very slow idioventricular rhythm and a faster independent atrial (sinus) rhythm.

by an *idioventricular pacemaker,* * producing wide QRS complexes (Fig. 15-5). As a general clinical rule, complete heart block with wide QRS complexes tends to be less stable than complete heart block with narrow QRS complexes, since the ventricular escape pacemaker is usually slower and less stable.

Complete heart block can occur for a number of reasons. It is most commonly seen in older patients who have chronic degenerative changes in their conduction systems *not* related to an acute myocardial infarction. Digitalis intoxication, which can cause first- and second-degree heart

block, may also lead to complete heart block (Chapter 16). Varying degrees of AV block, including some cases of complete block, have been reported with Lyme disease.

Complete heart block may be seen acutely as a complication of myocardial infarction. The course and therapy of complete heart block with MI depend to a large extent on whether the infarct is anterior or inferior. Transient AV conduction disturbances are commonly seen with acute inferior wall MI because of the common blood supply to the AV junction and inferior wall (via the right coronary artery). Occlusion of the right coronary artery with inferior MI also often leads to temporary ischemia of the AV node, sometimes resulting in complete heart block. (In addition, acute inferior MI may

---

*An idioventricular pacemaker may be located in the His-Purkinje system or the ventricular myocardium.

cause an increase in vagal tone.) Complete heart block occurring with inferior wall MI is often a transient and reversible complication that may respond to atropine and therefore not require a temporary pacemaker.

With acute anterior myocardial infarction and complete heart block, the situation is more serious. Patients with anterior wall and complete heart block generally have extensive myocardial damage. The idioventricular escape rhythm that develops is usually slow and unstable. Therefore, if complete heart block occurs with an acute anterior MI, cardiologists will insert a temporary pacemaker (and subsequently a permanent one).

Regardless of its cause, complete heart block is a serious and potentially life-threatening arrhythmia. If the ventricular rate becomes too slow, the cardiac output will drop and the patient may faint. Fainting spells associated with complete heart block (or other types of bradycardia) are referred to as *Stokes-Adams attacks*. In some patients complete heart block is a chronic and persistent finding. In others the block may occur transiently and be recognized only with more prolonged monitoring.

Complete heart block resulting from digitalis toxicity or acute inferior MI is often transient and can sometimes be treated medically without insertion of a pacemaker. However, chronic complete heart block (or intermittent complete heart block not due to some reversible cause) calls for an implanted (permanent) pacemaker (Chapter 20).

BIFASCICULAR BLOCKS AND COMPLETE HEART BLOCK

Cardiologists have been interested in developing criteria to predict which patients with acute myocardial infarction (particularly anterior wall infarcts) would develop life-threatening complete heart block. Current information suggests that certain high-risk patients can be identified. Specifically, it has been found that patients with an acute anterior wall MI and complete heart block often have other conduction disturbances before the onset of the block referred to as *bifascicular blocks*.

Recall, from Chapter 7, that the ventricular conduction system is trifascicular, consisting of the right bundle branch and the left bundle branch, the latter further dividing into left anterior and left posterior fascicles. Blockage of just the left anterior fascicle produces left anterior hemiblock with left axis deviation. Blockage of just the left posterior fascicle produces left posterior hemiblock with right axis deviation. Bifascicular block indicates blockage of any two of the three fascicles. For example, right bundle branch block with left anterior hemiblock produces a right bundle branch block pattern with marked left axis deviation (Figs. 8-20 and 15-6); right bundle branch block with left posterior hemiblock produces a right bundle branch block pattern with right axis deviation (provided other causes of right axis deviation are excluded). Similarly, a complete left bundle branch block may indicate blockage of both the anterior and the posterior fascicles.

Bifascicular blocks are significant because they make ventricular conduction dependent on the single remaining fascicle. Additional damage to this third remaining fascicle may completely block AV conduction, producing complete heart block (trifascicular block). Therefore the acute development of bifascicular block during an acute anterior wall MI is a warning signal of possible impending complete heart block. If a new bifascicular block occurs in the setting of acute anterior infarction (Fig. 8-20), cardiologists generally insert a temporary pacemaker as a prophylactic measure.

An important distinction must be made between *acute* bifascicular blocks occurring with anterior wall MI (Fig. 8-20) and *chronic* bifascicular blocks (Fig. 15-6). Many people without any symptoms at all may have ECGs resembling Figure 15-6. Patients with chronic bifascicular block do not generally require a pacemaker, unless they develop high-degree AV block. The risk of complete heart block in patients with chronic bifascicular block seems to be quite low. By contrast, patients with acute anterior infarction in whom bifascicular block suddenly occurs have a poor prognosis and are at much higher risk of complete heart block.

BIFASCICULAR BLOCK (RIGHT BUNDLE BRANCH BLOCK WITH LEFT ANTERIOR HEMIBLOCK)

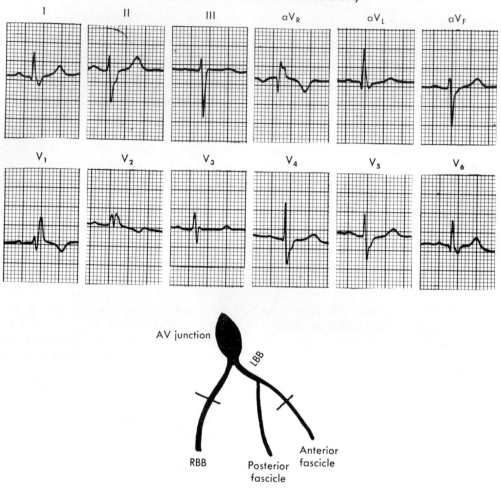

Fig. 15-6. Notice that the chest leads show the typical RBBB pattern (rSR′ in lead V_1 and qRS in V_6). The extremity leads show marked left axis deviation (mean QRS axis about $-60°$), consistent with left anterior hemiblock. Thus a bifascicular block, involving the right bundle branch and the anterior fascicle of the left bundle branch system, is present (as shown in the diagram).

AV DISSOCIATION (AVD)

Fig. 15-7. This type of AV dissociation is characterized by relatively independent atrial and ventricular rhythms, with the ventricular rate usually the same as (or slightly faster than) the atrial rate. Notice that the first and fifth P waves are partially hidden in the T waves and that the fourth and eighth P waves are lost in the QRS complexes. Notice also that some of the P waves here (e.g., the second and sixth) are probably conducted with a long PR interval, accounting for the slightly variable ventricular rate. See also Question 142, page 289.

AV DISSOCIATION

The term *"AV dissociation"* is used in two related, though not identical, ways by cardiologists. This classification continues to cause considerable (and understandable) confusion among students and clinicians.

AV dissociation is widely used as a *general* term to refer to any arrhythmia in which the atria and ventricles are controlled by independent pacemakers. The definition obviously includes complete heart block, discussed above, as well as some instances of ventricular tachycardia in which the atria remain in sinus rhythm (p. 225).

AV dissociation is also used as a *specific* term to describe a particular family of arrhythmias that are often mistaken for complete heart block. With this type of AV dissociation the SA node and AV junction appear to be "out of synch"; thus the SA node loses its normal control of the ventricular rate. As a result the atria and ventricles are paced independently—the atria from the SA node, the ventricles from the AV junction. This is similar to what occurs with complete heart block. *However, with AV dissociation the ventricular rate is the same as or slightly faster than the atrial rate.* When the atrial and ventricular rates are almost the same, the term *"isorhythmic"* AV dissociation is used.

The critical difference between AV dissociation (due to "desynchronization" of the SA and AV nodes) and complete heart block (due to conduction failure) is as follows: with AV dissociation a properly timed P wave can be conducted through the AV node whereas with complete heart block no P wave reaches the ventricles.

Thus AV dissociation (Fig. 15-7) can be regarded as a "competition" between the SA node and the AV node for control of the heartbeat. It may occur either when the SA node slows down (e.g., due to beta blocker or calcium-channel blocker drugs or with increased vagal tone) or when the AV node is accelerated (by ischemia or digitalis toxicity). Not uncommonly, isorhythmic AV dissociation is seen in healthy young individuals, particularly during sleeping hours.

Figure 15-7 presents an example of AV dissociation. Notice the P waves with a variable PR interval, because the ventricular (QRS) rate is slightly faster than the atrial rate. At times the P waves may merge with the QRS complexes and become imperceptible for several beats. If the sinus rate speeds up sufficiently (or the AV junctional rate slows), the stimulus may be able to penetrate the AV junction, reestablishing sinus rhythm.

REVIEW

There are three types of AV heart block:

1. *First degree*—the PR interval uniformly prolonged beyond 0.2 second
2. *Second-degree*—two major subtypes*:
   a. *Wenckebach (Mobitz type I) block*—increasing prolongation of the PR interval until a P wave is blocked and not followed by a QRS; this produces a distinctive clustering of QRS complexes separated by a pause resulting from the dropped beat (known as *group beating*)
   b. *Mobitz type II block*—sudden appearance of a nonconducted sinus P wave without prolongation of the preceding PR interval; also the PR interval following the nonconducted P wave is the same as the one before it

---

*A third subtype, called "advanced second-degree AV block," is sometimes listed. This refers to patterns in which there are several (two or more) consecutive nonconducted P waves (e.g., 3:1 or 4:1 block). (See page 314, Question 196.)

3. *Third-degree (complete)*—showing
   a. Atria and ventricles that beat independently because stimuli cannot pass through the AV junction
   b. An atrial rate faster than the ventricular rate
   c. A PR interval that is constantly changing

Complete heart block with acute anterior wall MI is sometimes preceded by the sudden appearance of *bifascicular block* (right bundle branch block with left anterior or posterior hemiblock or complete left bundle branch block). However, patients with *chronic* bifascicular block who have no symptoms usually do not require any special therapy.

The significance of complete heart block with acute MI depends on the location of the infarct. Complete heart block occurring with acute inferior wall MI is not uncommon, is usually transient, and can sometimes be managed without a pacemaker. By contrast, complete heart block with acute anterior wall MI is usually associated with a very poor prognosis and requires a pacemaker.

Complete heart block must be distinguished from other forms of *AV dissociation*. With "isorhythmic" AV dissociation the atria and ventricles beat independently; however, the ventricular rate is about the same as the atrial rate. AV dissociation is a minor, usually transient, arrhythmia.

Questions

True or false (1 to 5):
1. With first-degree AV block, the heart rate will be very slow.
2. Bifascicular block always leads to complete heart block.
3. The PR interval is constant in complete heart block.
4. Digitalis toxicity may cause complete heart block.
5. Complete heart block may occur with atrial fibrillation.
6. The rhythm strip below shows sinus rhythm with which of the following?
   a. Wenckebach type second-degree AV block
   b. Complete heart block
   c. 3:1 AV block
   d. AV dissociation
   e. Blocked premature atrial beats

7. In the rhythm strip below
   a. What is the approximate atrial (P wave) rate?
   b. What is the approximate ventricular (QRS) rate?
   c. Is the PR interval constant?
   d. What is the ECG abnormality shown?

Answers

1. False. The heart rate may be slow, fast, or normal.
2. False.
3. False.
4. True. Digitalis toxicity may cause any degree of AV block.
5. True. (See Figure 3-9.)
6. a. Wenckebach block. Notice the succession of P waves, with increasing PR intervals, followed by a dropped (nonconducted) P wave. This pattern leads to "group beating." Blocked premature atrial contractions can also cause group beating, but then the nonconducted P wave comes early, before the next sinus P wave is due. The P waves in this example come on time.
7. a. 100 beats/min.
   b. 42 beats/min.
   c. No.
   d. Sinus rhythm with complete heart block. Notice that some of the P waves are hidden in QRS or T waves.

16

Digitalis Toxicity

This chapter focuses on the arrhythmias and conduction disturbances caused by digitalis intoxication. There are several reasons for discussing this topic in an introductory textbook. The most important is that digitalis is a frequently prescribed drug and digitalis toxicity is still an important clinical problem. Furthermore, digitalis toxicity can cause fatal arrhythmias. Early recognition of digitalis toxicity therefore should be a preoccupation of everyone in clinical medicine. Finally, because digitalis toxicity can produce virtually any arrhythmia and all degrees of heart block, this topic provides a convenient review of material presented in previous chapters.

CLINICAL BACKGROUND

Digitalis refers to a class of cardiac drugs (glycosides) with specific effects on the mechanical and electrical function of the heart. The most commonly used digitalis preparation is digoxin.

Digitalis is used in clinical practice for two major reasons. First, in selected patients with dilated hearts and congestive heart failure it increases the strength of myocardial contractions. This is its *mechanical* action. Second, it affects the conductivity of certain heart tissues. This is its *electrical* action. Thus it is useful for treating selected arrhythmias. Its antiarrhythmic action results primarily from its slowing of conduction through the AV junction (node) due to an increase in vagal tone. Consequently, digitalis is used for controlling the ventricular response in atrial fibrillation and atrial

flutter, when there is excessive transmission of stimuli from the atria to the ventricles through the AV junction. It also is used in treating certain re-entrant types of paroxysmal supraventricular tachycardia (PSVT).*

Unfortunately, however, although it has wide use in the treatment of heart failure and selected arrhythmias, digitalis also has a relatively low margin of safety. The difference between therapeutic and toxic concentrations is very narrow.

SIGNS OF DIGITALIS TOXICITY

Digitalis toxicity can produce general systemic symptoms as well as specific cardiac arrhythmias and conduction disturbances. Common extracardiac symptoms include weakness, anorexia, nausea, and vomiting. Visual effects (altered color perception) and mental changes may occur. In this section we will concentrate on the arrhythmias and conduction disturbances produced by digitalis excess.

As a general clinical rule *virtually any arrhythmia and all degrees of AV heart block can be*

---

*The basic mechanisms involved in digitalis-related arrhythmias are complex and incompletely understood. Bradyarrhythmias may be due to excessive increases in vagal tone caused by digitalis. Increased automaticity and tachycardias may be due to the effects of toxic doses of digitalis on the sympathetic nervous system. The automaticity of cardiac cells in the atria, AV junction, and ventricles may also be directly enhanced by digitalis, leading to some of the arrhythmias described in this chapter.

Fig. 16-1. Ventricular bigeminy caused by digitalis toxicity. Ventricular ectopy is one of the most common signs of digitalis toxicity. The underlying rhythm in **A** is atrial fibrillation. In **B** each normal QRS is followed by a VPB.

BIDIRECTIONAL TACHYCARDIA

Fig. 16-2. This digitalis-toxic arrhythmia is a special type of ventricular tachycardia with QRS complexes that alternate in direction from beat to beat. No P waves are present.

produced by digitalis intoxication. Of all the arrhythmias we have discussed, atrial fibrillation and atrial flutter with a rapid ventricular response are the *least* likely to be caused by digitalis toxicity. However, there remain a number of arrhythmias that are commonly seen with digitalis toxicity.

Ventricular Arrhythmias

Ventricular premature beats (VPBs) are often the first sign of digitalis toxicity. Isolated VPBs may occur at first. Ventricular bigeminy (Fig. 16-1), with each normal beat followed by a VPB, is common. Ventricular tachycardia and fatal ventricular fibrillation may occur if the digitalis toxicity is not recognized and treated. (See Chapter 17.)

Bidirectional Ventricular Tachycardia

Bidirectional ventricular tachycardia (Fig. 16-2) resembles ventricular tachycardia, except that each successive beat in any lead alternates in direction. This distinctive tachyarrhythmia should always raise the question of digitalis intoxication.

AV Junctional (Nodal) Rhythms

AV junctional rhythms are frequently a sign of digitalis toxicity. Most AV junctional rhythms resulting from excessive digitalis have a rate of less than 120 beats/min.

Sinus Bradycardia and Sinoatrial (SA) Block

Sinus bradycardia may be one of the earliest signs of digitalis excess. SA block with sinus arrest may also occur.

Paroxysmal Atrial Tachycardia (PAT) with AV Block

PAT with block is another tachyarrhythmia that has not been discussed in earlier chapters. (An example appears in Figure 16-3.) PAT with block indicates an atrial tachycardia with P waves occurring at a rate usually between 150 and 250 beats/minute and, because of the AV block, a slower ventricular rate. Not uncommonly 2:1 AV block is present, so the ventricular rate will be half the atrial rate. Digitalis toxicity is an important, but not the only, cause of this arrhythmia. Superficially PAT with block may resemble atrial flutter; however, in PAT with block the baseline between P waves is isoelectric. Furthermore, when atrial flutter is present the atrial rate is faster (usually 250 to 350 beats/min).

AV Heart Block and AV Dissociation

Because digitalis slows conduction through the AV junction, it is not surprising that toxic doses can result in any degree of AV heart block.

First-degree block. With first-degree AV block there is uniform prolongation of the PR interval greater than 0.2 second. Some degree of PR lengthening may be expected with digitalis therapy. More marked widening of the PR interval suggests early digitalis toxicity.

Second-degree block. With higher doses of digitalis, first-degree AV block may progress to second-degree block of the Mobitz type I (Wenckebach) variety.

Complete heart block. Third-degree, or complete, heart block may also occur with digitalis toxicity.

In addition, digitalis toxicity may cause other types of AV dissociation. (See Chapter 15.)

Atrial Fibrillation or Flutter with Slow Ventricular Rate

Although atrial fibrillation and atrial flutter with a rapid ventricular response are two of the arrhythmias least likely to be caused by digitalis toxicity, digitalis toxicity can still occur in patients with atrial fibrillation or flutter. In such cases the toxicity is often shown by marked slowing of the ventricular rate (less than 50 beats/min) (Fig. 16-4) and/or the appearance of ventricular premature beats (VPBs). (In some cases the earliest sign of digitalis toxicity in a patient with atrial fibrillation may be a subtle *regularization* of the ventricular rate.)

Because of its frequency and potential lethality, digitalis toxicity should be suspected in any patient taking a digitalis preparation who has an unexplained arrhythmia until you can prove otherwise. The list below summarizes the most common and important arrhythmias and conduction disturbances seen with digitalis toxicity.

1. Ventricular ectopy: isolated VPBs, ventricular bigeminy, ventricular tachycardia, bidirectional ventricular tachycardia, ventricular fibrillation
2. AV junctional (nodal) rhythms
3. Sinus bradycardia and SA block
4. AV heart block (first, second, third degree) and AV dissociation
5. Atrial fibrillation with a slow or regularized ventricular response
6. PAT with block

FACTORS PREDISPOSING TO DIGITALIS TOXICITY

There are a number of factors that significantly increase the hazard of digitalis intoxication.

Hypokalemia. A low serum potassium concentration makes certain digitalis-induced arrhythmias (particularly ventricular ectopy and PAT with block) more likely. Hypokalemia is not uncommon in digitalized patients because these patients frequently receive diuretics for treatment of heart fail-

PAROXYSMAL ATRIAL TACHYCARDIA WITH BLOCK

Fig. 16-3. This rhythm strip shows atrial tachycardia (about 200 beats/min) with 2:1 block, producing a ventricular rate of about 100 beats/min.

Fig. 16-4. Atrial fibrillation with an excessively slow ventricular rate because of digitalis toxicity. Atrial fibrillation with a rapid ventricular rate is rarely caused by digitalis toxicity. However, in patients with underlying atrial fibrillation, digitalis toxicity is often manifested by excessive slowing or regularization of the QRS rate.

ure and edema. The serum potassium concentration must be checked periodically in any patient taking digitalis and in every patient suspected of having digitalis toxicity.

Hypomagnesemia and hypercalcemia. Hypomagnesemia is seen in a variety of settings—including alcoholism, intestinal malabsorption, and diuretic therapy. Hypercalcemia is seen with hyperparathyroidism and certain tumors, among other conditions.

Hypoxemia and chronic lung disease. Hypoxemia and chronic lung disease may also increase the risk of digitalis toxicity, particularly when associated with increased sympathetic tone.

Myocardial infarction. Patients with acute myocardial infarction or ischemia appear to be more sensitive to digitalis.

Old age. Elderly patients may be more susceptible to digitalis toxity, probably related in part to decreased excretion of the drug.

Renal insufficiency. Digoxin, the most widely used preparation of digitalis, is excreted primarily in the urine. Therefore any degree of renal insufficiency, as measured by increased blood urea nitrogen (BUN) and creatinine concentration, requires a lower maintenance dose of digoxin.

Hypothyroidism. Patients with hypothyroidism (myxedema) appear to be more sensitive to the effects of digitalis.

Other conditions. Even therapeutic levels of digoxin can be dangerous in certain patients. For example, digitalis may worsen the symptoms of patients with hypertrophic cardiomyopathy, an inherited heart condition associated with excessive cardiac contractility. Patients with heart failure due to amyloidosis are also extremely sensitive to digitalis. In addition, in patients with the Wolff-Parkinson-White syndrome and atrial fibrillation (p. 225), digitalis may cause extremely rapid transmission of impulses down the atrioventricular bypass tract, leading to a potentially lethal type of wide-complex tachycardia (Fig. 18-10, *A*).

TREATMENT OF DIGITALIS TOXICITY

The first step in treatment is prevention. Before starting any patient on a regimen of digoxin or related drug, you should obtain a baseline ECG, serum electrolytes, and BUN and creatinine measurements. Serum magnesium blood levels should also be considered, particularly if indicated by diuretic therapy, etc. In addition, take into consideration the patient's age, pulmonary status, and whether he or she is having an acute myocardial infarction. Early signs of digitalis toxicity (e.g., VPBs, sinus bradycardia, or increasing AV block) should be carefully checked. Furthermore, concomitant quinidine administration increases the digoxin level in patients taking both drugs. A similar effect occurs with other drugs including verapamil, amiodarone, and propafenone.

Definitive treatment of digitalis toxicity depends on the particular arrhythmia seen. In cases of minor arrhythmias (e.g., isolated VPBs, sinus bradycardia, first-degree or Wenckebach AV block) or AV junctional rhythms, stopping the digitalis and carefully observing the patient are usually adequate. More serious arrhythmias (e.g., prolonged ventricular tachycardia) may require suppression with an intravenous drug (lidocaine or procainamide). Potassium chloride should be given to raise the serum potassium level to well within normal limits. Patients with complete heart block from digitalis toxicity may require a temporary pacemaker to tide them over while the effect of the digitalis dissipates, particularly if they have symptoms of syncope, hypotension, or congestive heart failure. In other cases, complete heart block can be managed conservatively while the digitalis wears off.

Occasionally a patient will present with a large overdose of digitalis, taken either inadvertently or in a suicide attempt. In such cases the serum digoxin level will be markedly elevated and severe brady- or tachyarrhythmias may develop. In addition, massive digitalis toxicity may cause life-threatening *hyperkalemia* since the drug blocks the cell membrane mechanism that pumps potassium into the cells in exchange for sodium. Patients with a potentially lethal overdose of digitalis can be treated with a special digitalis-binding antibody (Digibind) given intravenously. A detailed account of the treatment of digitalis toxicity is given in selected references in the Bibliography.

Finally, it must be emphasized that electrical

cardioversion of arrhythmias in patients who have digitalis toxicity is extremely hazardous and may precipitate fatal ventricular tachycardia and fibrillation. Therefore you should not cardiovert electrically any patient who has PAT with block, atrial fibrillation, or atrial flutter and is suspected of having digitalis toxicity.

SERUM DIGOXIN LEVELS

The concentration of digoxin in the serum can be measured by means of radioimmunoassay. Therapeutic concentrations range from about 0.5 to 2 ng/ml in most laboratories. Concentrations exceeding 2 ng/ml are associated with a high incidence of digitalis toxicity. In ordering a test of digoxin level in a patient, it is important to recognize that therapeutic levels do not rule out the possibility of digitalis toxicity. Some patients, as mentioned, are more sensitive to digitalis. In other patients factors such as hypokalemia may produce digitalis toxicity despite a "therapeutic" serum level. Conversely, still other patients, particularly those in atrial fibrillation with a rapid ventricular response, will require *higher* levels of digitalis to control their ventricular rate. A high digoxin level therefore does not necessarily indicate digitalis

toxicity.* However, patients with high drug levels should be examined for evidence of digitalis excess, including extracardiac symptoms (e.g., gastrointestinal symptoms) and all the cardiac effects that have been discussed. (A spuriously high digoxin level may be obtained if blood is drawn within a few hours of when the last dose of the drug was given.)

DIGITALIS TOXICITY AND DIGITALIS EFFECT

Do not confuse digitalis toxicity (which refers to the arrhythmias and conduction disturbances produced by this drug) with digitalis effect. *Digitalis effect* (Fig. 10-1) refers to the distinct scooping of the ST-T complex seen in some patients taking digitalis. The presence of digitalis effect does not imply digitalis toxicity.

---

*The need for potentially toxic doses of digoxin to control the ventricular rate in atrial fibrillation has been obviated by the availability of other drugs (beta blockers, calcium-channel blockers) and AV nodal ablation procedures (Chapter 13).

REVIEW

Digitalis toxicity can produce almost any arrhythmia and all degrees of AV heart block. The following arrhythmias are commonly seen:

1. Ventricular ectopy (VPBs)—isolated at first, often followed by ventricular bigeminy (a VPB following each normal beat); fatal ventricular tachycardia and ventricular fibrillation can occur if digitalis toxicity is not recognized and treated
2. Bidirectional ventricular tachycardia—resembling conventional ventricular tachycardia, except that each successive beat in any lead points in the opposite direction
3. AV junctional (nodal) rhythms
4. Sinus bradycardia and SA block—actual sinus arrest may also occur
5. PAT with block (paroxysmal atrial tachycardia with AV block)
6. AV heart block—first-degree initially, sometimes followed by second-degree Wenckebach-type block; complete heart block or other types of AV dissociation may also be seen
7. Atrial fibrillation or flutter with a slow ventricular response—occurring when patients with atrial fibrillation or flutter are given excess digitalis; the ventricular rate may slow to 50 beats/min or less and will often become very regular

Atrial fibrillation or atrial flutter with a rapid ventricular response rarely occurs as a result of digitalis toxicity. Furthermore, digitalis toxicity does not produce bundle branch blocks.

Factors such as renal failure, hypokalemia, hypercalcemia, hypomagnesemia, hypoxemia, old age, and acute myocardial infarction may predispose to digitalis toxicity. Concomitant administration of drugs (e.g., quinidine, verapamil, amiodarone, or propafenone) will also increase serum digoxin levels.

Digitalis toxicity should not be confused with digitalis effect. *Digitalis effect* refers to the shortening of the QT interval and scooping of the ST-T complex produced by *therapeutic* doses of digitalis.

Questions

1. Name three factors that can potentiate digitalis toxicity.

True or false (2 to 5):
2. VPBs are a frequent manifestation of digitalis toxicity.
3. Atrial fibrillation with a rapid ventricular response is a common manifestation of digitalis toxicity.
4. Left bundle branch block may result from digitalis toxicity.
5. AV Wenckebach may be caused by digitalis toxicity.

Answers

1. Hypokalemia, hypomagnesemia, hypoxemia, acute myocardial infarction, renal failure. (See pages 204 and 206 for other answers.)
2. True.
3. False.
4. False.
5. True.

17

Cardiac Arrest

In the preceding chapters the major disorders of heart rhythm and atrioventricular conduction have been systematically discussed. In this chapter, instead of considering entirely new ECG patterns, we will review some earlier topics, placing them in a special clinical perspective. The subject of this chapter is the recognition of life-threatening arrhythmias causing cardiac arrest. By definition, *cardiac arrest occurs when the heart stops contracting effectively and ceases to pump blood.*

CLINICAL ASPECTS OF CARDIAC ARREST

The patient in cardiac arrest loses consciousness within seconds and may even have a seizure as a result of inadequate blood flow to the brain. Irreversible brain damage will usually occur within 4 minutes and sometimes sooner. Furthermore, shortly after the heart stops pumping, spontaneous breathing will also cease *(cardiopulmonary arrest)*. Sometimes, when respirations stop first (primary respiratory arrest), cardiac activity will stop very shortly thereafter.

The diagnosis of cardiac arrest should be made clinically even before the patient is connected to an electrocardiograph. Cardiac arrest should be recognized immediately in any unconscious person who does not have palpable pulses. The patient is quickly examined by trying to feel for pulses in the carotid arteries. The patient in cardiac arrest will become cyanotic (bluish gray) from lack of oxygenated blood. No heart tones will be audible

with a stethoscope on the chest, and the blood pressure will, of course, be unobtainable. The arms and legs become cool; and if the brain becomes severely hypoxic, the pupils will be fixed and dilated. Seizure activity may occur. *The absence of pulses in an unconscious person, however, is the major diagnostic sign of cardiac arrest.*

When cardiac arrest is recognized, cardiopulmonary resuscitation (CPR) must be started without delay. In capsule form the initial treatment of any cardiac arrest consists of the following four steps:

A—Establish an *Airway.*

B—Breathe for the patient, either by mouth-to-mouth or mouth-to-mask methods or by manually compressing a bag-valve device, forcing air into the patient's nose or mouth.

C—Maintain *Circulation* by external cardiac compression.

D—Begin *Definitive* treatment with whatever intravenous or endotracheal drugs are needed, with electrical defibrillation, or with a temporary pacemaker when indicated.*

The details of CPR, including drug dosages, use of defibrillators, and so on, lie outside the scope of this book but are discussed in selected references in the Bibliography. In this chapter we will

---

*While the above steps are being done by two or more rescuers, another rescuer can raise the patient's lower extremities to a vertical position and keep them elevated for 15 seconds. This may help return blood to the central circulation.

concentrate primarily on the particular ECG patterns seen during cardiac arrest and on the clinical implications of these patterns.

It is important to reemphasize that initial treatment of the patient with ventilation and external cardiac compression should **never** *be delayed while the patient is being connected to the electrocardiograph.*

THE THREE BASIC ECG PATTERNS IN CARDIAC ARREST

There are only three basic ECG patterns seen with cardiac arrest, and they have been mentioned in earlier chapters. Cardiac arrest may be associated with

1. Ventricular tachyarrhythmia (ventricular fibrillation or a sustained type of ventricular tachycardia)
2. Ventricular standstill (brady-asystolic patterns)
3. Electromechanical dissociation

We will review each of these patterns briefly, stressing the clinical implications of each in cardiac arrest (Figs. 17-1 to 17-7).

Ventricular Tachyarrhythmia

With ventricular fibrillation (VF) the ventricles do not contract but instead twitch rapidly in a completely ineffective way. There is no cardiac output, and the patient loses consciousness within seconds. The characteristic ECG pattern, with its unmistakable, fast, oscillatory waves, is illustrated in Figure 17-1.

Of the three basic ECG patterns seen with cardiac arrest, ventricular fibrillation is the most common one initially encountered. It may appear spontaneously, although (as noted in Chapter 14) it often is preceded by another ventricular arrhythmia (usually ventricular tachycardia or premature ventricular beats). Figure 17-2 shows a ventricular tachycardia degenerating into ventricular fibrillation during cardiac arrest.

Treatment of ventricular fibrillation was mentioned in Chapter 12. The patient should be immediately defibrillated with a DC *defibrillator (cardioverter)* used to administer a direct-current electric shock to the heart by means of paddles placed on the chest wall (p. 184). Figure 17-7, *D,* shows an example of a successful defibrillation.

Success in defibrillating any patient depends on a number of factors. The single most important is haste. The less delay in defibrillation, the greater will be the chance of succeeding.

Sometimes it may take repeated shocks before the patient is successfully defibrillated. In other cases all attempts will fail. Finally, it is important to stress that external cardiac compression must be continued between attempts at defibrillation.

Cardiac arrest may also occur during a sustained episode of other ventricular tachyarrhythmias, including conventional ventricular tachycardia, torsade de pointes, and ventricular flutter. These arrhythmias are described in Chapter 14.*

Ventricular Standstill (Brady-Asystolic Patterns)

Ventricular standstill and escape rhythms are described in Chapter 11. The normal pacemaker of the heart is the sinus node, located in the right atrium. Failure of the sinus node to function (sinus arrest) will lead to ventricular standstill (asystole) if no other subsidiary pacemaker (for example, in the atria, AV junction, or ventricles) takes over. In such cases the ECG will record a *straight-line pattern* (Fig. 17-3), indicating asystole. Whenever you encounter a straight-line pattern, confirm this finding in at least two leads and check to see that all the electrodes are connected to the patient. They often become disconnected during a cardiac arrest, leading to the mistaken diagnosis of asystole. Very low-amplitude ventricular fibrillation may also mimic a straight-line pattern.

Treatment of ventricular standstill also requires continued external cardiac compression. Sometimes spontaneous cardiac electrical activity will resume. Drugs such as epinephrine may help stimulate cardiac activity. Patients with refractory ventricular standstill will require a *temporary pace-*

---

*At this point it should be mentioned that sometimes a strong thump on the sternum with your fist ("thump version") may itself restore normal rhythm during cardiac arrest, particularly if the patient is having a sustained run of VT or VF (Fig. 14-13) and a defibrillator is not immediately available.

Fig. 17-1. Ventricular fibrillation causing cardiac arrest.

VT   VF

Fig. 17-2. Ventricular tachycardia *(VT)* and ventricular fibrillation *(VF)* recorded during cardiac arrest. The rapid sine-wave type of ventricular tachycardia seen here is sometimes referred to as ventricular flutter.

Fig. 17-3. Complete ventricular standstill (asystole) producing a straight-line pattern during cardiac arrest.

maker, inserted (in an emergency) at the bedside. As described in Chapter 20, a temporary *transvenous* pacemaker is a special catheter wire electrode inserted usually through a vein into the right ventricle and connected to a battery outside the body. More recently a new type of *external* temporary pacemaker has become commercially available that does not require intravenous insertion. This noninvasive *(transcutaneous)* pacemaker utilizes special electrodes that are pasted on the chest wall.

Not uncommonly with ventricular standstill, you will also see occasional QRS complexes appearing at infrequent intervals against the back-ground of the basic straight-line rhythm. These are *escape beats* (Chapter 11) and represent the attempt of intrinsic cardiac pacemakers to restart the heart's beat. Examples of escape rhythms with underlying ventricular standstill are shown in Figure 17-4. In some cases the escape beats are narrow (Fig. 17-4, *A*), indicating their origin from either the atria or the AV junction. In others they come from a lower focus in the ventricles, producing a slow *idioventricular* rhythm with wide QRS complexes (Fig. 17-4, *B*). The term *"brady-asystolic pattern"* is sometimes used to describe this type of cardiac arrest ECG.

Escape beats should not be confused with *arti-*

Fig. 17-4. Escape rhythms with underlying ventricular standstill: **A,** junctional escape rhythm with narrow QRS complexes; **B,** idioventricular escape rhythm with wide QRS complexes. Treatment should include the use of intravenous atropine and, if needed, sympathomimetic drugs in an attempt to speed up these bradycardias, which cannot support the circulation. If hyperkalemia is present, it should be vigorously treated.

Fig. 17-5. External cardiac compression artifact. External cardiac compression during a resuscitation produces artifactual ECG complexes (marked *C*), which may be mistaken for actual QRS complexes.

Fig. 17-6. Sinus rhythm with electromechanical dissociation (EMD). Although the ECG showed sinus rhythm, the patient had no pulse or blood pressure. In this case the EMD was a result of depressed myocardial function after a cardiac arrest.

facts produced by external cardiac compression. Artifacts are large wide deflections that occur with each compression (Fig. 17-5). Their size varies with the strength of the compression, and their direction varies with the lead in which they appear (negative in leads I, II, III, and aV_F, positive in aV_R and aV_L).

Electromechanical Dissociation

The large majority of patients with cardiac arrest will have an ECG showing either a sustained ventricular tachyarrhythmia or ventricular standstill (sometimes with escape beats). Occasionally, however, the ECG of a patient in cardiac arrest will, surprisingly, continue to show identifiable QRS complexes at a normal rate. The actual heart rhythm in such cases may be a sinus rhythm, AV junctional (nodal) rhythm, or heart block. However, despite the presence of regularly recurring QRS complexes and even P waves on the ECG, the patient is unconscious and does not have a palpable pulse or blood pressure. In other words, the patient has cardiac electrical activity but no mechanical heart contractions to effectively pump blood. The term *"electromechanical dissociation"* (EMD) is used in such cases.*

Electromechanical dissociation can arise in a number of settings. When assessing a patient with EMD, it is essential to consider the potentially *reversible* causes first. One of the most important of these is pericardial effusion (in which the pericardial sac fills up with an excessive amount of blood or other fluid). The term *"pericardial tamponade"* is used to describe situations in which pericardial effusion produces decreased cardiac output and ultimately cardiac arrest. Pericardial tamponade can be treated by removal of some of the fluid from the pericardial sac with a special needle inserted through the chest wall (pericardiocentesis). Because the disease process is primarily extracardiac (involving the pericardium), the ECG generally shows relatively normal electrical activity, despite the impaired mechanical function of the heart.

Tension pneumothorax and massive pulmonary embolism are two other potentially reversible causes of EMD.

Probably the most common setting in which EMD occurs is when the myocardium has sustained severe generalized injury that may not be reversible (e.g., myocardial infarction). In such cases, even though the heart's conduction system may be intact enough to generate a relatively normal rhythm, there is not sufficient functional ventricular muscle to respond to this electrical signal with an adequate contraction. Sometimes the myocardial depression will be temporary and reversible ("stunned myocardium") and the patient may respond to resuscitative efforts.

Figure 17-6 shows an example of EMD in which there was sinus rhythm and yet no pulse or blood pressure following severe depression of myocardial contractility.

• • •

The three basic ECG patterns seen with cardiac arrest—ventricular tachyarrhythmia, ventricular standstill, and electromechanical dissociation—have all been described separately. However, during the course of resuscitating any patient, it is not unusual to see two or even all three of these ECG patterns at different times during the arrest.

Figure 17-7 shows an actual "ECG history" of a cardiac arrest.

CLINICAL CAUSES OF CARDIAC ARREST

Cardiac arrest associated with any of the three electrical mechanisms—ventricular tachyarrhythmia, ventricular standstill, electromechanical dissociation—may occur in numerous settings. It can be due to any type of organic heart disease. For example, a patient with an acute MI may have cardiac arrest for several reasons. Myocardial ischemia and increased ventricular irritability may precipitate ventricular fibrillation. Damage to the conduction system may result in ventricular standstill. Finally, electromechanical dissociation may occur with extensive myocardial injury. Occasionally, actual rupture of the infarcted ventricular wall will

---

"Pulseless electrical activity" (PEA) is another term sometimes used to describe cardiac arrest with frank EMD or a profound brady-asystolic pattern.

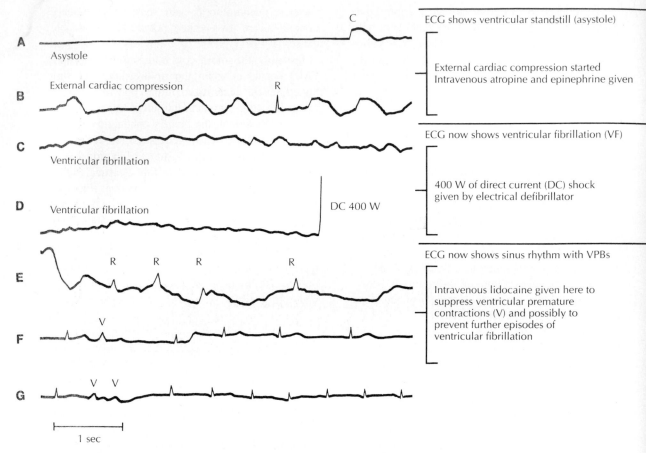

Fig. 17-7. ECG history of cardiac arrest and successful resuscitation. The left panel shows the ECG sequence during an actual cardiac arrest. The right panel shows sequential therapy appropriate for the different ECG patterns. Initially, **A** and **B**, there is ventricular standstill (asystole) with a straight-line pattern, treated by external cardiac compression. This is followed, **C** and **D**, by ventricular fibrillation. Sinus rhythm, **E** to **G**, appears after defibrillation with 400 watt-seconds of direct-current electric shock. *C* is an external cardiac compression artifact; *R* is an R wave from the spontaneous QRS complex; *V* is a ventricular premature beat.

occur, leading to fatal pericardial tamponade.

Cardiac arrest also occurs in people with electrical instability associated with *chronic* heart disease (e.g., due to previous infarction, valvular abnormalities, hypertension, or a cardiomyopathy).

Lightning strike or electric shock may produce cardiac arrest in normal hearts. Cardiac arrest may also occur during surgical procedures, particularly in patients with underlying heart disease. Drugs such as epinephrine can produce ventricular fibrillation. Quinidine and related drugs may lead to torsade de pointes (described in Chapter 14). Excessive digitalis can also lead to fatal ventricular arrhythmias. Recognition of arrhythmias caused by digitalis intoxication was discussed in the preceding chapter. Other cardiac drugs may precipitate sustained ventricular tachyarrhythmias through their so-called *proarrhythmic effect* (Chapter 14).

The recreational use of *cocaine* has been reported to precipitate fatal arrhythmias.

Marked elevation of the serum potassium concentration (Chapter 10) will ultimately lead to cardiac arrest with ventricular standstill. A very low serum potassium may cause fatal ventricular arrhythmias, especially in a patient taking digitalis, quinidine, or related drugs. Hypokalemia (as well as hypomagnesemia and hypocalcemia) can also lead to torsade de pointes.

Brady-asystolic cardiac arrest may occur with the sick sinus syndrome (Chapters 11 and 18) or with high-degree AV block (Chapter 15).

Following successful resuscitation of the patient in cardiac arrest, an intensive search for the cause must be started. Serial 12-lead ECGs, along with serum cardiac enzymes, will help diagnose MI. A complete blood count and serum electrolytes should be obtained, as well as an arterial blood gas sample. A portable chest x-ray unit and, if needed, an echocardiograph machine can be brought to the bedside. In addition, a pertinent medical history should be obtained from every available source, with particular attention to drug usage (digitalis, antiarrhythmic therapy, etc.) and previous cardiac problems.

Sudden Cardiac Death

The term *"sudden cardiac death"* is used to describe the situation in which an individual who sustains a cardiac arrest and is not resuscitated dies instantly or within an hour or so of the development of symptoms. Over 400,000 such deaths occur each year in the United States. Sudden cardiac death is most often initiated by a ventricular tachyarrhythmia, less commonly by a brady-asystolic mechanism or electromechanical dissociation. Most individuals have underlying structural heart disease. An estimated 20% of patients with acute myocardial infarction die suddenly before reaching the hospital. Another important substrate for sudden death is severe left ventricular dysfunction from previous myocardial infarctions or dilated cardiomyopathy. Other patients with sudden cardiac death have structural heart disease with valvular abnormalities or myocardial disease, associated for example with aortic stenosis, hypertrophic cardiomyopathy, or myocarditis. Some patients with sudden cardiac death do not have mechanical cardiac dysfunction, but may have intrinsic electrical instability due to the long QT syndrome (predisposing to torsade de pointes), Wolff-Parkinson-White preexcitation syndrome, or conduction system disease causing heart block. As noted, drugs such as cocaine or cardiac antiarrhythmic agents may induce arrhythmias. Finally, a small subset of individuals will sustain a cardiac arrest without any demonstrable structural or electrophysiologic abnormality. The identification and management of patients at high risk of sudden death are central areas of investigation in cardiology today. The role of *implantable cardioverter-defibrillator* (ICD) devices in preventing sudden death in high risk patients is mentioned in Chapter 14.

REVIEW

Cardiac arrest occurs when the heart stops pumping blood. The diagnosis should be made clinically even before the patient is connected to an electrocardiograph. The major clinical sign of cardiac arrest is the absence of pulses in an unconscious patient.

Cardiac arrest may be associated with one or more of the following ECG patterns:

1. *Ventricular tachyarrhythmia*—ventricular fibrillation, sustained typical ventricular tachycardia, torsade de pointes, or ventricular flutter
2. *Ventricular standstill (asystole)* or *brady-asystolic pattern*—a straight-line pattern, sometimes with interruptions by junctional or ventricular escape beats

3. *Electromechanical dissociation* (EMD)—regularly recurring QRS complexes, sometimes even P waves, not associated with a palpable pulse or blood pressure; usually caused by diffuse myocardial injury, although may be due to pericardial tamponade, tension pneumothorax, or massive pulmonary embolism

During the course of resuscitating a patient, you may see any or all of the above patterns.

In addition, the ECG with cardiac arrest may show distinctive *artifacts* caused by external cardiac compression (wide complexes that should not be mistaken for the intrinsic electrical activity of the heart).

The term *"sudden cardiac death"* is used in reference to individuals who sustain a cardiac arrest and, unless resuscitated, die instantly or within an hour or so of the development of symptoms.

Questions

1. Would a pacemaker be of any value in treating a patient with cardiac arrest and electromechanical dissociation (EMD)?

2. The rhythm strip below was obtained from a patient during the course of a cardiac arrest and attempted resuscitation.
   a. What is the basic rhythm?
   b. What are the complexes marked X caused by?

3. Name four drugs that can produce cardiac arrest associated with a sustained ventricular tachyarrhythmia (ventricular fibrillation, typical ventricular tachycardia, torsade de pointes, or ventricular flutter).

Answers

1. No. By definition, patients with EMD have relatively normal electrical activity. The problem is that this electrical activity is not associated with adequate mechanical (pumping) action, usually because of diffuse myocardial injury, pericardial tamponade, or severe loss of intravascular volume. A pacemaker would not be of help in this situation because the patient already has adequate electrical stimulation.

2. a. Idioventricular escape rhythm.
   b. External cardiac compression artifacts.

3. Digitalis (digoxin), epinephrine, cocaine, quinidine (also procainamide, disopyramide, and other antiarrhythmic agents).

18

Bradycardias and Tachycardias
REVIEW AND DIFFERENTIAL DIAGNOSIS

The preceding chapters have described the major arrhythmias and AV conduction disturbances. There are numerous ways of classifying these abnormalities. In this section we will simply divide them into two groups, bradycardias and tachycardias, and discuss the differential diagnosis of each group.

BRADYCARDIAS (BRADYARRHYTHMIAS)

We have discussed several arrhythmias and conduction disturbances associated with a slow heart rate. The term *"bradycardia"* or *"bradyarrhythmia"* is used to refer to arrhythmias and conduction abnormalities producing a heart rate of less than 60 beats/min. Fortunately, the differential diagnosis of a patient with a relatively slow pulse is relatively simple since there are only a handful of possible causes. Specifically, we can cite five general classes of bradyarrhythmias.

Sinus bradycardia. Sinus bradycardia (Fig. 18-1) is sinus rhythm with a rate less than 60 beats/min.* Each QRS is preceded by a P wave, and the P wave is negative in lead aV_R and positive in lead II, indicating that the sinus node is the pacemaker. Some patients may have a sinus bradycardia as slow as 40 beats/min or less.

---

*Some cardiologists reserve the term *"sinus bradycardia"* for rates less than 50 beats/min.

Sinus bradycardia, including SA block
AV junctional (nodal) escape rhythm
AV heart block (second or third degree) or AV dissociation
Atrial fibrillation or flutter with a slow ventricular response
Idioventricular escape rhythm

Sinus bradycardia may be related to a decreased firing rate of the sinus node pacemaker cells or to actual SA block. The most extreme example is sinus node arrest (Chapter 11).

AV junctional (nodal) escape rhythm. With a slow junctional escape rhythm (Fig. 18-2) either the P waves (appearing just before or just after the QRS complexes) are *retrograde* (inverted in lead II, upright in lead aV_R) or else no P waves are apparent if the atria and ventricles are stimulated simultaneously.

AV heart block (second or third degree) or AV dissociation (Fig. 18-3). A slow ventricular rate of 60 beats/min or less (even as low as 20 beats/min) is the rule with complete heart block, owing to the slow intrinsic rate of the junctional or idioventricular pacemaker. Patients with second-degree AV block (either Wenckebach or

SINUS BRADYCARDIA

Fig. 18-1. Sinus bradycardia with a slight sinus arrhythmia.

AV JUNCTIONAL ESCAPE RHYTHM

Monitor lead

Fig. 18-2. The heart rate is about 43 beats/min. The baseline between complexes is perfectly flat (no P waves evident).

COMPLETE HEART BLOCK

Fig. 18-3. The atrial (P wave) rate is about 80 beats/min. The ventricular (QRS) rate is about 43 beats/min. The atria and ventricles are beating independently, so the PR intervals are variable. The QRS complex is wide because the ventricles are paced by an idioventricular pacemaker.

ATRIAL FIBRILLATION WITH A SLOW VENTRICULAR RATE

Fig. 18-4. Regularization and excessive slowing of the ventricular rate with atrial fibrillation are sometimes a sign of digitalis toxicity or AV node disease. (See Chapter 16).

Mobitz type II) also often have a bradycardia because of the dropped beats (Fig. 15-3 and Table 15-1). Isorhythmic AV dissociation, which may be confused with complete heart block (p. 198), is also often associated with a heart rate of less than 60 beats/min.

Atrial fibrillation or flutter with a slow ventricular rate (Fig. 18-4). Paroxysmal atrial fibrillation is generally associated with a rapid ventricular rate, which may become excessively slow (less than 50 to 60 beats/min) because of drug effects or toxicity (beta blocker, calcium channel blocker, digitalis) or if the patient has underlying disease of the AV junction. In such cases the ECG shows the characteristic atrial fibrillatory waves with a slow ventricular (QRS) rate. The f waves may be very fine and easily overlooked. (A very slow regularized ventricular response in atrial fibrillation suggests the presence of complete AV heart block; see page 195.)

Idioventricular escape rhythm. In some cases, when the SA nodal and AV junctional escape pacemakers fail to function, a very slow pacemaker in the ventricular conduction (His-Purkinje) system may take over. This rhythm is referred to as an idioventricular escape rhythm. The rate is usually very slow (<45 beats/min) and the QRS complexes are wide without any preceding P wave (Fig. 17-4, *B*). Hyperkalemia should always be excluded in such cases.

Clinical Significance

With the exception of sinus bradycardia, which is a common normal variant, the other bradycar-

dias are often abnormal.* The possible causes of AV junctional rhythms, heart block, and atrial fibrillation were all described in earlier chapters.

It is worth reemphasizing that in any patient with a bradycardia the possibility of digitalis excess or other drug toxicity (e.g., beta blockers and calcium-channel blockers) must always be considered. Hyperkalemia (Chapter 10) is another important, reversible, life-threatening cause of bradyarrhythmias.

Patients with any of the bradycardias just discussed may have no symptoms or may complain of light-headedness or fainting due to decreased cardiac output. Treatment depends on the particular arrhythmia and the clinical setting.

To summarize: Most patients with an ECG heart rate of less than 60 beats/min will have one of the five following classes of arrhythmia: sinus bradycardia (including SA block), AV junctional rhythm, AV heart block (or AV dissociation), atrial fibrillation or flutter with a very slow ventricular rate, or idioventricular escape rhythm.†

TACHYCARDIAS (TACHYARRHYTHMIAS)

At the opposite end of the spectrum from bradyarrhythmias are the tachycardias (i.e., rhythm disturbances producing a heart rate faster

---

*Occasionally normal subjects (in particular, athletes with increased vagal tone at rest) may show a slow junctional rhythm or even AV Wenckebach.

†Bradycardia can also be due to a wandering atrial pacemaker (Fig. 18-15).

than 100 beats/min). They can be usefully divided into two general groups: (1) those with a "narrow" (normal) QRS duration and (2) those with a "wide" QRS duration. "Narrow"complex tachycardias are almost invariably *supra*ventricular (i.e., the focus of stimulation is within or *above* the AV junction). Wide-complex tachycardias, by contrast, are either ventricular or supraventricular with aberrant ventricular conduction (SVT with aberrancy).

There are four major classes of supraventricular tachyarrhythmia*: sinus tachycardia, paroxysmal supraventricular tachycardia (PSVT), atrial flutter, and atrial fibrillation. With each the site(s) of cardiac activation is located in either the atria or the AV junction (node), above the ventricles (hence *supra*-ventricular). This is in contrast to ventricular tachycardia; with VT the stimulus starts in the ventricles themselves. VT is simply a run of three or more consecutive premature ventricular depolarizations (Fig. 14-5). The QRS complexes are always wide because the ventricles are not being stimulated simultaneously. The rate of VT is usually between 100 and 200 beats/min. With supraventricular arrhythmias, by contrast, the ventricles are stimulated normally (simultaneously) so the QRS complexes are narrow (unless a bundle branch block is also present).

The first step in analyzing a tachyarrhythmia is to look at the width of the QRS complex in all 12 leads if possible. If the QRS is narrow (0.1 sec or less), you are dealing with some type of supraventricular arrhythmia and not VT. If it is very wide (particularly if greater than 0.14 sec), then consider the rhythm to be VT unless it can be proved otherwise.

*Be aware of the following possible confusion in terminology. "Supraventricular tachycardia" (SVT) is used in two related, but different, ways by cardiologists. First, it refers most generally to any arrhythmia originating in the AV junction, atria, or sinus node area, above the ventricular conduction system (hence *supra*ventricular). Second, it is also used more specifically to refer to a class of often paroxysmal tachycardias (PSVTs) originating in the atria or AV junction (node) regions. These PSVTs, due to reentry or automaticity, are distinct from sinus tachycardia, atrial fibrillation, or atrial flutter. (See Chapter 12 for a discussion of PSVTs.)

Differential Diagnosis of Narrow-Complex Tachyarrhythmias

The four most common types of supraventricular tachyarrhythmias have already been mentioned. They are (1) sinus tachycardia, (2) PSVT, (3) atrial fibrillation, and (4) atrial flutter.

The characteristics of these tachyarrhythmias have been described in previous chapters. *Sinus tachycardia* in adults generally produces a heart rate between 100 and 180 beats/min. Finding a narrow-complex tachycardia with a rate of 180 beats/min or more in a resting individual means that you are almost certainly dealing with one of the other three types of arrhythmias mentioned above. *PSVT* and *atrial fibrillation* can be distinguished on the basis of their regularity. PSVT due to AV nodal reentry or a concealed bypass tract is usually an almost perfectly regular tachycardia with a ventricular rate between 140 and 250 beats/min. Atrial fibrillation, on the other hand, is distinguished by its irregularity. Remember that with rapid atrial fibrillation (Fig. 18-5) the fibrillatory waves may not be clearly visible but the diagnosis of atrial fibrillation can be made in almost every case by noting the absence of P waves and the haphazardly irregular QRS complexes. *Atrial flutter* (Fig. 18-6) is characterized by sawtooth flutter waves between QRS complexes. However, when atrial flutter is present with 2:1 block (e.g., when the atrial rate is 300 beats/min and the ventricular response is 150 beats/min), the flutter waves are often hidden. Atrial flutter at 150 beats/min therefore can be confused with sinus tachycardia, PAT, or atrial fibrillation (Fig. 18-7). Atrial fibrillation can be excluded because atrial flutter with 2:1 conduction is generally very regular.

Nevertheless, the differential diagnosis of sinus tachycardia, PSVT with a ventricular rate of about 150 beats/min, atrial fibrillation, and atrial flutter can be a problem (Fig. 18-7). One way of separating them is to use carotid sinus massage*

*However, carotid sinus massage is not without risks, particularly in elderly patients. For details regarding this maneuver as well as the use of adenosine in the differential diagnosis of tachycardias, readers should consult the Bibliography.

ATRIAL FIBRILLATION WITH A RAPID VENTRICULAR RATE

Fig. 18-5. The ventricular rate is about 130 beats/min (13 QRS cycles/6 sec). Notice the characteristic haphazardly irregular rhythm.

Fig. 18-6. This strip shows atrial flutter with 2:1 conduction.

(CSM). Pressure on the carotid sinus produces a reflex increase in vagal tone. The effects of CSM on sinus tachycardia, reentrant-types of PSVT, and atrial flutter are described next.

Sinus tachycardia. Sinus tachycardia generally slows slightly with CSM. However, there is usually no abrupt change in heart rate. Slowing of sinus tachycardia may make the P waves more evident. Sinus tachycardia generally begins and ends gradually, not abruptly.

PSVT. PSVT due to AV nodal reentry or reentry involving a concealed bypass tract usually has an *all-or-none* response to CSM. In successful cases it will break suddenly and sinus rhythm resumes following the CSM (Fig. 12-7). Other times CSM will have no effect and the tachycardia continues at the same rate.

Atrial flutter. CSM will often increase the degree of block in atrial flutter, converting flutter with a 2:1 response to 3:1 or 4:1 flutter with a ventricular rate of 100 or 75 beats/min. Slowing of the ventricular rate will unmask the characteristic flutter waves (Fig. 13-2).*

• • •

Another type of SVT, which has not yet been discussed, is *multifocal atrial tachycardia* (MAT). An example is shown in Figure 18-8. This tachyarrhythmia is characterized by multiple ectopic

---

*An increase in the degree of AV block also may occur with paroxysmal atrial tachycardia (PAT), unmasking a rapid series of nonconducted P waves (at a rate of usually less than 250 beats/min).

Fig. 18-7. Four look-alike narrow-complex tachyarrhythmias: **A,** sinus tachycardia; **B,** atrial fibrillation; **C,** PSVT due to AV nodal reentrant tachycardia; **D,** atrial flutter with 2:1 block. When the ventricular rate is about 150 beats/min, these four arrhythmias may be difficult if not impossible to tell apart with the standard ECG. In this example of sinus tachycardia the P waves can barely be seen. Notice that the irregularity of the atrial fibrillation is very subtle. In PSVT the rate is quite regular without evident P waves here. In atrial flutter the F waves cannot be seen clearly in this lead.

MULTIFOCAL ATRIAL TACHYCARDIA

Fig. 18-8. The P waves show variable shapes or variable PR intervals, or both.

foci stimulating the atria. To diagnose it requires finding three or more P waves with different shapes. The PR intervals often will vary. MAT is usually seen in patients with chronic lung disease. Because the ventricular rate is irregular and rapid, this arrhythmia is most likely to be mistaken for atrial fibrillation. It is due to multiple atrial pacemakers firing in an unpredictable fashion. This is in contrast to classical PAT (Chapter 12), which typically involves only a single ectopic pacemaker in the atrium.

Differential Diagnosis of VT

Tachycardias are divided into SVTs and VT. This section describes the differential diagnosis of VT. A tachycardia with widened QRS complexes indicates two possible diagnoses. The first and more important is VT, a potentially life-threatening arrhythmia. As noted, VT is a consecutive run of three or more VPBs at a rate generally between 100 and 200 or more beats/min. It is usually very regular. The second possible cause of a tachycardia with widened QRS complexes is so-called "SVT with aberration." The term *aberration* simply means that some abnormality in ventricular activation is present and causing widened QRS complexes.

Differential Diagnosis of "SVT with Aberrancy" from VT

There are only two major mechanisms for aberrancy with an SVT: (1) a bundle branch block and (2) the Wolff-Parkinson-White (WPW) preexcitation syndrome.

SVT with a bundle branch block. If a patient has any of the SVTs just listed in association with a bundle branch block, the ECG will show a wide-complex tachycardia that may be mistaken for VT. For example, a patient with sinus tachycardia, atrial fibrillation, atrial flutter, or PSVT who also has a right or left bundle branch block will have a wide-complex tachycardia.

Figure 18-9, *A*, shows atrial fibrillation with a rapid ventricular response occurring with LBBB. Figure 18-9, *B*, shows an example of VT. There is an obvious resemblance, making it difficult to

Fig. 18-9. Supraventricular tachycardia with bundle branch block compared to ventricular tachycardia. **A,** Atrial fibrillation with LBBB pattern. **B,** Ventricular tachycardia. It may be difficult and sometimes impossible to tell from the ECG if a patient has actual ventricular tachycardia or a supraventricular tachycardia with bundle branch block.

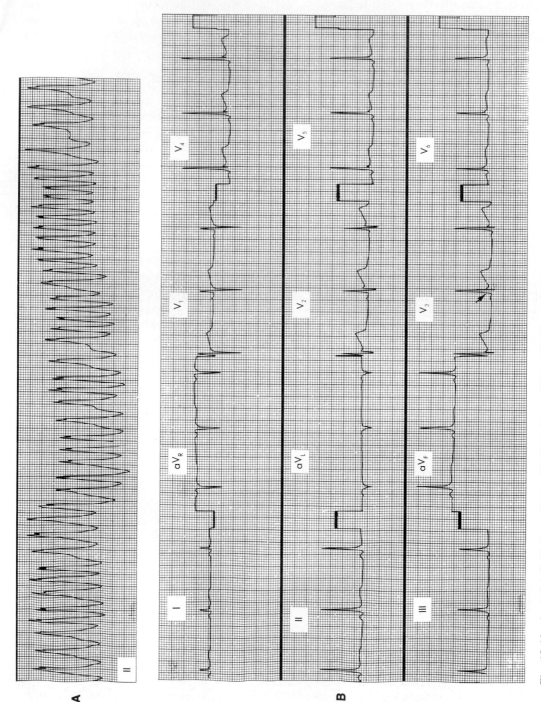

Fig. 18-10. A, Atrial fibrillation with the Wolff-Parkinson-White (WPW) syndrome may lead to a wide-complex tachycardia with very rapid rate. Notice that some of the **RR** intervals are less than 0.20 second. Irregularity is due to the underlying atrial fibrillation. **B,** After conversion to sinus rhythm the classic WPW triad is visible but subtle: relatively short PR interval, wide QRS, and delta wave (*arrow* in V_3).

tell these patterns apart. The major distinguishing feature is the irregularity of the atrial fibrillation as opposed to the regularity of the VT. However, in some cases VT may be irregular.

It is important to recognize that in some cases of SVT with aberration, the bundle branch block is seen only during the episodes of tachycardia. Such rate-related bundle branch blocks are said to be "tachycardia dependent."

SVT with the WPW syndrome. The second mechanism responsible for a wide-complex tachycardia is SVT with the WPW syndrome (described in Chapter 10). As noted, patients with WPW pre-excitation have an accessory pathway connecting the atria and ventricles, thus bypassing the AV node. Such patients are especially prone to a re-entrant type of PSVT with narrow (normal) QRS complexes for the reason described on page 136. Sometimes, however, particularly if atrial fibrillation (or atrial flutter) develops, a wide-complex tachycardia may result from conduction down the bypass tract at very high rates. This kind of wide-complex tachycardia will also, obviously, mimic VT. An example of WPW with atrial fibrillation is shown in Figure 18-10.

The diagnosis of WPW with atrial fibrillation should be strongly suspected if you encounter a wide-complex tachycardia that is irregular and has a very high rate (very short RR intervals). In particular, RR intervals of 0.20 second or less are rarely seen with conventional atrial fibrillation and are also rare with ventricular tachycardia. They relate to the ability of the bypass tract (in contrast to the AV node) to conduct impulses in extremely rapid succession (Fig. 18-10, *A*).

The recognition of WPW with atrial fibrillation is of considerable clinical importance because digitalis may, paradoxically, enhance conduction down the bypass tract. As a result the ventricular response may increase, leading to possible myocardial ischemia and in some cases to ventricular fibrillation. A similar effect has been reported with intravenous verapamil.

• • •

An important clue that may be helpful in differentiating SVT with aberrancy from VT is the *presence of AV dissociation.*

Recall from Chapter 15 that with AV dissociation, as implied by the name, the atria and ventricles are paced from separate sites. Some patients with VT, though not all, will also have AV dissociation; in other words, the ventricles will be paced from an *ectopic* site at a rapid rate while the atria continue to be paced independently by the sinus node. In such cases you may be able to see P waves occurring at a slower rate than the rapid wide QRS complexes shown in Figure 18-11. Some of the P waves may be "buried" in the QRS complexes and be difficult to discern. Unfortunately, only a minority of the cases of VT clearly show AV dissociation. Therefore the absence of AV dissociation does not exclude VT. However, the presence of AV dissociation in a patient with wide complexes at a rapid rate is virtually diagnostic of VT. Furthermore, in some cases of VT with AV dissociation the sinus node may transiently "capture" the ventricles, producing a beat with normal QRS duration ("capture beat") or a "fusion beat," in which case the sinus beat and

Fig. 18-11. Ventricular tachycardia with AV dissociation. Note the independent atrial rate (75/ min) and ventricular rate (140/min).

Fig. 18-12. Ventricular tachycardia with AV dissociation producing fusion *(F)* and capture *(C)* beats. Leads I and II were recorded simultaneously.

Fig. 18-13. A, Ventricular tachycardia at a rate of about 200/min. Notice the wide QRS complexes with a right bundle branch block morphology. The QRS in leads V_1 and V_2 shows a broad R wave. **B,** Following conversion to sinus rhythm the pattern of an underlying anterior wall MI and ventricular aneurysm becomes evident. There are Q waves and ST elevations in V_1 to V_3 with ischemic T wave inversions in V_4 to V_6. Note also that the QRS is wide (0.12 sec) due to an intraventricular conduction delay with left axis deviation (left anterior hemiblock). The prominent negative P waves in V_1 are due to left atrial abnormality.

ventricular beat will coincide to produce a hybrid complex. Figure 18-12 illustrates capture and fusion beats in a case of VT.

What other ECG clues are helpful in distinguishing SVT with aberration from VT? Over the years cardiologists have tried to develop more precise criteria to assist in this important differential diagnosis. Unfortunately, no single criterion has proved absolutely reliable. Nevertheless, in addition to AV dissociation, the following will be helpful if you are confronted with a wide-complex tachycardia (see Josephson and Wellens, 1990):

1. When the QRS shape resembles a right bundle branch block pattern, an rsR' in V_1 suggests SVT and a single broad R wave or a qR, QR, or RS complex in that lead suggests VT (Fig. 18-13).
2. When the QRS shape resembles a left bundle branch block pattern, a prominent R wave in V_1 or V_2 or a QR complex in V_6 strongly suggests VT.

At times it will be impossible to distinguish reliably between VT and SVT with aberration from the 12-lead ECG. In such cases clinical judgment must be used. For example, if the patient is hypotensive the tachycardia is generally treated as VT (Table 18-1). On the other hand, remember that not all patients with VT will be hypotensive. Indeed, occasional patients may have minimal symptoms at rest when they are in sustained VT.

*Caution: Intravenous verapamil should **not** be used in undiagnosed wide-complex tachycardias. It may cause hemodynamic collapse in patients with VT or atrial fibrillation with WPW.*

Clinical Significance

As mentioned earlier, the first question to ask in looking at any tachyarrhythmia is whether the rhythm is VT. If sustained VT is present, then emergency treatment is required (as described in Chapter 14).

With narrow-complex tachycardias therapy depends on the clinical setting. In the case of sinus tachycardia (Chapter 11) treatment is directed at the underlying cause (e.g., fever, sepsis, congestive heart failure, or hyperthyroidism). Similarly

Table 18-1. Major Tachyarrhythmias: Simplified Classification

Narrow QRS Complexes	Wide QRS Complexes
Sinus tachycardia	Ventricular tachycardia
Paroxysmal supraventricular tachycardias (PSVTs)*	Supraventricular tachycardia (SVT) with aberration due to either Bundle branch block or Wolff-Parkinson-White (WPW) preexcitation
Atrial flutter	
Atrial fibrillation	

*The three most common types of PSVTs are AV nodal reentrant tachycardias (AVNRTs), bypass tract tachycardias, and atrial tachycardias (including PAT and MAT) as discussed in Chapter 12. Other *non*paroxysmal supraventricular tachycardias may also occur, including types of so-called *incessant* atrial, junctional, and bypass tract tachycardias. (See the Bibliography for further details.)

treatment of multifocal atrial tachycardia (MAT) should be directed at the underlying problem (usually chronic pulmonary disease). Electrical cardioversion should *not* be used with MAT, since it is not likely to be helpful and may induce serious ventricular arrhythmias. The calcium-channel blocker verapamil can be used to slow the ventricular response in MAT.

In assessing any patient with a narrow-complex tachycardia, you should ask the following three key questions related to the effects of the tachycardia on the heart and circulation:

1. Is the patient's blood pressure abnormally low? In particular, is he or she in shock?
2. Is the patient having an acute myocardial infarction or severe ischemia?
3. Is the patient in severe congestive heart failure (pulmonary edema)?

Patients in any one of these categories with atrial fibrillation or atrial flutter with a rapid ventricular response or a PSVT will require emergency therapy. If they do not respond promptly to initial drug administration, then electrical cardioversion should be considered.

Another major question to ask about any patient having a tachyarrhythmia (or any arrhythmia for that matter) is whether digitalis or other drugs are

Fig. 18-14. Brady-tachy (sick sinus) syndrome. This rhythm strip shows a narrow-complex tachycardia (probably atrial flutter) followed by a sinus pause, an AV junctional escape beat *(J)*, and then sinus rhythm.

Fig. 18-15. Wandering atrial pacemaker. Notice the variability of P wave configuration in this lead II rhythm strip caused by shifting of the pacemaker site. (From Phibbs B: *The cardiac arrhythmias,* ed 3, St Louis, 1978, Mosby.)

part of the therapeutic regimen. Some arrhythmias (e.g., PAT with block) may be digitalis-toxic rhythms, disturbances for which electrical cardioversion is contraindicated (Chapter 16). Finally, in the case of atrial fibrillation you should check to see whether the arrhythmia is chronic or acute, remembering that, although chronic atrial fibrillation can sometimes be converted to normal sinus rhythm, the rhythm often reverts to atrial fibrillation (Chapter 13).

SICK SINUS SYNDROME AND THE BRADY-TACHY SYNDROME

We continue this discussion of arrhythmias with an interesting group of patients who have bradyarrhythmias sometimes alternating with episodes of tachyarrhythmias.

The term *"sick sinus syndrome"* has been coined to describe patients with sinus node dysfunction that causes marked sinus bradycardia, sinus arrest, or junctional escape rhythms, which may lead to symptoms of light-headedness and even syncope.

In some patients with the sick sinus syndrome these bradycardia episodes are interspersed with paroxysms of tachycardia (usually atrial fibrillation or flutter or some type of PSVT). Sometimes the bradycardia will occur immediately after spontaneous termination of the tachycardia. The term *"brady-tachy syndrome"* has been used to describe this subset of patients with sick sinus syndrome who have tachyarrhythmias as well as bradyarrhythmias (Fig. 18-14).

Diagnosis of the sick syndrome and, in particular, the brady-tachy variant often requires monitoring the patient's heartbeat over several hours or even days. A single ECG strip may be normal or may reveal only the bradycardic or tachycardic episode. Only long-term monitoring may reveal both sides of these patients' problem: the bradyarrhythmias and tachyarrythmias. The use of continuous ECG (Holter) monitoring in evaluating elderly patients with light-headedness and syncope has shown a surprisingly high frequency of sick sinus syndrome. Treatment generally requires a permanent pacemaker to prevent sinus arrest and antiarrhythmic drugs to control the tachycardias after the pacemaker has been inserted.

WANDERING ATRIAL PACEMAKER

We conclude this chapter with another arrhythmia, wandering atrial pacemaker, that has not been mentioned to this point because it is somewhat difficult to classify. As shown in Figure 18-15, wandering atrial pacemaker is characterized by multiple P waves of varying configuration with a relatively normal or slow heart rate. This pattern reflects shifting of the pacemaker between the sinus node, other atrial sites, and sometimes the AV junction. Wandering atrial pacemaker may be seen in a variety of settings. Occasionally it develops in normal subjects (particularly during sleep), and it may be seen with digitalis excess or other drug toxicity, with the sick sinus syndrome, as well as with a variety of different types of organic heart disease.

Wandering atrial pacemaker is distinct from MAT (p. 221), another arrhythmia with multiple different P waves. In wandering atrial pacemaker the rate is normal or slow. In MAT it is rapid.

REVIEW

Arrhythmias can be grouped into *bradycardias* (with a heart rate *slower* than 60 beats/min) and *tachycardias* (with a heart rate *faster* than 100 beats/min).

Bradycardias include five major classes of arrhythmias or conduction disturbances: (1) sinus bradycardia, (2) AV junctional (nodal) escape rhythm, (3) second- or third-degree heart block or AV dissociation, (4) atrial fibrillation (or flutter) with a slow ventricular rate, and (5) idioventricular escape rhythm. Digitalis or other drug toxicity or hyperkalemia may be responsible for any of these arrhythmias.

Tachycardias can be subdivided into (1) those with *narrow* QRS complexes and (2) those with *wide* QRS complexes. The narrow-QRS tachycardias are always *supraventricular* in origin—the four most common being (1) sinus tachycardia, (2) paroxysmal supraventricular tachycardias (PSVTs), including atrial tachycardias and reentrant tachycardias involving the AV node or a concealed bypass tract, (3) atrial fibrillation, and (4) atrial flutter. Carotid sinus massage is sometimes helpful in differentiating these arrhythmias at the bedside. Tachycardias with a wide QRS complex may be either *ventricular* or any of the SVTs associated with a *bundle branch block* or *Wolff-Parkinson-White* mechanism.

The term *"sick sinus syndrome"* describes patients with sinus node dysfunction who may have a marked sinus bradycardia, sometimes with sinus arrest or slow junctional rhythms, that causes light-headedness or syncope. Some patients with the sick sinus syndrome will have periods of tachycardia alternating with the bradycardia *(brady-tachy syndrome)*.

Wandering atrial pacemaker is an arrhythmia characterized by multiple P waves of varying configuration, usually with a relatively normal or slow heart rate.

Questions

1. Answer the following questions concerning the lead II rhythm strip below:
   a. Is the rate regular or irregular?
   b. Are there discrete P waves present?
   c. What is this arrhythmia?

2. What is the most likely diagnosis for the arrhythmia shown below (monitor lead)?

3. A 40-year-old man complaining of occasional palpitations with a fast heartbeat is found to have runs of narrow QRS complex tachycardia at a rate of 200 beats/min without evident P waves on his Holter monitor tracing. The rhythm is very regular. What is the most likely diagnosis?

4. What is the cause of the bradycardia in the rhythm strip shown below?

5. Name three readily reversible causes of bradycardia.

Answers

1. a. Irregular.
   b. No. The baseline shows an irregular fibrillatory pattern.
   c. Atrial fibrillation.
2. VT.
3. PSVT (Probably AV nodal reentrant tachycardia; see Chapter 12).
4. Sinus rhythm with 2:1 AV block, with a sinus rate of about 74/min and a ventricular rate of about 37/min.
5. Digitalis toxicity, hyperkalemia, excess beta blocker, excess calcium-channel blocker, hypothyroidism.

19

Limitations and Uses of the ECG

Throughout this book the clinical uses of the ECG have been stressed. The purpose of this review chapter is threefold: to underscore some important *limitations* of the ECG, to reemphasize its *utility,* and to review some common *pitfalls* in its interpretation.

IMPORTANT LIMITATIONS OF THE ECG

Like most clinical tests, the ECG yields both *false-positive* and *false-negative* results. A false-positive result is an apparently abnormal ECG in a normal subject. For example, prominent precordial voltage may occur in the absence of LVH (p. 67). Furthermore, Q waves may occur as a normal variant and therefore do not always indicate heart disease (p. 100). False-negative results, on the other hand, occur when the ECG fails to show evidence of some cardiac abnormality. For example, some patients with acute MI may not show diagnostic ST-T changes, or patients with severe coronary artery disease may not show diagnostic ST depressions during stress testing.

The diagnostic accuracy of any test is determined by the percentages of these false-positive and false-negative results. The *sensitivity* of a test is a measure of the percentage of patients with a particular abnormality that can be identified by an abnormal test result. For example, a test with 100% sensitivity will not have any false-negative results. The more false-negative results, the less sensitive is the test. The *specificity* of a test is a measure of the percentage of false-positive results.

The more false-positive test results, the less specific is the test. As just noted, both the sensitivity and the specificity of the ECG in diagnosing a variety of conditions, including MI, are limited. It is of great importance for those in clinical practice to be aware of these diagnostic limitations.

Following is a list of a number of important problems that *cannot* be excluded simply because the ECG is normal or shows only nondiagnostic abnormalities:

1. Prior MI
2. Acute MI*
3. Severe coronary artery disease
4. Significant LVH
5. Significant RVH
6. Intermittent arrhythmias (e.g., ventricular tachycardia and complete heart block)
7. Acute pulmonary embolism
8. Pericarditis

UTILITY OF THE ECG: SPECIAL CASES

Despite these important limitations, the ECG is an extremely useful test that often helps in the diagnosis of specific cardiac conditions and sometimes can aid in the evaluation and management of general medical problems (e.g., electrolyte dis-

---

*The pattern of acute MI may also be masked in patients with LBBB, Wolff-Parkinson-White preexcitation, or electronic pacemakers.

orders). The following list indicates some of the particular areas in which the ECG may be helpful:

1. Significant hyperkalemia, a life-threatening electrolyte abnormality, virtually always produces ECG changes, beginning with T wave peaking, loss of P waves, QRS widening, and finally asystole (p. 126).
2. LVH is seen in most patients with critical aortic stenosis.
3. Most patients with a moderate to large atrial septal defect have an RBBB pattern.
4. Persistent ST elevations several weeks after an MI should suggest a ventricular aneurysm.
5. Low QRS voltage in a patient with elevated central venous pressure (distended neck veins) and sinus tachycardia suggests possible pericardial tamponade. Sinus tachycardia with electrical alternans (Fig. 10-13) is virtually diagnostic of pericardial effusion with tamponade.
6. ST segment elevation in a right chest precordial lead (e.g., V_{4R}) in a patient with acute inferior infarction indicates associated right ventricular ischemia or infarction (Chapter 8). Clinically, check carefully for elevated central venous pressure on examination of the neck veins.
7. Frequent VPBs and nonspecific ST-T changes, particularly in a younger patient, should prompt a search for mitral valve prolapse.
8. Unexplained atrial fibrillation should prompt a search for occult mitral valve disease, hyperthyroidism, or cardiomyopathy.
9. A new S_1Q_{III} or RBBB pattern, particularly in association with sinus tachycardia, should suggest the possibility of pulmonary embolism (Fig. 10-15).
10. Most patients with acute MI show diagnostic ECG changes (new Q waves, ST elevations, hyperacute T waves, ST depressions, or T wave inversions). However, in the weeks and months following an acute MI these changes may become less apparent and, in some cases, disappear.
11. The combination of left atrial enlargement and right ventricular hypertrophy on the ECG should suggest the possibility of mitral stenosis (Fig. 19-1).
12. The combination of low voltage and sinus bradycardia should suggest possible hypothyroidism.
13. The combination of low voltage and poor precordial R wave progression is commonly seen with chronic lung disease.
14. The triad of relatively low limb lead voltage, prominent precordial voltage, and poor R wave progression suggests an underlying cardiomyopathy (Fig. 10-17).

COMMON APPLICATIONS OF THE ECG

The ECG may also provide very important clues in the evaluation of certain major medical problems, such as syncope, coma, shock, and weakness.

Syncope

Fainting can result from primary cardiac factors as well as from a variety of noncardiac causes. The noncardiac causes include neurogenic mechanisms (e.g., vasovagal attacks), orthostatic (postural) hypotension, and brain dysfunction from vascular insufficiency or metabolic derangements (alcohol, hypoglycemia). The primary cardiac causes, in turn, can be divided into mechanical obstructions (aortic stenosis, primary pulmonary hypertension, atrial myxoma) and electrical problems (brady- or tachyarrhythmias).

Patients with syncope resulting from aortic stenosis generally show LVH on their resting ECG. Primary pulmonary hypertension is most common in young and middle-aged adult women. The ECG generally shows RVH. The presence of frequent VPBs may be a clue to intermittent ventricular tachycardia. A severe bradycardia (usually from heart block or sick sinus syndrome) in a patient with syncope constitutes the Stokes-Adams syndrome (p. 197). In some cases serious arrhythmias can be detected only when long-term monitoring is performed. Syncope in a patient with ECG evidence of bifascicular block (e.g., RBBB with left

Fig. 19-1. This ECG from a 45-year-old woman with severe mitral stenosis shows multiple abnormalities. The rhythm is sinus tachycardia. Right axis deviation and a tall R in V_1 indicate right ventricular hypertrophy. The prominent biphasic P wave in V_1 indicates left atrial enlargement. The tall P waves in lead II may indicate concomitant right atrial enlargement. There are also nonspecific ST-T changes and an incomplete right bundle branch block. The combination of right ventricular hypertrophy and left atrial enlargement is highly suggestive of mitral stenosis.

LEAD REVERSAL

ARM ELECTRODES
REVERSED

CORRECTED ECG

Fig. 19-2. Whenever the QRS axis is unusual, it is important to check for limb lead reversal. Most commonly, the left and right arm electrodes get switched so lead I shows a negative P wave and negative QRS complex.

anterior hemiblock) should prompt a search for intermittent second- or third-degree heart block or other arrhythmias. Syncope in patients taking quinidine may be caused by drug toxicity. These persons often have QT prolongation or prominent U waves and thus are prone to torsade de pointes, which may occur despite the fact that the serum quinidine level is in the "therapeutic" or even "subtherapeutic" range.

Selected patients with *unexplained syncope* may benefit from invasive electrophysiologic testing. During these studies placement of intracardiac electrodes permits more direct and controlled assessment of sinus node function, atrioventricular conduction, and the susceptibility to sustained ventricular or supraventricular tachycardia.

Coma

An ECG should be obtained on all comatose patients. If coma is from MI with subsequent cardiac arrest, diagnostic ECG changes related to the infarct are usually seen. Subarachnoid hemorrhage may cause very deep T wave inversions (Fig. 9-10), simulating the changes of MI. Patients with coma associated with hypercalcemia will often show a short QT interval. Myxedema coma generally presents with ECG evidence of sinus bradycardia and low voltage. Widening of the QRS in a comatose patient should raise the possibility of drug overdose (phenothiazine or tricyclic antidepressant) or hyperkalemia.

Shock

An ECG should be obtained promptly on any patient with severe hypotension, because MI is a major cause of shock (cardiogenic shock). In other cases hypotension may be caused or worsened by a brady- or tachyarrhythmia. Finally, some patients with shock from noncardiac causes (e.g., hypovolemia, diabetic ketoacidosis) may have myocardial ischemia and sometimes infarction as a consequence of their initial problem.

Weakness

An ECG may be helpful in evaluating patients with unexplained weakness. Elderly patients, in particular, may have relatively "silent" MIs with minimal or atypical symptoms, such as the onset of fatigue or general weakness. A prolonged QT interval may be an important clue to unsuspected hypocalcemia, an important metabolic cause of weakness. Hypokalemia may cause weakness along with characteristic ECG changes, including ST depression, T wave flattening, and prominent U waves. In other cases weakness may result from a brady- or tachyarrhythmia. Digitalis toxicity (with or without arrhythmias) may also cause weakness or fatigue.

COMMON PITFALLS IN ECG INTERPRETATION

You can minimize errors in interpreting ECGs by taking care to analyze *all* the points listed on p. 250 in Chapter 21. Many mistakes result from the failure to be systematic (see box). Other mistakes result from confusing ECG patterns that are "look-alikes."

Some common pitfalls (caveats) in ECG interpretation are listed in the accompanying box.

1. Limb lead reversal. Inadvertent reversal of limb lead electrodes will cause diagnostic confusion unless recognized and corrected. For example (Fig. 19-2), reversal of the left

---

SOME IMPORTANT REMINDERS

Check standardization

Exclude limb lead reversal (negative P with negative QRS in lead I suggests left/right arm electrode switch)

Look for hidden P waves: AV block, blocked APBs, PAT with block

Regular narrow-complex tachycardia at about 150/min: consider atrial flutter with 2:1 block, in addition to PSVT and sinus tachycardia

Group beating (clusters of QRS complexes): think of Wenckebach vs blocked APBs

Wide QRS with short PR: consider Wolff-Parkinson-White

Wide QRS without P waves or with AV block: think of hyperkalemia and right arm electrodes will cause an apparent rightward QRS axis shift as well as an abnormal P wave axis that simulates an ectopic atrial or junctional rhythm. *As a general rule, when lead I shows a negative P wave and a negative QRS, suspect that the left and right arm electrodes have been reversed.*

2. Failure to check standardization. Many an ECG is mistakenly thought to show "high" or "low" voltage when, in fact, the voltage is normal but the standardization marker is set at $2\times$ or $\frac{1}{2}\times$.

3. Atrial flutter with 2:1 block (conduction). This is one of the most commonly missed diagnoses. The rhythm is often misdiagnosed as either sinus tachycardia (mistaking part of a flutter wave for a P wave) or paroxysmal supraventricular tachycardia (PSVT). *When you see a narrow-complex tachycardia with a ventricular rate of about 150/min, you should always consider atrial flutter.* (See Figure 13-2.)

4. Coarse atrial fibrillation vs atrial flutter. When the fibrillatory waves are prominent (coarse), the rhythm is commonly mistaken for atrial flutter. However, with atrial fibrillation the ventricular rate is completely erratic and the atrial waves are not exactly consistent from one segment to the next. With pure atrial flutter, on the other hand, even when the ventricular response is variable, the atrial waves will be identical from one moment to the next. (See Figure 19-3.)

5. Wolff-Parkinson-White (WPW) pattern. The WPW pattern is frequently mistaken for a bundle branch block, hypertrophy, or infarction pattern because the preexcitation results in a wide QRS and may cause increased QRS voltage, T wave inversions, and pseudoinfarction Q waves. (See Figure 10-20.)

6. Isorhythmic AV dissociation vs complete heart block. With isorhythmic AV dissociation the sinus and AV node pacemakers become "desynchronized" and the QRS rate

is the same as or slightly faster than the P wave rate (p. 198). With complete heart block the atria and ventricles also beat independently but the ventricular rate is much slower than the atrial (sinus) rate. Isorhythmic AV dissociation is usually a minor arrhythmia, although it may reflect conduction disease or drug toxicity (e.g., digitalis, cardizem, verapamil, and beta blockers). Complete heart block is always a major arrhythmia and generally requires pacemaker therapy.

7. Normal-variant vs pathologic Q waves. Do not forget (p. 100) that Q waves may be a normal variant as part of QS waves in leads aV_R, aV_L, aV_F, III, V_1, and occasionally V_2. Small q waves, as part of qR waves, may occur in leads I, II, III, aV_L, and aV_F as well as the left chest leads (V_4 to V_6). These "septal" q waves are less than 0.04 second in duration. On the other hand, small pathologic Q waves may be overlooked because they are not always very deep. In some cases it may not be possible to state definitively whether or not a Q wave is pathologic.

8. AV Wenckebach. In this commonly missed diagnosis an important clue is the appearance of "group beating" (p. 193). The QRS complexes become grouped in clusters due to the intermittent failure of AV nodal conduction.

9. Hidden ("buried") P waves. These may lead to mistakes in the diagnosis of a number of arrhythmias, including blocked atrial premature beats (APBs), PAT with block, and second- or third-degree (complete) AV block. It is important therefore to search in the ST segment and T wave for buried P waves. (See Figure 16-3.)

10. Multifocal atrial tachycardia (MAT) and atrial fibrillation. These are often confused because the ventricular response in both is usually rapid and irregular. With MAT, look for multiple different P waves. With atrial fibrillation, be careful not to mistake

Fig. 19-3. Atrial flutter with variable block, **A,** and coarse atrial fibrillation, **B,** are often confused. Notice that with atrial fibrillation the ventricular rate is completely erratic and the atrial waves are not identical from segment to segment.

the sometimes "coarse" fibrillatory (f) waves for actual P waves.

11. Left bundle branch block (LBBB). This may be mistaken for infarction because it is associated with poor R wave progression and often ST segment elevation in the right chest leads.

12. U waves. These are sometimes overlooked. While small U waves are a physiologic finding, large U waves (which may be apparent in only the chest leads) are sometimes an important marker of hypokalemia or drug toxicity (e.g., quinidine). Large U waves may be associated with increased risk of *torsade de pointes,* a potentially lethal ventricular arrhythmia (Chapter 14).

13. Severe hyperkalemia. Severe hyperkalemia must always be considered immediately in any patient with an unexplained wide QRS, particularly if P waves are not apparent. Delay in making this diagnosis has proved fatal, because severe hyperkalemia may lead to asystole and cardiac arrest while the clinician is waiting for the report from the laboratory. (See Figures 10-5 to 10-7.)

REVIEW

Like most clinical tests, the ECG yields both *false-positive* and *false-negative* diagnoses. For example, not all Q waves indicate MI and not all subjects with actual MI show diagnostic ECG changes. A normal or nondiagnostic ECG also does not exclude LVH, RVH, intermittent life-threatening brady- or tachyarrhythmias, pulmonary embolism, or pericarditis. Despite these limitations in sensitivity and specificity, the ECG does have major uses in a wide range of clinical situations. Besides its obvious utility in assisting cardiac diagnosis, the ECG may also help in evaluating some major medical problems (e.g., syncope, coma, weakness, and shock).

Questions

1. Which arrhythmias can lead to syncope (fainting)?

True or false (2 and 3)
2. A normal exercise tolerance test excludes significant coronary disease.
3. The more false-positive results associated with a particular test, the less sensitive the test is.

Answers

1. Syncope can be caused by a variety of brady- or tachyarrhythmias (including excessive sinus bradycardia, or sinus arrest, AV junctional escape rhythms, second- or third-degree AV block, atrial fibrillation with an excessively slow ventricular response, ventricular tachycardia, paroxysmal supraventricular tachycardias, and atrial fibrillation or flutter with a rapid ventricular response).
2. False.
3. False. The sensitivity of a test is a measure of how well the test can detect a given abnormality. False-positive results (abnormal results in normal subjects) will lower the specificity, not the sensitivity, of the test.

20

Pacemakers: An Introduction

The purpose of this chapter is to provide a brief overview of an important aspect of clinical electrocardiography, electronic cardiac pacemakers. Particular emphasis will be placed on the different types of pacemakers, major indications for pacemaking, and recognition of pacemaker malfunction.

DEFINITIONS

Pacemakers are battery-powered devices designed to electrically stimulate the heart. Pacemakers are used primarily when the patient's own heart rate is excessively slow (bradyarrhythmias, Chapter 18).

A pacemaker has two major components: a battery, which serves as the power source, and wire electrodes attached to the heart chamber(s) being stimulated.

There are two basic types of pacemakers: *temporary* and *permanent (implanted)*. With temporary pacemakers the pacing wire is connected to a battery outside the body. With long-term implanted pacemakers, the battery is inserted subcutaneously, usually under the chest wall. With both, the pacemaker wire is usually threaded through a vein into the right ventricular cavity so the pacemaker electrode can then stimulate the endocardium of the right ventricle (Fig. 20-1). Occasionally, *epicardial* pacemaker wires are used. In such cases the wire is sewn directly into the epicardium of the left or right ventricle and the battery is implanted under the skin of the abdomen. In addi-

tion to ventricular pacing, atrial pacing can be performed. Finally, many patients benefit from a *dual-chambered* pacemaker with electrodes in both the right atrium and the right ventricle.

PACEMAKER ECG PATTERNS

When a ventricular pacemaker fires, it produces a sharp vertical deflection (pacemaker spike) followed by a QRS complex (representing depolarization of the ventricle). Can you predict what the ECG will show with a functioning right ventricular pacemaker? The ECG should show an LBBB pattern (Fig. 7-8). Recall that the pacemaker is stimulating the right ventricle initially and therefore left ventricular depolarization will be delayed. Figures 7-8 and 20-2 show examples of typical pacemaker tracings. The vertical line preceding each QRS complex is the pacemaker spike, followed by a wide QRS with an LBBB morphology (QS in V_1 and wide R wave in V_6). What pattern would you predict with an epicardial pacemaker stimulating the left ventricle? It would be that of an RBBB.

An atrial pacemaker will produce a spike followed by a P wave (Fig. 20-3).

PACEMAKER BATTERIES

There are a variety of battery units that can be used to power implanted pacemakers. Early pacemaker batteries used mercury-zinc cells. However, because of their relatively short life span, these units have been supplanted by lithium batteries,

239

Fig. 20-1. Implanted pacemaker generator (battery) with a wire electrode inserted through the left subclavian vein into the right ventricle.

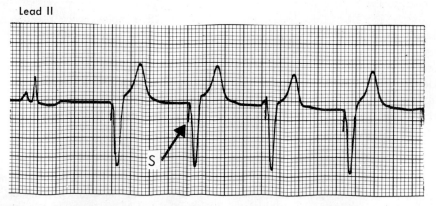

Fig. 20-2. Pacemaker beats. The first QRS is from a normal sinus beat. It is followed by four pacemaker beats. Notice the pacemaker spike *(S)* preceding each paced beat. Pacemaker beats are wide and resemble bundle branch block beats.

Fig. 20-3. With the pacemaker electrode placed in the right atrium, notice the pacemaker spike *(A)* before each P wave. The QRS is normal since there is no electronic ventricular pacemaker.

which may last for 5 or more years. As the power cells of conventional pacemakers wear out, the pacemaker rate will usually start to slow.

VENTRICULAR PACING: FIXED-RATE AND DEMAND PACEMAKERS

There are two modes of pacemaker function: (1) *fixed rate* and (2) *demand*. A fixed-rate pacemaker is one that fires at a specific preset rate, regardless of the patient's own heart rate. The earliest pacemakers were fixed-rate devices. Contemporary pacemakers are demand units. A demand pacemaker literally functions "on demand," that is, only when the patient's heart rate falls below a preset value. Therefore, a demand pacemaker has two distinct aspects: first, a *sensing* mechanism designed so the pacemaker will be inhibited when the heart rate is adequate; second, a *pacing* mechanism designed to trigger the pacemaker when no intrinsic QRS complexes occur within a predetermined period. By contrast, fixed-rate pacemakers lack a sensing mechanism. Demand units can be temporarily converted to fixed-rate mode by placing a special magnet on the chest wall over the battery. The magnet test is routinely performed when the pacemaker rate is being checked. Present-day demand-type pacemakers are also "programmable"; that is, the pacing rate can be adjusted once the pacemaker is implanted (p. 243). Adjustment of rate is accomplished by placing a special telemetry device on the chest wall to allow communication with the pacemaker.

Demand ventricular pacemakers usually are QRS (R wave) inhibited. They emit pulses only when the spontaneous heart rate falls below the escape rate of the pacemaker (e.g., 70/min) (Figs. 20-4 and 20-5). They do not emit pulses when the patient's spontaneous heart rate is faster than the escape rate of the pacemaker. Each time a QRS-inhibited pacemaker senses a spontaneous QRS complex, formation of a pacemaker pulse is inhibited. Therefore these pacemakers show pacemaker spikes only when the spontaneous heart rate is slower than the escape rate of the pacemaker. The spikes appear before each QRS complex.

The QRS-inhibited pacemaker also has a *refractory* period (e.g., 0.4 sec) that begins whenever the pacemaker senses a QRS or emits a pulse (Fig. 20-6). During the refractory period the pacemaker cannot sense another R wave. However, if spontaneous ventricular beats or ventricular premature complexes occur during the refractory period, they will not be inhibited but appear on the ECG. The refractory period is followed by an *alert* period, during which the pacemaker can sense an R wave. If no QRS is sensed by the end of the alert period, the pacemaker emits another pulse (Fig. 20-6). However, if a spontaneous QRS occurs, the pacemaker will be recycled into another refractory period and then into another alert period.

DUAL-CHAMBER PACING

In dual-chamber pacemakers, electrodes are inserted into the right atrium as well as the right ventricle. With most models, the circuitry permits sensing and pacing in both the atrium and the ven-

Fig. 20-4. A ventricular demand (QRS-inhibited) pacemaker will emit an electronic pulse only when the intrinsic heart rate falls below the escape rate of the pacemaker.

Fig. 20-5. QRS-inhibited pacing (lead II). In beats *1* and *2* the rhythm is normal sinus. In beat *3* the ventricular rate has slowed slightly so a pacemaker spike appears at approximately the same time as the regular stimulus spreads through the ventricles from the AV node. The result is a fusion beat. In beats *4* through *12* the pacemaker is functioning because the patient's spontaneous heart rate has slowed below the pacemaker escape rate (in this case, 70/min). Then the patient's spontaneous ventricular rate becomes more rapid, so beat *13* is a fusion beat and beat *14* again shows regular sinus rhythm. P waves merge into QRS complexes in beats *4* through *7* and then reemerge in beats *12* to *14*.

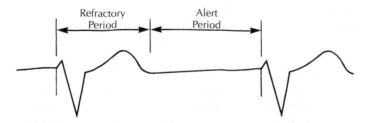

Fig. 20-6. During the refractory period a ventricular demand pacemaker will not sense any electrical activity. This is followed by the alert period. If no QRS is sensed by the end of the alert period, the pacemaker will emit an escape pulse.

DUAL CHAMBER (DDD) PACEMAKER FUNCTIONS

A. Atrial sensing
   Ventricular pacing

B. Atrial pacing
   Ventricular pacing

C. Atrial pacing
   Ventricular sensing

D. Atrial and ventricular
   sensing

Fig. 20-7. Dual-chamber (DDD) pacemakers sense and pace in both the atria and the ventricles. The pacemaker emits a stimulus (spike) whenever a native P wave or QRS is not sensed within some programmed time interval.

tricle. Thus the atrial lead is able to sense the patient's intrinsic P waves and, when the atrial rate becomes too slow, to stimulate the right atrium. The circuitry is designed to allow for a physiologic delay between atrial stimulation and ventricular stimulation. This *AV delay* (interval between the atrial pacemaker spike and the ventricular pacemaker spike) is analogous to the PR interval seen in normal conduction.

With the type of dual-chamber pacemaker that allows for both atrial sensing and atrial pacing as well as ventricular sensing and pacing, a variety of ECG patterns may be seen depending on the patient's intrinsic electrical activity. A schematic of these pacemaker patterns appears in Figure 20-7.

Dual-chamber pacing is helpful in maintaining physiologic timing between atrial systole and ventricular systole. When ventricular pacing alone is used, such physiologic timing will be lost. In some patients the loss of timed atrial contractions causes a marked reduction in cardiac output. Dual-chamber pacing will produce a significant improvement in the cardiac performance of these persons. It may also be desirable in selected patients

in permitting a physiologic increase in ventricular rate during exercise. For example, consider the patient with complete heart block and underlying sinus rhythm whose ventricular rate with a ventricular pacemaker is constant (e.g., 72/min) regardless of the atrial (P wave) rate. With a dual-chamber pacemaker the ventricular rate will be able to increase in tandem with the sinus rate during exercise, further increasing cardiac output.

Dual-chamber pacemakers, however, are not without their disadvantages. Atrial electrodes are more likely than ventricular electrodes to become dislodged. Furthermore, dual-chamber pacemakers may facilitate tachycardias in some patients. In addition, they are considerably more expensive than simple ventricular pacemakers. Finally, atrial sensing or pacing is obviously of no use in the setting of atrial fibrillation or atrial flutter.

PROGRAMMABILITY

In the early days of cardiac pacing the pacemaker rate was not adjustable once the unit had been inserted. A major advance was the introduction of programmable pacemakers, in which the pacemaker rate could be externally changed.* In modern pacemakers multiple other parameters in addition to the rate can be externally programmed—including the voltage of the pacemaker discharge, the sensitivity of the electrode to the intrinsic beats, the pacemaker refractory period, and the duration of the pacemaker spike. For discussion of multi-programmable pacemakers the reader is referred to the Bibliography.

INDICATIONS FOR CARDIAC PACING
Implanted (Permanent) Pacemakers

There are numerous indications for electronic pacemakers. As noted before, *the major reason for implanting a pacemaker is the presence of a symptomatic bradyarrhythmia.*

For example, permanent pacemakers are indicated in patients with syncope, light-headedness, weakness, or congestive failure caused by complete heart block, second-degree AV block, marked sinus bradycardia or sinus pauses (sick sinus syndrome), slow junctional rhythms, or atrial fibrillation or flutter with an excessively slow ventricular response.

Temporary Pacemakers

There are two major types of temporary pacemakers: transvenous and transcutaneous (p. 211). With *transvenous* pacemakers the battery is connected to a pacing electrode that has been threaded through a vein into the right ventricle. With *transcutaneous* temporary pacing specially designed electrodes are pasted on the chest wall. Although this technique is not successful in all patients and may cause some discomfort, it has proved highly useful and may spare the patient the need for inserting a transvenous pacemaker. (See page 211.)

Temporary pacemakers are often employed during cardiac emergencies (e.g., MI), when an extremely slow heart rate occurs. For example, they may be used immediately after open heart surgery or during cardiac arrest (Chapter 17), when the ECG shows asystole or a slow escape rhythm that does not respond to drug therapy. Occasionally they will be needed with digitalis or other drug toxicities causing profound bradycardia.

As noted, temporary (and permanent) pacemakers are usually employed when the heart rate is too slow. Rarely one will be implanted to treat a tachyarrhythmia (e.g., ventricular tachycardia). The use of temporary pacing in the treatment of atrial flutter is mentioned in Chapter 13.

PACEMAKER MALFUNCTION

Pacemaker malfunctions occur when either the sensing or the pacing function is impaired.

For example, when the pacemaker battery runs down, the pacemaker rate generally slows and *failure to sense* may occur. Failure to sense can be diagnosed by observing pacemaker spikes despite the patient's own adequate rate (Fig. 20-8). The most common causes of failure to sense are dislodgment of the pacemaker wire or excessive fibrosis around the tip of the pacing wire.

Pacemaker malfunction can also result from *failure to pace.* Failure to pace is diagnosed either by observing pacemaker spikes without subsequent QRS complexes (failure to "capture") (Fig. 20-9) or by the complete absence of pacemaker spikes despite an excessively slow heart rate (Fig. 20-10). Failure to pace can also be caused by dislodgment of the pacemaker wire or by fibrosis around the tip of the pacing wire. In such cases pacemaker spikes will occur without associated QRS complexes. In other cases (particularly with a broken electrode wire, a short-circuit in the pacing circuit, or electrical interference from the muscles of the chest wall) failure to pace will occur without any pacemaker spike.

Pacemaker malfunction in patients with temporary pacemakers should always prompt a search for loose connections between the battery and the pacing wire, a faulty battery, or a dislodged wire.

---

*Some newer rate-responsive pacemakers are designed with special sensors to detect muscle activity or other changes that correlate with increased activity. The pacing rate automatically increases with exercise to accommodate for the increased cardiac output.

Fig. 20-8. Pacemaker malfunction: failure to sense. Notice that after the first two paced complexes there is a series of sinus beats with first-degree AV block. Failure of the pacemaker unit to sense these intrinsic QRS complexes leads to inappropriate pacemaker spikes (*), which fall on T waves. Three of these spikes do not capture the ventricle because they occur during the refractory period of the cardiac cycle. (From Conover MH: *Understanding electrocardiography,* ed 4, St Louis, 1984, Mosby.)

Fig. 20-9. Pacemaker malfunction: failure to pace. Notice that beats *1, 3,* and *4* show the pacemaker spikes *(s)* and normally paced QRS complexes and T waves. The remaining beats show only pacemaker spikes. *R* represents the patient's slow spontaneous QRS complexes.

Fig. 20-10. Pacemaker malfunction: failure to pace (no pacemaker spikes). The underlying rhythm is second degree (2:1) AV block. Despite a slow heart rate, the pacemaker fails to function.

COMPLICATIONS OF PACEMAKER THERAPY

Pacemakers are not without potential harm. Therefore careful thought should be given before inserting a temporary or, particularly, a permanent pacemaker. Infection may occur at the pacemaker site. The electrode may perforate the ventricular wall. The pacemaker itself may cause serious arrhythmias. For example, certain dual-chamber pacemakers may initiate runs of supraventricular tachycardia ("endless loop" arrhythmias). Occasionally the pacemaker will also pace the muscles of the chest wall or the diaphragm, resulting in patient discomfort.

DIAGNOSIS OF MI WITH PACEMAKERS

The ECG diagnosis of MI may be difficult or impossible in patients with functioning pacemakers in which all beats are paced. In such cases (with a right ventricular electrode) the ECG will show an LBBB configuration. As described in Chapter 8, LBBB generally masks both the QRS and the ST-T changes of MI. Therefore, unless you see spontaneous QRS-T complexes, the diagnosis of acute or prior MI may not be possible from the ECG alone.

Finally, it is important to recognize that pacemakers may also produce ECG changes simulating MI. Following periods of electronic ventricular pacemaking the ECG may show deep noninfarctional T waves in the patient's spontaneous beats. These *post-pacemaker T wave inversions* can be mistaken for primary ischemic ST-T changes.

APPENDIX: PACEMAKER CODE

A three-position pacemaker code is often used to describe what a particular pacemaker's functions and mode of response are. As shown on page 247, the letter in the first position indicates the chamber(s) being paced—which may be the *atrium* (A), the *ventricle* (V), or *both* (D). The letter in the second position indicates the chamber(s) where sensing occurs—again the atrium (A), ventricle (V), or both (D). Finally, the letter in the third position refers to the mode of response of the pacemaker (p. 241). In the earlier, and in many current, pacemaker models the pacing mode was either *inhibited* (I) or *triggered* (T). The mode of response is labeled D *(double)* in the case of the newer, more advanced, *dual-chamber* pacemakers, which are engineered so the pacemaker responds to atrial electrical activity by delivering a ventricular spike (provided, or course, a spontaneous QRS has not already occurred). There is a fourth mode of response, designated R, which stands for *reverse*. A pacemaker in the reverse mode will pace during periods of tachycardia rather than bradycardia. Such pacemakers are used for their antiarrhythmic action. (See the Bibliography.)

The most widely used pacemakers today are still VVI units; that is, they are single-chamber pacemakers that both pace (V) and sense (V) exclusively in the *ventricle* and are *inhibited* (I) by the patient's own QRS complexes.

The most versatile pacemakers are DDD units. These are dual-chamber pacemakers that can pace the atrium or ventricle (D) and sense in the atrium or ventricle (D). In addition, the mode of response is double (D): atrial pacing can be inhibited by the patient's P waves and a ventricular pacer spike will be triggered by the patient's P waves if a native QRS does not appear within a preset time because of AV block.

Three-Position Pacemaker Code

Position	I	II	III
Category	Chamber(s) paced	Chamber(s) sensed	Mode of response(s)
Letters used	V—Ventricle	V—Ventricle	T—Triggered
	A—Atrium	A—Atrium	I—Inhibited
	D—Dual (A + V)	D—Dual (A + V)	D—Dual (T + I)*
	O—None	O—None	O—None
		O—None	

Double mode of response. This refers to dual-chamber pacemakers in which atrial pacing may be inhibited by the patient's own P waves and a ventricular spike may be triggered by the patient's P wave if AV block is present.

Sensing + Stimulation

The basic three-letter pacemaker code has been expanded to five letters, reflecting rapid advances in pacemaker electronics over the past decade. The fourth letter indicates the *programming* features of the pacemaker, including rate-responsiveness. (See footnote on page 244.) The fifth letter indicates *special antiarrhythmic features* that are available in certain pacemakers. Further discussion of these technical areas lies beyond the scope of this brief introduction.

REVIEW

Pacemakers are battery-powered devices used to stimulate the heart electrically, particularly in cases where the patient's own heart rate is excessively slow. When the pacemaker wire is attached to the right ventricular endocardium, the ECG will show an LBBB pattern as a result of delayed left ventricular stimulation. Each QRS will be preceded by a pacemaker spike. Cardiac pacing can be done in a *fixed-rate* or *demand* mode. Demand pacemakers are inhibited when the heart rate is faster than the escape rate of the pacemaker.

A temporary pacemaker is a unit with an external battery. Temporary pacing wires can be inserted during cardiac emergencies (for example, cardiac arrest caused by asystole or MI complicated by high-degree heart block or sinus arrest). An implanted permanent pacemaker, in which the battery is inserted subcutaneously, usually in the chest wall, is indicated for patients with symptomatic second- or third-degree AV block or other major bradyarrhythmias (such as sinus arrest or slow junctional escape rhythm) leading to inadequate cardiac output.

Dual-chamber (atrial and ventricular) pacemakers were developed to maintain physiologic timing between atrial and ventricular contractions, thus increasing cardiac output.

When the pacemaker battery starts to run down, the pacemaker rate will slow. Dislodgment of the pacemaker wire or excessive fibrosis around the tip of the wire can cause failure to sense or failure to pace. Pacing failure in permanent units can also be caused by electrode fracture, short-circuits, or electrical interference from skeletal muscles.

Pacemakers may obscure the ECG diagnosis of MI. Conversely, following electronic pacing of the ventricles, deep noninfarctional T wave inversions may appear in spontaneous QRS complexes *(post-pacemaker T wave pattern)*.

Questions

1. The major indication for *permanent* pacemakers is
   a. History of multiple prior MIs
   b. Symptomatic bradyarrhythmia
   c. Digitalis toxicity
   d. Ventricular bigeminy
   e. Paroxysmal supraventricular tachycardia (PSVT)
2. The following rhythm strip shows
   a. Failure to sense
   b. Failure to pace
   c. Normal pacemaker function with a VPB
   d. Failure to sense and pace

3. What does the following rhythm strip show?

Answers

1. b
2. b. This is an example of intermittent failure to pace, when the fourth pacemaker spike is not followed by a QRS. The two most common causes of failure to pace, with a pacemaker spike that does not capture, are dislodgment of the electrode wire and fibrosis around the pacing wire tip. Pacemaker failure may also occur in which no pacing spikes are seen (Fig. 20-10).
3. Atrial pacing. Notice the sharp pacemaker spike before each P wave followed by a normal QRS. (See Figure 20-3.)

21

How to Interpret an ECG

In Parts I and II the fundamentals of the normal ECG and the major abnormal patterns and arrhythmias were described. Part III is a collection of test questions to help you review these topics. We will conclude Part II with a brief summary of how systematically to approach any ECG.

ECG INTERPRETATIONS

Accurate interpretation of ECGs requires, above all, thoroughness and care. Therefore it is essential to develop a systematic method of reading ECGs that is applied in every case. Many of the most common mistakes are errors of omission: failure to note certain subtle but critical findings. For example, overlooking a short PR interval may result in missing the important diagnosis of the Wolff-Parkinson-White pattern. Marked prolongation of the QT interval, a potential precursor of torsade de pointes (Chapter 14) and sudden death, sometimes goes unnoticed. These and other common pitfalls in ECG diagnosis are reviewed in Chapter 19.

There are 14 features that should be analyzed on every ECG.

1. Standardization (calibration) and technical quality
2. Heart rate
3. Rhythm
4. PR interval
5. P wave size
6. QRS width (interval)
7. QT interval
8. QRS voltage
9. Mean QRS electrical axis
10. R wave progression in chest leads
11. Abnormal Q waves
12. ST segments
13. T waves
14. U waves

Standardization and technical features (p. 8). Make sure that the electrocardiograph has been properly calibrated so the standardization mark is 10 mm tall (1 mV = 10 mm).* Also check for limb lead reversal (p. 235) and ECG artifacts (p. 252).

Heart rate (p. 15). Calculate the heart rate. If the rate is faster than 100 beats/min, then a tachycardia is present. A rate slower than 60 beats/min means a bradycardia is present.

Be particularly careful not to overlook hidden P waves, seen, for example, in some cases of second-or-third-degree AV block, paroxysmal atrial tachycardia (PAT) with block, and blocked APBs. Also, whenever the ventricular rate is about 150/min, always consider the possibility of atrial flutter since the flutter waves may mimic the P waves of sinus or atrial tachycardia.

Rhythm. The rhythm is usually (1) normal sinus (or a sinus variant such as sinus bradycardia or tachycardia), (2) sinus with extra (ectopic) beats

---

*In special cases the ECG may be intentionally recorded at ½ standardization (1 mV = 5 mm) or 2× standardization (1 mV = 20 mm).

such as atrial or ventricular premature beats (APBs or VPBs), or (3) an entirely ectopic (non-sinus) mechanism such as atrial fibrillation or flutter, ventricular tachycardia, or an AV junctional escape rhythm.

PR interval. The normal PR interval (measured from the beginning of the P wave to the beginning of the QRS) is 0.12 to 0.2 second. A uniformly prolonged PR interval is referred to as *first-degree AV block*. A short PR interval with sinus rhythm and with a wide QRS and a delta wave is seen with the Wolff-Parkinson-White syndrome. A short PR interval with sinus rhythm and with a normal width QRS may represent Lown-Ganong-Levine type of preexcitation. By contrast, a short PR with retrograde P waves (negative in lead II) generally indicates an ectopic (atrial or AV junctional) pacemaker.

P wave size. Normally the P wave does not exceed 2.5 mm amplitude and is less than 3 mm wide in all leads. Tall peaked P waves may be a sign of right atrial enlargement (P pulmonale). Wide P waves are seen with left atrial abnormality.

QRS width (interval). Normally the QRS width is 0.1 second (100 msec) or less in all leads. The differential diagnosis of a wide QRS complex is described on page 140.

QT interval. A prolonged QT interval may be a clue to electrolyte disturbances (hypocalcemia, hypokalemia), drug effects (quinidine, procainamide), or myocardial ischemia. Shortened QT intervals are seen with hypercalcemia and digitalis effect.

QRS voltage. Look for signs of right or left ventricular hypertrophy (pp. 64, 67). Remember that thin-chested people and young adults frequently show tall voltage without left ventricular hypertrophy. Do not forget about low voltage (p. 133), which may result from pericardial effusion, myxedema, emphysema, obesity, or myocardial disease.

Mean QRS electrical axis. Estimate the mean QRS axis in the frontal plane. Decide by inspection whether the axis is normal (between $-30°$ and $+100°$) or whether left or right axis deviation is present.

R wave progression in chest leads. Inspect leads V_1 to V_6 to see if the normal increase in R waves is seen as you move across the chest. Poor R wave progression (small or absent R waves in V_1 to V_3)* may be a sign of myocardial infarction, but it may also be seen with left ventricular hypertrophy, chronic lung disease, left bundle branch block, and other conditions in the absence of infarction.

Abnormal Q waves (Chapter 8). Prominent Q waves in leads II, III, and aV_F may indicate inferior wall infarction. Prominent Q waves in the anterior leads (I, aV_L, and V_1 to V_6) may indicate anterior wall infarction.

ST segments. Look for abnormal ST segment elevations or depressions.

T waves. Inspect the T waves. Normally they are positive in leads with a positive QRS complex. They are also normally positive in leads V_3 to V_6 in adults, negative in lead aV_R, and positive in lead II. The polarity of the T waves in the other extremity leads depends on the QRS electrical axis. (T waves may be normally negative in lead III even in the presence of a vertical QRS axis.)

U waves. Also look for prominent U waves, which may be a sign of hypokalemia or drug effect or toxicity (as with quinidine).

• • •

After you have analyzed these 14 points, you should formulate an overall interpretation.†

The final ECG reading actually consists of two sections: (1) a list of notable findings and (2) an interpretive summary that attempts to integrate or explain these findings. For example, the ECG might show a prolonged QT interval and promi-

---

*The term *"reversed R wave progression"* is used to describe abnormally tall R waves in V_1 that progressively decrease in amplitude. This pattern may occur with a number of conditions, including right ventricular hypertrophy, posterior (or posterolateral) infarction, and dextrocardia.

†Students looking for a mnemonic to help recall the key features of the ECG can try using "IR WAX." *I* is for the four major Intervals (RR [heart rate], PR, QRS, QT); *R* is for Rhythm; *W* is for the five Waves (P, QRS, ST, T, U); and *AX* is for Axis.

nent U waves. The interpretation could state: "Repolarization abnormalities consistent with drug effect or toxicity (quinidine, procainamide, etc.) or hypokalemia. Clinical correlation suggested." Another ECG might show wide P waves, right axis deviation, and a tall R wave in lead V_1 (Fig. 19-1). The interpretation could state: "Findings consistent with left atrial abnormality (enlargement) and right ventricular hypertrophy. This combination is highly suggestive of mitral stenosis." In yet a third case the interpretation might simply be: "Within normal limits."

Thus the ECG is analogous to a newspaper account that consists, first, of the hard facts and, second, of the editorial comment. Like the editorialist, the ECG interpreter may sometimes offer suggestions, such as "Serial tracings advisable to evaluate possible evolving ischemic T-wave changes." Figure 21-1 illustrates this systematic approach, and Part III contains other examples for practice.

Remember: Every ECG abnormality you identify should summon up a list of differential diagnostic possibilities. You should search for an explanation of every abnormality found. For example, if the ECG shows sinus tachycardia, then the next question to ask is what caused this arrhythmia? Is it a result of anxiety, hyperthyroidism, congestive heart failure, hypovolemia, sympathomimetic drugs, alcohol withdrawal, or other causes? If you find ventricular tachycardia, what are the diagnostic possibilities? Is it due to myocardial infarction or some promptly reversible cause such as hypoxemia, digitalis toxicity, toxic effects of another drug, hypokalemia, or hypomagnesemia? If you see signs of left ventricular hypertrophy, what is the likely cause: valvular heart disease, hypertensive heart disease, or cardiomyopathy? In this way the interpretation of an ECG becomes an integral part of clinical diagnosis and patient care.

Computerized ECG Interpretations

Use of computerized ECG systems is becoming increasingly widespread. These systems provide interpretation and storage of ECG records. In recent years the computer programs (software) for ECG analysis have become more sophisticated and accurate.

However, despite these advances, computer ECG analyses have important limitations and, not infrequently, are subject to error. Diagnostic errors are most likely with arrhythmias or with more complex abnormalities. Therefore computerized interpretations (including measurements of basic ECG intervals and electrical axes) must never be accepted without careful review.

ECG Artifacts

This section will conclude with a brief discussion of some important ECG artifacts. The ECG, like any other electronic recording, is subject to numerous artifacts that may interfere with accurate interpretation. Some of the most common of these are described here.

60-Hertz (cycle) interference. Interference from alternating-current generators produces the characteristic pattern shown in Figure 21-2. Notice the fine-tooth comb 60 hertz (Hz) artifacts. By switching the electrocardiograph plug to a different outlet or by turning off other electrical appliances in the room, you can usually eliminate 60 Hz interference.

Muscle tremor. Involuntary muscle tremor (e.g., parkinsonism) (Fig. 21-3) can produce undulations in the baseline that may be mistaken for atrial flutter or fibrillation.

Wandering baseline. Upward or downward movement of the baseline may produce spurious ST segment elevations or depressions (Fig. 21-4).

Poor electrode contact or patient movement. Poor electrode contact or patient movement (Fig. 21-5) can produce artifactual deflections in the baseline that may obscure the underlying pattern or be mistaken for abnormal beats.

Improper standardization. The electrocardiograph, as mentioned, should be standardized before each tracing so a 1 mV pulse produces a square wave 10 mm high (Fig. 2-5). Failure to standardize properly will result in complexes that are either spuriously low or spuriously high. Furthermore, most electrocardiographs are equipped with half standardization and double standardization settings. Unintentional recording of an ECG on either of these settings will also result in misleading low or high voltage.

Fig. 21-1. ECG for interpretation:

1. Standardization: proper (1 mV = 10 mm); mark recorded at the end of leads I, V_1, and V_6 (The standardization mark need be recorded only once when taking an ECG.)
2. Heart rate: 88 beats/min
3. Rhythm: normal sinus
4. PR interval: 0.16 second
5. P waves: normal size
6. QRS width: 0.08 second (normal)
7. QT interval: 0.36 second (normal for rate)
8. QRS voltage: normal
9. Mean QRS axis: about −30° (biphasic QRS complex in lead II with positive QRS in lead I)
10. R wave progression in chest leads: early precordial transition with relatively tall R in V_2
11. Abnormal Q waves: leads II, III, and aV_F
12. ST segments: slightly elevated in leads II, III, and aV_F
13. T waves: inverted in leads II, III, aV_F, and V_6
14. U waves: not prominent

Impression: This ECG is consistent with an inferolateral (or inferoposterolateral) wall MI of indeterminate age. Comment: You cannot determine the age of an infarct from the ECG. The changes here (Q waves and ST-T abnormalities) could have been caused by an infarct that occurred the day before or the year before. The relatively tall R in V_2 could reflect loss of lateral potentials or actual posterior wall involvement.

Fig. 21-2. A common ECG artifact is that produced by 60-hertz (Hz) interference. **A,** Fast oscillations of the baseline. **B,** Same recording without the artifact.

Fig. 21-3. Another common artifact is that produced by muscle tremor. **A,** Wavy baseline simulating atrial flutter. **B,** Same recording without the artifact showing normal P waves.

Fig. 21-4. Wandering baseline resulting from patient movement.

Fig. 21-5. Deflections simulating ventricular premature beats produced by patient movement. 60 Hz artifact is also present.

REVIEW

The following 14 points should be evaluated on every ECG:
1. Standardization
2. Heart rate
3. Rhythm
4. PR interval
5. P wave size
6. QRS width (interval)
7. QT interval
8. QRS voltage
9. Mean QRS axis
10. R wave progression in chest leads
11. Abnormal Q waves
12. ST segments
13. T waves
14. U waves

Any ECG abnormality should be related to the clinical status of the patient. The ECG can also be affected by numerous artifacts, including 60 Hz interference, patient movement, poor electrode contact, and muscle tremor.

Computer interpretations of ECGs are subject to error and must be carefully reviewed.

SELF-ASSESSMENT PROBLEMS

This third and final section of the text is intended for self-assessment. Numerous review questions and practice examples are included based entirely on the material covered in Parts I and II. The review begins with a number of short-answer questions followed by actual ECGs for interpretation. Unless otherwise indicated, the ECGs have been standardized so 1 mV = 10 mm.

QUESTIONS

1. The P wave represents _____ _____ *(two words)*.
2. The QRS complex represents _____ _____ *(two words)*.
3. The T wave represents _____ _____ *(two words)*.
4. The normal range of the PR interval in adults is between _____ and _____ second.
5. Lead V_1 is obtained by placing the chest electrode to the right of the sternum in the _____ intercostal interspace.
6. With hypocalcemia the QT interval_____.
7. A *delta* wave is seen in what syndrome?
8. Name three drugs that may prolong the QT interval.
9. Name three causes of low-voltage QRS complexes.
10. Name at least three arrhythmias associated with digitalis toxicity.
11. A wide rSR' complex in lead V_1 with sinus rhythm most likely indicates_____.
12. Name three ECG patterns that may be seen with acute pulmonary embolism.
13. If the P wave in lead aV_R is −2 mm and the P wave in lead aV_L is −3 mm, then what must the amplitude of the P wave in lead aV_F be?
14. Two factors that may potentiate digitalis toxicity are _____ and _____.
15. Digitalis *(increases? decreases? has no effect on?)* conduction of impulses through the AV node.
16. What metabolic or drug-related factor may prolong the QRS duration?
17. Prominent U waves are often seen with what electrolyte abnormality?
18. Tall peaked P waves in leads II, III, and aV_F are suggestive of_____.
19. With normal sinus rhythm the P wave is virtually always negative in lead _____ and positive in lead_____.

20. Draw the hexaxial diagram showing the six extremity (frontal plane) leads.
21. Normally the R/S ratio in lead V_1 (in adults) is less than_____.
22. Atrial fibrillation is sometimes seen in which endocrine disorder?
23. Name the three basic ECG patterns that may be seen in cardiac arrest.
24. Names three causes of sinus tachycardia.
25. Syncope associated with complete heart block or other profound bradycardias is called the_____ _____ syndrome.
26. Define ventricular tachycardia.
27. Tall, peaked T waves are characteristic of which electrolyte disturbance?
28. Name three causes of ST segment elevations.
29. A patient experiencing typical angina pectoris with exertion may show what ECG pattern in lead V_5 as a sign of subendocardial ischemia?
30. Right bundle branch block is always a sign of serious organic heart disease *(true or false)*.
31. Atrial fibrillation is always a sign of serious organic heart disease *(true or false)*.
32. Left bundle branch block is often a sign of serious organic heart disease *(true or false)*.
33. The *early repolarization* pattern is a normal variant *(true or false)*.
34. Prinzmetal's angina is characterized by ST segment elevations *(true or false)*.
35. With acute transmural *anterior* wall ischemia, leads II, III, and aV_F are likely to show reciprocal ST segment _____.
36. Wide (> 0.12 sec) P waves in lead II suggest _____ _____.
37. Draw a QS complex.
38. A wide (>0.12 sec) QS complex in lead V_1 with sinus rhythm is seen with _____.
39. Name five causes of ventricular ectopy.
40. A 20-year-old college student complaining of light-headedness and palpitations is found to have a regular tachycardia with normal QRS complexes at a rate of 190 beats/min without evident P waves. The arrhythmia terminates abruptly during carotid sinus massage. What is the most likely diagnosis?
41. A patient is found to have a pulse rate of 35 beats/min. The ECG is most likely to show one of five basic classes of rhythms. Name them.
42. Left axis deviation is defined as an axis more negative than $-$_____ °.
43. Name three causes of sinus bradycardia.
44. Name three causes of atrial fibrillation.
45. Persistent ST segment elevations several weeks following an acute myocardial infarct suggest a possible_____ _____.
46. Which of the following tachyarrhythmias is most likely to terminate abruptly following carotid sinus massage: sinus tachycardia, atrial fibrillation, AV nodal reentrant tachycardia, or ventricular tachycardia?
47. A wide biphasic P wave in lead V_1 may indicate _____.
48. Which of the following drugs may shorten the QT interval: digitalis, quinidine, procainamide, furosemide (Lasix)?
49. Normally the QRS width is equal to or less than 0._____ second.
50. A qR complex is normally seen in which lead: V_1, V_6, or aV_R?

Define the Following Terms

51. "R on T" phenomenon (p. 181)
52. Ectopic beat (p. 156)
53. Current of injury (p. 89)
54. Bypass tract (p. 137)
55. Escape beat (p. 151)
56. Bifascicular block (p. 197)
57. Frontal plane leads (p. 28)
58. Horizontal plane leads (p. 28)
59. Hyperacute T wave (p. 91)
60. Vertical QRS axis, horizontal QRS axis (p. 42)

Draw the QRS-T Pattern You Would Expect to See in Lead V_6 *(for nos. 61 to 65)*

61. Normal pattern
62. Left bundle branch block
63. Right bundle branch block
64. Left ventricular hypertrophy with "strain"
65. Digitalis effect
66. What life-threatening metabolic abnormality caused the ECG findings in this patient?

67. What drug could have produced these ST-T changes?

68. What ventricular conduction disturbance is present here?

69. What is this abnormal heart rhythm?

70. What is X?

II

71. Calculate the approximate mean QRS axis in *A* and *B*.

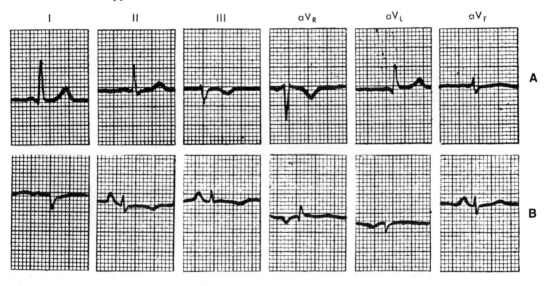

I   II   III   aVR   aVL   aVF

A

B

72. Calculate the approximate mean QRS axis in these leads.

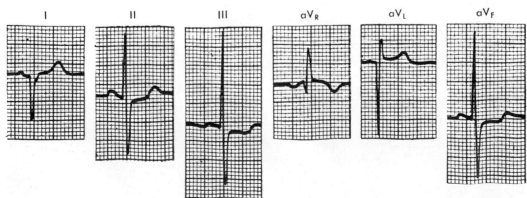

I   II   III   aVR   aVL   aVF

73. Is the mean QRS axis in this example normal, right, or left?

74. a. What is the major abnormality shown here?
    b. What factors can produce it?

75. What is the heart rhythm?

76. a. What is the approximate sinus (P wave) rate?
    b. What type of AV conduction disturbance is present?
    c. What abnormality is indicated by the P waves?

77. a. What is the approximate heart rate?
    b. What arrhythmia is present here?

78. What type of AV conduction disturbance is present?

79. Identify beats *A* and *B*.

80. a. What arrhythmia is present?
    b. Of what symptom might this patient be complaining?

81. Look at the first and second halves of this rhythm strip. What are the rhythms?
    What syndrome do they suggest?

82. What is the arrhythmia shown here? Name three conditions that might lead to it.

83. What type of ventricular conduction disturbance is present here?

Identify the Rhythm in Each Case
(for nos. 84 to 111)

84.

85.

86.

87.

88.

89.

90.

91.

aV$_R$

92.

II

93.

II

94.

Monitor lead

95.

II

96.

aV$_R$

97.

II

98.

Monitor lead

99.

100.

101.

Monitor lead

102.

103.

II

104.

II

V₁

105.

II

106.

II

107.

aV$_R$

108.

V$_1$

109.

MONITOR LEAD

110.

aV$_L$

111.

112. What two abnormalities are present here?

113. A 50-year-old patient complained of palpitations during the time this Holter monitor record was being obtained. What arrhythmia is shown?

114. What two abnormalities are present?

115. What abnormality is present here in addition to the VPB?

116. What ventricular conduction disturbance is present?

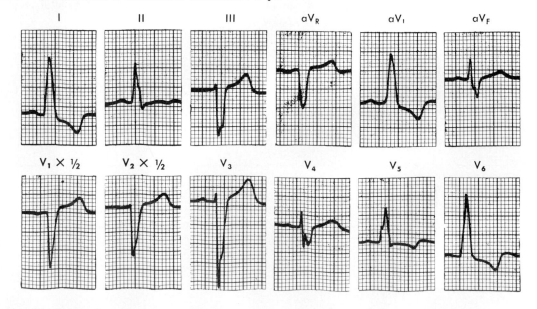

Interpret These ECGs Fully According to the Method Suggested in Chapter 21
(for nos. 117 to 121)

117.

118.

119.

120.

121.

122. What is the major ECG diagnosis here?

123. The following rhythm strip shows
    a. Sinus rhythm with frequent premature atrial beats
    b. Sinus rhythm with complete heart block
    c. Sinus rhythm with 3:2 AV Wenckebach
    d. Multifocal atrial tachycardia
    e. Sinus arrhythmia

124. Answer these questions about the following ECG:
     a. Is it properly standardized?
     b. What is the heart rate?
     c. Is sinus rhythm present?
     d. What is the mean QRS axis?
     e. Is axis deviation present?
     f. Is the QRS voltage normal?
     g. What is the major abnormality?

125. Answer these questions about the following ECG:
    a. What is the approximate heart rate?
    b. What evidence is there of myocardial infarction?

126. The following rhythm strip shows
    a. Atrial fibrillation
    b. Paroxysmal atrial tachycardia
    c. Multifocal atrial tachycardia
    d. Atrial bigeminy

127. The ECG strip below, obtained during an exercise test, shows
    a. Ventricular tachycardia
    b. ST changes consistent with acute transmural infarction
    c. ST changes consistent with Prinzmetal's angina
    d. ST changes consistent with acute subendocardial ischemia

128. Answer these questions from the following ECG:
    a. What waveform is abnormally prominent here?
    b. What are the major causes for this finding?

129. A 46-year-old man presented complaining of having had 4 hours of chest pain. What is the diagnosis? Note: V_{4R} to V_{6R} are right precordial leads.

130. What wave does the arrow in V_5 point to, and what is the significance of this wave?

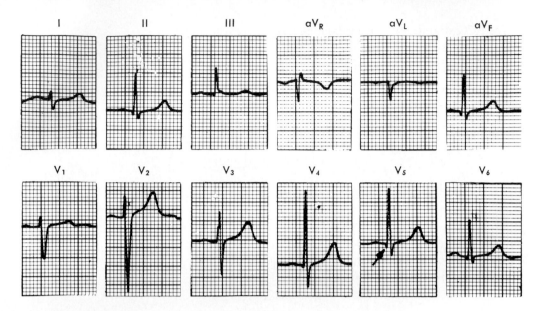

131. A patient complaining of severe chest pain had abnormally elevated cardiac enzymes. Using the ECG shown below, what is the clinical diagnosis?

132. What is this rhythm?

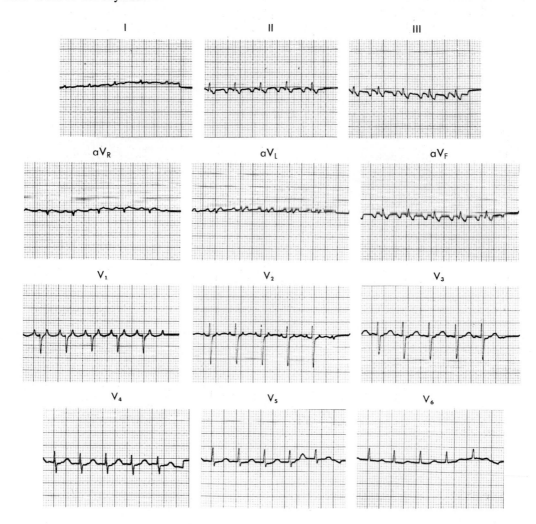

133. What arrhythmia is present here?

134. A 50-year-old man is complaining of chest pain. What is the likely cause of his complaint?

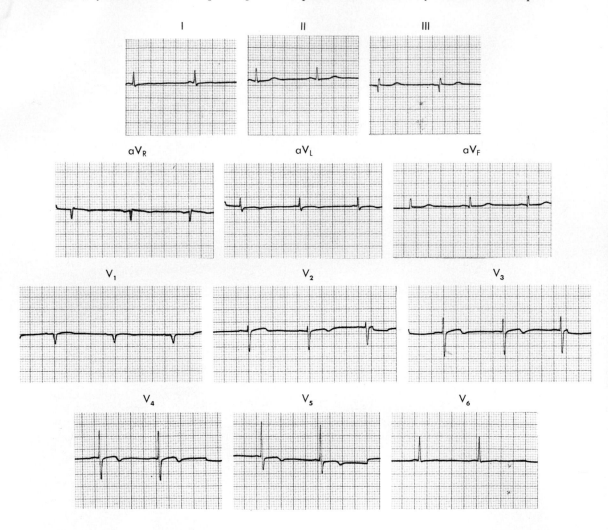

135. A patient presenting with palpitations received carotid sinus massage. What is the arrhythmia?

136. This patient's ECG was normal 3 days ago. What is the diagnosis from this repeat ECG?

137. This lead II rhythm strip shows what three abnormalities?

138. What is the major ECG diagnosis?

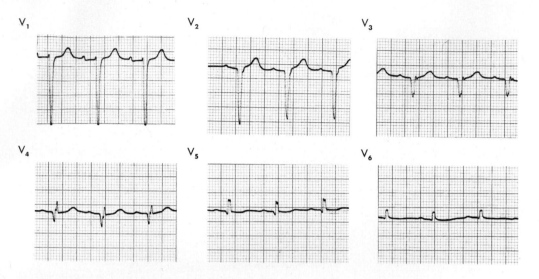

139. Name the major abnormalities here.

140. What is this subtle rhythm disturbance in a patient on digoxin therapy for congestive heart failure?

II

141. A 41-year-old man is complaining of "indigestion." What is the diagnosis?

| I | II | III | aV$_R$ | aV$_L$ | aV$_F$ |

| V$_1$ | V$_2$ | V$_3$ | V$_4$ | V$_5$ | V$_6$ |

142. What is this rhythm?

Lead II: continuous

143. What is this rhythm?

V₁

144. Name the major abnormalities here.

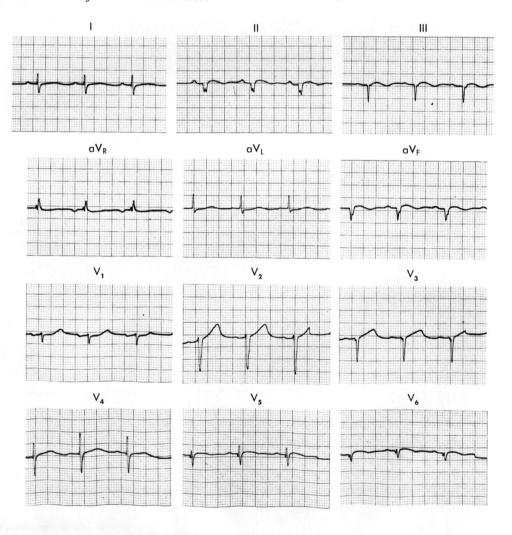

145. Name the major abnormalities here.

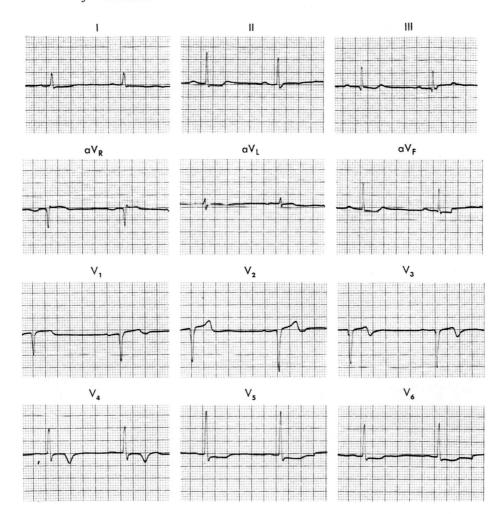

146. What is this arrhythmia?

147. What is the cause of the "dropped" P wave here?

148. Following is the preoperative ECG of an athletic 45-year-old man. What is the diagnosis?

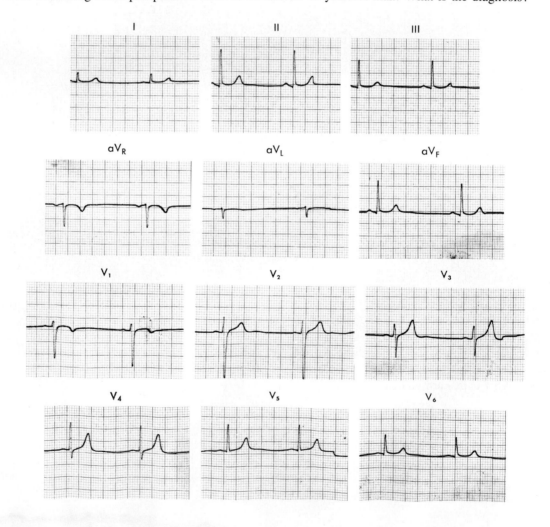

149. Following is the preoperative ECG of a 65-year-old woman. What is the diagnosis?

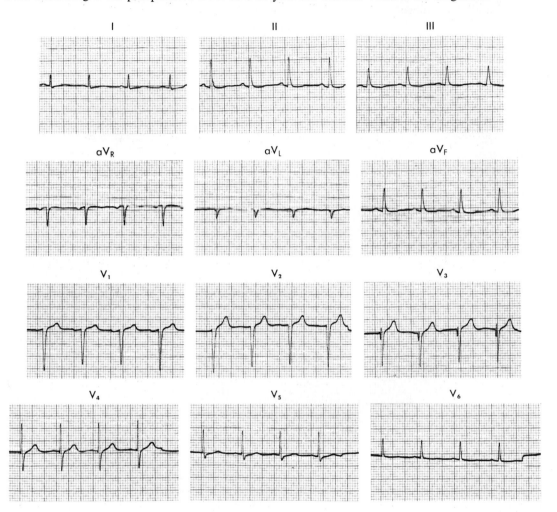

150. What caused this patient's syncope?

Monitor lead

151. The following ECG is from a 60-year-old man with severe hypertension.
     What are the findings?

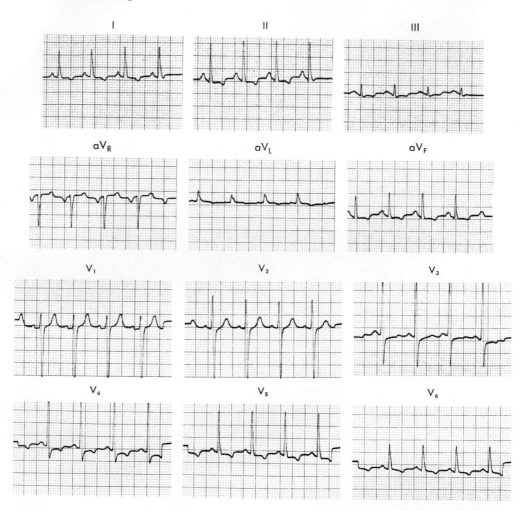

152. What is this arrhythmia?

153. The following ECG is from a 24-year-old healthy male medical student.
     What is the diagnosis?

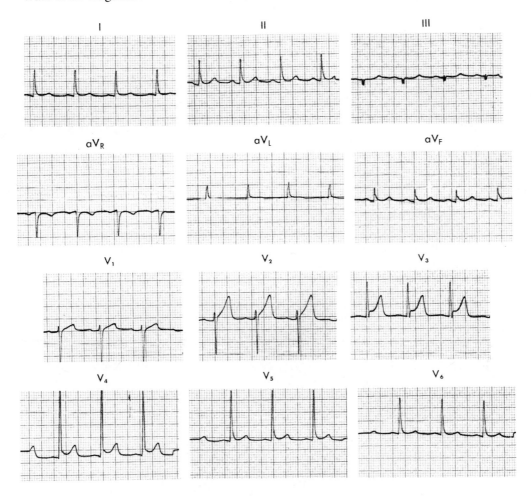

154. What is the cause of the wide QRS complexes?

155. The following ECG is from a 50-year-old dialysis patient complaining of sharp pleuritic chest pain. What is the cause of his complaint?

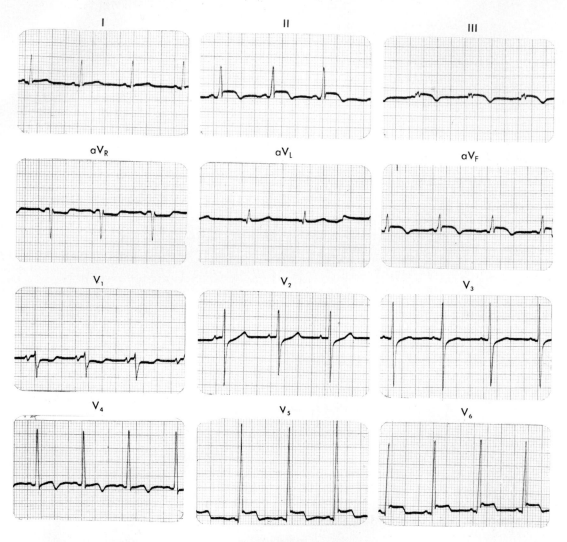

156. What is this rhythm and what clinical condition do you suspect?

157. The following ECG is from a 62-year-old man. Describe the major abnormalities.

158. What is this subtle arrhythmia and what type of drug toxicity do you suspect?

159. The following ECG is from a 59-year-old woman. Describe the major findings.

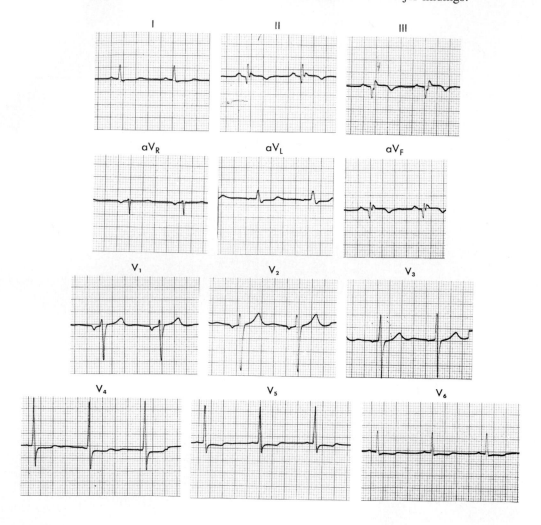

160. What is this rhythm?

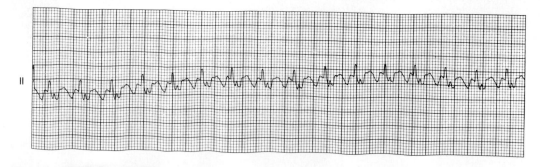

161. The following ECG is from a 50-year-old woman with suspected recurrent pulmonary emboli. What are the major abnormalities?

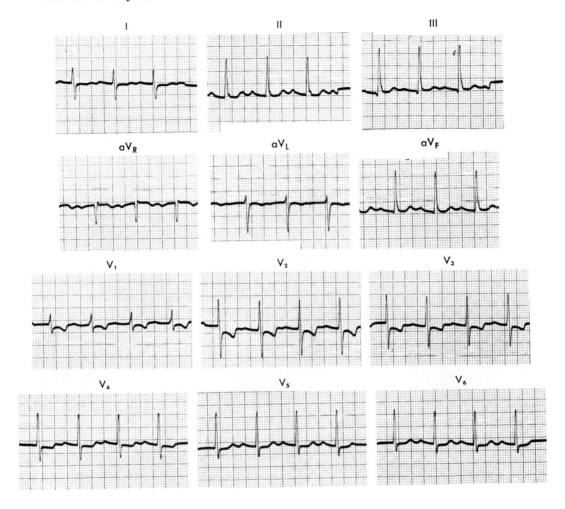

162. What is this rhythm?

163. The following ECG is from a 20-year-old woman with sharp chest pain. What is the diagnosis?

164. What are the notable findings here?

165. What arrhythmia is causing this patient's palpitations?

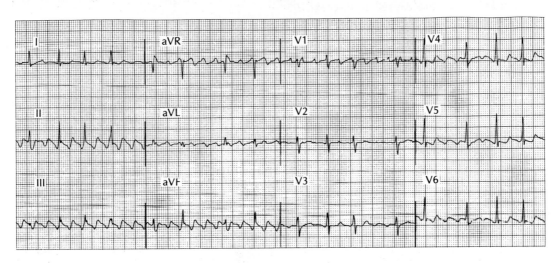

166. What factor is most likely to have caused the change from *A* to *B?*
   a. Hypocalcemia
   b. Hyperkalemia
   c. Hypokalemia
   d. Digitalis

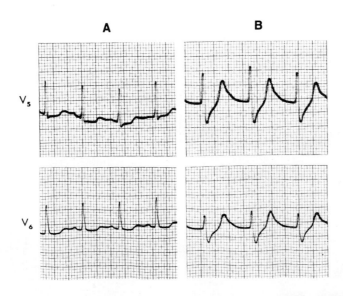

167. What metabolic problem was corrected in this patient, accounting for the marked change on the ECG from one day, *A*, to the next, *B?*

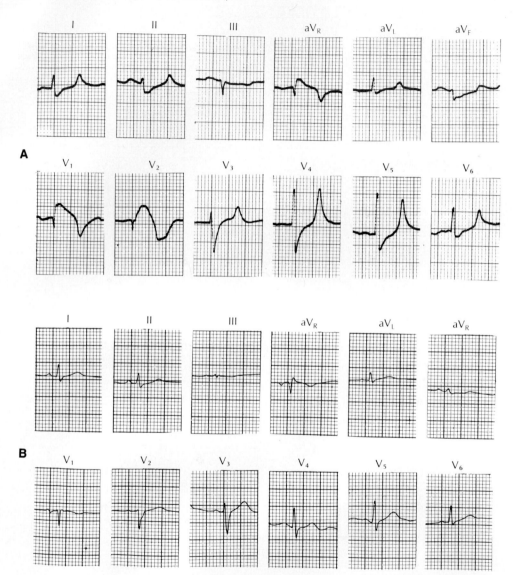

168. A 76-year-old woman complains that her "heart skips beats." What does her rhythm strip show?

169. What type of conduction disturbance is present here?

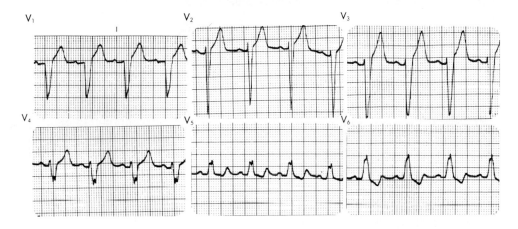

170. This patient's bradycardia is associated with what subtle arrhythymia?

171. A patient with an evolving inferior infarction has intermittent wide QRS complexes. What are these beats?

172. A 44-year-old woman with a history of intermittent atrial fibrillation complains of palpitations. What drug is she probably taking, and what is the arrhythmia?

173. A 70-year-old man taking propranolol for hypertension comes to the emergency room complaining of light-headedness and weakness for the past week. What does his monitor lead rhythm strip show?

MONITOR LEAD

174. A 70-year-old man was given verapamil for treatment of angina. What does his rhythm strip show?

175. This patient with pulmonary edema that developed over 2 days is being seen in the emergency room. What are the major ECG findings?

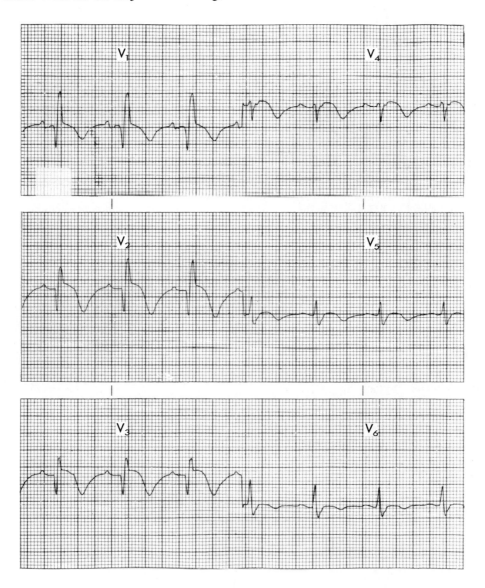

176. A 48-year-old man complains of intermittent palpitations.
What arrhythmia does he have?

177. An acute left hemiparesis developed in a 72-year-old man.
What etiology does his ECG suggest?

178. A 92-year-old man loses consciousness while eating dinner.
What does his rhythm strip indicate?

179. A 54-year-old psychiatrist complains of sudden palpitations after an argument with a "signifi-cant other." What does his ECG show?

180. A 60-year-old man is admitted with severe congestive heart failure. His ECG is identical to one recorded 6 months earlier. Cardiac enzymes are normal. What is the likely diagnosis?

181. A 27-year-old man is told he has "congenital heart disease." Except for some mild exertional fatigue, he feels fine. He is not cyanotic on physical examination. A loud systolic ejection murmur is heard with fixed splitting of the second heart sound. What does his ECG show, and what is the likely clinical diagnosis?

182. A 37-year-old man presents with intermittent palpitations. What does his ECG show?

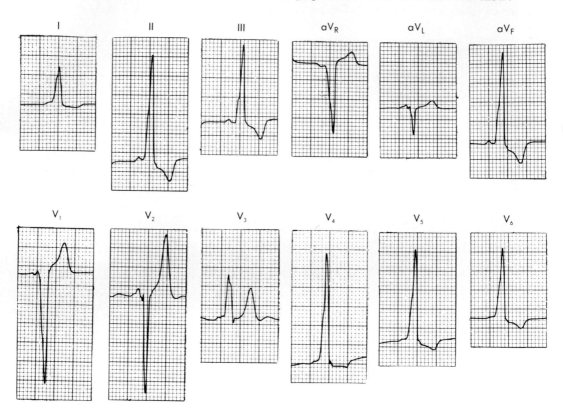

183. A 75-year-old woman treated with quinidine for atrial arrhythmias has a cardiac arrest 4 days later. This rhythm strip was obtained. What does it show?

MONITOR LEAD

184. The ECG was initially misinterpreted as showing "accelerated idioventricular rhythm." What is the correct diagnosis?

185. An 80-year-old woman complained of light-headedness. The following rhythm strip was obtained in the coronary care unit. What conduction disturbance is present?

MONITOR LEAD

186. The following Holter monitor recording shows sinus rhythm with intermittent
    a. Ventricular tachycardia
    b. Left bundle branch block
    c. Accelerated idioventricular rhythm (AIVR)
    d. Wolff-Parkinson-White pattern
    e. Ventricular paced rhythm

187. This ECG gives an important clue to a life-threatening electrolyte abnormality. (The serum K^+ was normal.) What is the likely diagnosis?

188. This ECG shows
    a. Sinus tachycardia
    b. Atrial flutter with 3:1 conduction
    c. Paroxysmal atrial tachycardia (PAT) with block
    d. Multifocal atrial tachycardia
    e. None of the above

189. What life-threatening metabolic disturbance does this ECG most strongly suggest?
    a. Hyperkalemia
    b. Hypokalemia
    c. Hypercalcemia
    d. Hypocalcemia
    e. Hyponatremia

190. This patient was thought to have atrial fibrillation on examination. What is the actual finding accounting for the erratic pulse on this Holter monitor recording?

191. What does this patient have to account for this ECG pattern?

192. A 54-year-old woman complained of palpitations. The monitor lead recorded this episode. What is the diagnosis?

MONITOR
LEAD

193. Two simultaneous leads were recorded during Holter monitoring of a patient with frequent APBs. What does the *arrow* point to? What is this arrhythmia?

194. Two simultaneous leads were recorded during Holter monitoring. The rhythm is sinus brady-cardia. What subtle conduction abnormality is present? What is the anatomic substrate for this finding?

195. A 54-year-old woman presented with chronic obstructive pulmonary disease. Does the ECG fit in with this diagnosis?

196. A Holter monitor recorded this strip from a patient complaining of intermittent lightheadedness. What arrhythmia is present?

197. A 77-year-old woman complains of shortness of breath and palpitations. What is the rhythm?

198. A 76-year-old insulin-requiring diabetic man with coronary artery disease became hypotensive during a hypoglycemic episode. Cardiac enzymes were normal. What are the major ECG findings?

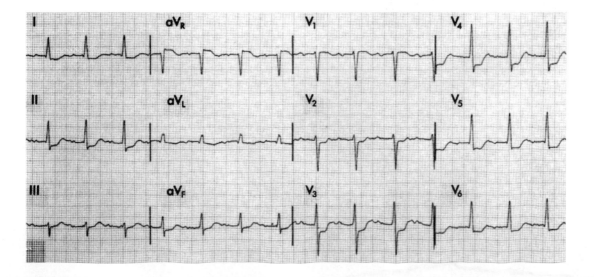

199. A 65-year-old woman had chest pain 3 days earlier. What are the major findings?

200. Finale.

ANSWERS

1. Atrial depolarization (stimulation).
2. Ventricular depolarization (stimulation).
3. Ventricular repolarization (recovery).
4. 0.12 and 0.2.
5. Fourth.
6. Lengthens.
7. Wolff-Parkinson-White syndrome.
8. Quinidine, procainamide, disopyramide, sotalol, amiodarone, and others
9. Pericardial effusion, emphysema, and obesity. Also extensive myocardial fibrosis or infiltration with substances like amyloid. Low voltage may also be a normal variant.
10. Ventricular ectopy (VPBs, ventricular bigeminy, ventricular tachycardia, ventricular fibrillation, bidirectional tachycardia), sinus bradycardia and SA block, junctional rhythms, PAT with block, and so on. (See page 204.)
11. RBBB.
12. Right axis shift, S_1Q_{III} pattern, RBBB, sinus tachycardia and other arrhythmias, right ventricular strain. (See page 135 for other patterns.)
13. +5 mm. Recall that the summed voltages of each of the waveforms in $aV_R + aV_L + aV_F$ must equal 0.
14. Hypokalemia and renal insufficiency; also hypoxia, hypercalcemia, hypomagnesemia, old age, and others. (See pages 204 and 206.)
15. Decreases.
16. Hyperkalemia, quinidine, procainamide, disopyramide, tricyclic antidepressants, phenothiazines, etc.
17. Hypokalemia.
18. P pulmonale (right atrial enlargement).
19. aV_R, II.
20. See page 48.
21. 1.
22. Hyperthyroidism.
23. Ventricular fibrillation (and related ventricular tachyarrhythmias), asystole (with or without escape beats), and electromechanical dissociation.
24. Fever, excitement, and congestive heart failure. (See page 150 for other causes.)
25. Stokes-Adams.
26. Three or more consecutive VPBs.
27. Hyperkalemia.
28. Acute myocardial infarction, acute pericarditis, Prinzmetal's angina; also ventricular aneurysm.
29. ST segment depressions.
30. False. Some normal people will have an RBBB pattern.

31. False. Atrial fibrillation, although often seen in people with organic heart disease (coronary, hypertensive, valvular, etc.), may occur in people with normal hearts. It may also be associated with metabolic factors (hyperthyroidism) or excessive alcohol consumption ("holiday heart syndrome").

32. True.

33. True. (See page 133.)

34. True.

35. Depressions (reciprocal to the ST elevations seen in the anterior leads).

36. Left atrial abnormality (enlargement).

37. See page 12.

38. LBBB.

39. Myocardial ischemia, digitalis toxicity, hypokalemia, hypoxia, pulmonary embolism, and congestive heart failure. (See page 183 for additional causes.)

40. Paroxysmal supraventricular tachycardia (PSVT), probably due to AV nodal reentry. See also Question 100.

41. Sinus bradycardia, AV junctional rhythm, AV heart block (second or third degree) or AV dissociation, atrial fibrillation or flutter with a slow ventricular response, or idioventricular escape rhythm.

42. $-30°$.

43. Normal variant, beta blockers such as propranolol, calcium channel blockers (verapamil, diltiazem), digitalis toxicity, increased vagal tone caused by myocardial ischemia, and so on.

44. Coronary artery disease, hypertensive heart disease, and mitral valve disease.

45. Ventricular aneurysm.

46. AV nodal reentrant tachycardia.

47. Left atrial abnormality (enlargement).

48. Digitalis.

49. 0.1 second.

50. V_6.

51-60. See the pages listed.

61-65. See diagrams below.

V_6 61   62   63   64   65

66. Hyperkalemia. Notice the tall "tented" T waves. First degree AV block is also present.
67. Digitalis.
68. RBBB is present with wide rSR′ complexes in V_1. (In addition, first-degree AV block is present.)
69. Sinus rhythm with a brief nonsustained (five-beat) run of ventricular tachycardia.
70. Ventricular premature beat.
71. *A.* 0°.
    B. +180°.
    In both *A* and *B,* lead aV_F shows a biphasic RS-type complex; thus the mean QRS axis must be directed at right angles to the axis of lead aV_F, which is at +90°. In example *A* lead I shows a positive R wave deflection, so the axis must be pointed in that direction (at 0°). In example *B* the mean QRS axis is directed at right angles to aV_F, away from I, and toward leads III and aV_R, or at +180° (marked right axis deviation).
72. +150°. Lead II shows a biphasic RS complex; thus the mean QRS axis must be directed at right angles to the axis of lead II, which is at +60°. Therefore the axis must be either −30° or +150°. Obviously, since I is negative and II and aV_R are mainly positive, the axis must be +150°. This indicates marked right axis deviation.
73. Left.
74. a. The QT interval is prolonged (0.48 sec) with a sinus bradycardia at 55/min.
    b. QT prolongation may be caused by numerous factors, including hypocalcemia (present here, note the long ST segment), hypokalemia (often with large U waves), and drugs such as quinidine or procainamide (with wide flattened T waves).
75. Atrial flutter. Notice the characteristic sawtooth flutter waves. The atrial (flutter) rate is approximately 300 beats/min, while the ventricular (QRS) rate is about 75 beats/min; thus 4:1 flutter is present.
76. a. About 70/min.
    b. AV Wenckebach. Notice the repeating cycles in which the PR intervals get progressively longer until the P wave is not conducted. (The fifth and ninth P waves are not conducted.)
    c. The wide notched P waves indicate left atrial abnormality (enlargement).
77. a. About 130 beats/min. (There are 13 QRS cycles/6 sec.) (See page 15.)
    b. Atrial fibrillation. Often, as in this case, with rapid atrial fibrillation, the fibrillation waves are not well seen. The diagnosis of atrial fibrillation is then made by finding a haphazardly irregular rhythm with no discrete P waves.
78. First-degree AV block (PR interval about 0.22 sec). Notice that the QRS is somewhat wide, 0.11 second, indicating some type of intraventricular conduction disturbance as well.
79. *A* is an atrial premature beat (APB). *B* is a junctional escape beat.
80. a. Complete heart block. To analyze this arrhythmia, you need to label each P wave and each QRS complex. The ventricular rate is about 40 beats/min. Looking at the P waves (some of which are hidden by QRS complexes and T waves), you can see that the atrial rate is 90 to 100 beats/min and the PR intervals are completely variable. Therefore complete heart block is present. The QRS complexes are abnormally wide probably because the ventricles are being paced by an idioventricular focus located below the AV junction.
    b. The patient complained of light-headedness and fainting spells (Stokes-Adams syndrome).

81. The first part of the rhythm strip shows *coarse atrial fibrillation,* which then spontaneously converts to a marked *sinus bradycardia.* This sequence suggests the *brady-tachy variant* of the *sick sinus syndrome.*

82. Atrial fibrillation with a rapid ventricular rate. This may be due to multiple conditions, including coronary artery disease, hypertension, valvular disease, cardiomyopathy, alcohol consumption, and hyperthyroidism.

83. RBBB.

84. Atrial paced rhythm. Notice the pacemaker spike before each P wave.

85. Atrial fibrillation.

86. Sinus arrhythmia.

87. Sinus rhythm with a multiform ventricular couplet.

88. Sinus tachycardia. (Nonspecific ST-T changes are also present.)

89. Ventricular fibrillation.

90. Ventricular tachycardia.

91. Atrial fibrillation.

92. Sinus rhythm with first-degree AV block.

93. Sinus rhythm with atrial premature beats. (The third, sixth, and ninth beats are APBs; therefore this is atrial *trigeminy.*)

94. Sinus rhythm with ventricular premature beats. (The second and sixth beats are VPBs.)

95. Sinus bradycardia. (Notice also the abnormal ST-T segment because of left ventricular strain or ischemia.)

96. AV junctional rhythm. (Notice the absence of visible P waves with a normal-duration QRS complex. AV junctional rhythms with rates between about 70 and 120 are sometimes referred to as nonparoxysmal AV junctional tachycardias or accelerated junctional rhythms.)

97. Sinus tachycardia with a short burst of ventricular tachycardia. (The ninth beat is also a VPB.)

98. Sinus rhythm with an APB (fourth beat).

99. Sinus rhythm with a run of accelerated idioventricular rhythm (AIVR). Notice that the second and ninth beats are *fusion* beats.

100. Paroxysmal supraventricular tachycardia (PSVT) at a rate of about 190/min. Given the absence of visible P waves (which are probably occurring during the QRS), this most likely represents AV nodal reentrant tachycardia.

101. Ventricular bigeminy.

102. Coarse atrial fibrillation with incomplete RBBB (note the rSR' in lead V_1).

103. Idioventricular (slow ventricular escape) rhythm.

104. Atrial flutter with variable block.

105. Ventricular trigeminy. Every second sinus beat is followed by a VPB.

106. Coarse atrial fibrillation.

107. Accelerated junctional rhythm (nonparoxysmal AV junctional tachycardia). Notice the absence of visible P waves. (See Question 96.)

108. Ventricular paced rhythm. Notice the pacemaker spike before each QRS and the nonconducted P waves (some hidden). The latter indicate underlying complete heart block.

109. Ventricular fibrillation (recorded during cardiac arrest).

110. Ventricular tachycardia.
111. Atrial flutter with 2:1 block (atrial rate, about 300 beats/min; ventricular rate, about 150 beats/min).
112. Lead II rhythm strip showing marked ST elevations (caused by acute inferior wall infarction) with a junctional (or ectopic atrial) rhythm. (Notice the retrograde P waves immediately preceding each QRS.)
113. Sinus rhythm with a three-beat run of paroxysmal atrial tachycardia (PAT). Notice that complexes 5 to 7 are atrial premature beats (APBs).
114. Atrial flutter with variable block; incomplete RBBB.
115. Pacemaker rhythm with pacemaker malfunction. Notice the pacemaker spike in the center of the strip, which is not followed by a QRS (owing to pacemaker failure).
116. LBBB.
117. a. *Analysis*
     (1) Standardization: 1 mV = 10 mm (mark as shown).
     (2) Heart rate: about 60 beats/min.
     (3) Rhythm: normal sinus.
     (4) PR interval: about 0.16 second (normal).
     (5) P wave size: broad and biphasic in V_1, suggesting possible left atrial abnormality, although in other leads within normal limits.
     (6) QRS width: 0.1 second (upper limits of normal).
     (7) QT interval: about 0.4 second (normal for rate).
     (8) QRS voltage: R wave in aV_L is abnormally tall (15 mm).
     (9) Mean QRS axis: about $-60°$. The R wave in aV_L equals the S wave in aV_F, so the mean QRS axis must lie between the positive pole of aV_L ($-30°$) and the negative pole of aV_F ($-90°$). Therefore the mean QRS axis must be approximately $-60°$.
     (10) R wave progression in chest leads: poor, with QS complexes in V_1 to V_3.
     (11) Abnormal Q waves: V_1 to V_3 show abnormal QS complexes. Notice the bizarre W-shaped QS in V_3.
     (12) ST segment elevation in V_2 with slight depression in V_3 to V_6.
     (13) T waves: inverted in I, aV_L, and V_4 to V_6, with some scooping of the ST segment in I and aV_L.
     (14) U waves: normal.
    b. *Interpretation*
    Abnormal ECG. Left axis deviation consistent with left anterior hemiblock.
    QS complexes in V_1 to V_3 consistent with anteroseptal infarction of indeterminate age.
    Left ventricular hypertrophy by voltage.
    Left atrial abnormality.
    Abnormal ST-T changes consistent with left ventricular strain and/or ischemia, and possibly with digitalis effect (with scooping of ST-T in I and aV_L). (The ST-T changes on this ECG are somewhat complicated. As noted, the T wave inversions and slight ST depressions in V_3 to V_6 may reflect a combination of left ventricular strain and/or lateral wall ischemia. The scooping of the ST-T segment in I and aV_L may also reflect strain or

ischemia but is suggestive of the classic pattern of digitalis effect as well. Finally, notice the high takeoff of the ST segment in V_2, suggesting acute infarction. However, in cases of LVH the right precordial leads may show such ST elevation as a persistent finding in the absence of acute ischemia.)

118. a. *Analysis*
   (1) Standardization: 1 mV = 10 mm (mark not shown).
   (2) Heart rate: approximately 40 beats/min.
   (3) Rhythm: sinus bradycardia.
   (4) PR interval: about 0.18 second.
   (5) P wave size: biphasic in V_1, suggesting possible left atrial abnormality.
   (6) QRS width: 0.1 to 0.11 second.
   (7) QT interval: 0.52 second (within normal limits for rate).
   (8) QRS voltage: tall in chest leads ($S_{V_1} + R_{V_6}$ = more than 35 mm).
   (9) Mean QRS axis: about +30°. R waves are of equal amplitude in I and II so the mean QRS axis must be directed between these leads.
   (10) R wave progression in chest leads: delayed, with the transition zone between V_4 and V_5.
   (11) Abnormal Q waves: none.
   (12) ST segments: isoelectric.
   (13) T waves: inverted in I, II, aV_L, V_5, and V_6.
   (14) U waves: small in V_1 to V_4.

   b. *Interpretation*
   Abnormal ECG.
   Marked sinus bradycardia.
   Left ventricular hypertrophy by voltage. ST-T changes are consistent with left ventricular "strain" and possibly ischemia.
   Possible left atrial abnormality.
   In this case the left ventricular hypertrophy and atrial abnormality resulted from hypertensive heart disease. The marked sinus bradycardia was caused by one of the drugs (beta blocker) that the patient was taking for high blood pressure.

119. a. *Analysis*
   (1) Standardization: 1 mV = 10 mm (mark not shown).
   (2) Heart rate: approximately 75 beats/min.
   (3) Rhythm: ectopic atrial. (Notice the retrograde P waves in II with biphasic P waves in aV_R.)
   (4) PR interval: 0.1 (short because of the ectopic atrial rhythm).
   (5) P wave size: normal.
   (6) QRS width: 0.08 second.
   (7) QT interval: 0.35 second (normal for rate).
   (8) QRS voltage: tall in aV_L (R wave = 16 mm).
   (9) QRS axis: approximately −45°. The R wave in I is about equal to the S wave in aV_F. Therefore the mean QRS axis must lie midway between the positive pole of I (0°) and the negative pole of aV_F (−90°), making the axis −45°. Furthermore, by inspection, you can tell that left axis deviation is present (axis more negative than −30°), since

lead II shows an rS complex with the S wave deeper than the r wave is tall. (See page 55.)

(10) R wave progression in the chest leads: delayed with QS complexes in V_1 to V_3.

(11) Abnormal Q waves: QS complexes in leads V_1 to V_3. Abnormally wide in aV_L. (Notice that this Q wave is 0.04 second wide, making it abnormal even though it is not very deep.)

(12) ST segments: slightly elevated in V_2 to V_4.

(13) T waves: deeply inverted and symmetric in I, II, aV_L, and V_2 to V_6.

(14) U waves: normal.

b. *Interpretation*

Abnormal ECG.

Ectopic atrial rhythm.

LVH by voltage.

Left axis deviation consistent with left anterior hemiblock.

Abnormal Q waves and T wave inversions consistent with anterior wall infarction (possibly recent or evolving).

   The exact age of the infarct cannot be deduced from the ECG. In this case it was 1 week old.

120. a. *Analysis*

(1) Standardization: 1 mV = 10 mm (mark shown in V_1).

(2) Heart rate: approximately 75 beats/min, with slight irregularity.

(3) Rhythm: normal sinus, with both premature atrial beats (in I, aV_F, V_2, and V_6) and premature ventricular beats (third beat in V_1).

(4) PR interval: 0.12 second (lower limits of normal).

(5) P wave size: broad and biphasic in V_1 (suggesting left atrial abnormality).

(6) QRS width: 0.12 to 0.13 second. The RSR′ in V_1 indicates RBBB.

(7) QT interval: 0.36 second (normal for rate).

(8) QRS voltage: normal.

(9) Mean QRS axis: +90°. Biphasic RS wave in I.

(10) R wave progression in chest leads: normal.

(11) Abnormal Q waves in II, III, and aV_F.

(12) ST segments: normal.

(13) T waves: slight inversion in II, III, and aV_F.

(14) U waves: normal.

b. *Interpretation*

Abnormal ECG.

Sinus rhythm with atrial and ventricular ectopy.

RBBB.

Left atrial abnormality.

Inferior wall infarct of indeterminate age.

121. a. *Analysis*
    (1) Standardization: 1 mV = 10 mm (mark not shown).
    (2) Heart rate: 55 to 60 beats/min.
    (3) Rhythm: sinus bradycardia.
    (4) PR interval: 0.16 second.
    (5) P wave size: normal.
    (6) QRS width: 0.08 second.
    (7) QT interval: 0.4 second (normal for rate).
    (8) QRS voltage: upper normal limits.
    (9) QRS axis: +30°.
    (10) R wave progression in chest leads: normal.
    (11) Abnormal Q waves: none.
    (12) ST segments: isoelectric in the extremity leads; slightly elevated J point in V_2 and V_3.
    (13) T waves: normal.
    (14) U waves: normal.

    b. *Interpretation*
    Normal electrocardiogram. The ST elevation in the chest leads represents a normal "early repolarization" variant. (The subject was a healthy 25-year-old man.)

122. Major findings are ST elevations and hyperacute T waves in the anterior chest leads (V_1 to V_5) with reciprocal ST depressions in II, III, and aV_F. (This patient was having an acute anterior wall infarction.)

123. c.

124. a. Yes. (Notice that the standardization mark in I is 10 mm tall.)
    b. 60 beats/min.
    c. Yes.
    d. +30°.
    e. No.
    f. Yes.
    g. Ischemic T wave inversions in I, aV_L, and V_2 to V_6. (Clinically the patient had an evolving non–Q wave MI.)

125. a. 60 beats/min.
    b. Prominent Q waves in II, III, and aV_F with ST segment elevations in those leads and reciprocal ST depressions in I, aV_L, and V_2 to V_3; deep T wave inversions in II, III, aV_F, and V_4 to V_6. (This pattern is consistent with an evolving inferolateral infarct.)

126. c.

127. d.

128. a. Prominent U waves.
    b. The two major causes are hypokalemia and drug effect (particularly, quinidine, procainamide, and disopyramide). This patient was hypokalemic. Patients who have markedly prolonged repolarization with large U waves from any cause are at risk of developing torsade de pointes (p. 188).

129. Acute inferior wall and right ventricular infarction. Note the ST elevations and Q waves in II, III, and aV$_F$ as well as the ST elevations in the right precordial leads. ST depressions in I and aV$_L$ are consistent with reciprocal changes.

130. This is a normal "septal" q wave, representing left-to-right spread of septal depolarization forces. (Notice its low amplitude and short duration [less than 0.04 second].)

131. Subendocardial infarction. (Notice the diffuse marked ST depressions [I, II, III, aV$_F$, and V$_3$ to V$_6$] with ST elevation in aV$_R$. These changes indicate subendocardial ischemia or non–Q wave infarction. The elevated enzymes confirm infarction.)

132. Atrial flutter with 2:1 AV conduction. (The atrial rate is about 300/min, and the ventricular rate about 150/min. Notice the positive flutter waves in V$_1$ and the negative flutter waves in II. The classic sawtooth configuration may not be seen in all leads [e.g., V$_1$ here]. Low voltage in the limb leads is also present.)

133. Atrial bigeminy.

134. This shows abnormal T wave inversions in aV$_L$ and V$_3$ to V$_5$, suggesting myocardial ischemia, with or without actual infarction.

135. Paroxysmal supraventricular tachycardia (PSVT) converting abruptly to normal sinus rhythm. (Notice the sudden slowing of heart rate and the appearance of normal P waves.)

136. Acute anterior wall MI. (Pathologic Q waves in V$_1$ to V$_5$ and aV$_L$, with ST segment elevations in these leads and reciprocal ST depressions in II, III, and aV$_F$.)

137. a. Left atrial abnormality (enlargement).
     b. First-degree AV block (PR = 0.24 sec).
     c. One VPB. In addition, there is axis deviation. (Notice the RS complex in II with the S wave > R wave. Therefore the axis must be more negative than −30° or more positive than +150°. You need two frontal plane leads to know if the axis is markedly leftward or rightward.)

138. Prior anterior wall MI. (There is a loss of normal R wave progression, with pathologic Q waves in V$_2$ to V$_5$.)

139. a. RBBB.
     b. Borderline first-degree AV block. (The PR is about 0.2 second.)
     c. Nonspecific ST-T abnormalities. With "pure" RBBB you would expect to see T wave inversions in leads with an rSR′ complex, so-called *secondary* ST-T changes. However, the ST segments here are also abnormally depressed in I, II, aV$_F$, and V$_3$ to V$_6$. These *primary* ST-T changes are nonspecific and could have been caused by ischemia, digitalis effect, or some other condition. (See page 74.)

140. Paroxysmal atrial tachycardia (PAT) with 2:1 block. Notice the two P waves for every QRS, with an atrial rate of about 190/min and a ventricular rate of 95/min. This arrhythmia was due to digitalis toxicity.

141. Diffuse subendocardial ischemia. (Notice the horizontal or downward sloping ST segment depression, best seen in I, II, aV$_F$, and V$_3$ to V$_6$, with ST elevation only in aV$_R$.)

142. Isorhythmic AV dissociation. (The atrial and ventricular rates are about equal, with P waves moving "in" and "out" of the QRS.) (See page 198.)

143. Sinus tachycardia with atrial quadrigeminy (i.e., every fourth beat an APB).

144. a. Prior inferior and anterolateral MIs, with Q waves in II, III, aV_F, V_5, and V_6 as well as T wave inversions in the left chest leads.
    b. Borderline first-degree AV block (PR about 0.2 sec).
    c. QT prolongation. (The interval is 0.4 second, which is somewhat long for a heart rate of about 77 beats/min. The patient was taking quinidine, a drug that may prolong the QT.)
    d. Marked left axis deviation.
145. a. Evolving anterior wall MI with Q waves in V_1 to V_3 and deep T wave inversions in V_3 and V_4. (The ST-T changes in the inferolateral leads are also suggestive of ischemia.)
    b. First-degree AV block.
    c. Probable left atrial abnormality (enlargement) with broad P waves.
146. Complete heart block. Notice the independent atrial and ventricular complexes, with an atrial rate of about 100/min and a ventricular rate of about 40/min.
147. Sinus rhythm with AV Wenckebach. Notice the increased length of the PR interval preceding the nonconducted P wave. The PR interval *following* this P wave is shorter than the one preceding.
148. Sinus bradycardia (a common finding in athletes). Within normal limits.
149. Prior anteroseptal infarction. Abnormal Q waves in V_1 to V_3.
150. Complete heart block. (Notice the independent atrial and ventricular complexes, with the ventricles being paced by a slow indioventricular pacemaker [wide QRS]. The combination of heart block and syncope is called Stokes-Adams syndrome.)
151. LVH with associated ST-T abnormalities. (Notice the prominent chest lead voltage [S_{V_1} and R_{V_5} greater than 35 mm] with "strain" pattern. P waves are prominent, broad, and notched in III [consistent with left atrial abnormality]. Notice also the relatively tall P waves in II. This combination may be due to biatrial enlargement. Notice that the patient also has sinus tachycardia, which can cause slightly peaked P waves without actual right atrial overload.)
152. Ventricular tachycardia (rapid, monomorphic).
153. Normal variant "early repolarization." (Notice the ST segment elevations [without reciprocal ST depressions] in V_2 to V_4.)
154. Wolff-Parkinson-White pattern. (Notice the triad of wide QRS, short PR interval, and slurring on the QRS upstroke [delta wave].)
155. a. Acute pericarditis. (Notice the ST elevations in I, II, III, aV_F, and V_4 to V_6, with T wave inversions in most of these leads. Diffuse distribution of ST elevations [present in I, II, and III] supports the clinical diagnosis of pericarditis. Notice also the LVH by voltage with left atrial abnormality. The patient was hypertensive as a result of chronic renal disease and had uremic pericarditis.)
156. Multifocal atrial tachycardia (MAT), which is most commonly associated with chronic obstructive lung disease.
157. a. Inferior wall MI of indeterminate age with Q waves in II, III, and aV_F and T wave inversions.
    b. Anterior wall MI of indeterminate age with loss of R waves in V_1 to V_3 and Q waves in V_3 to V_5, as well as deep ischemic T wave inversions in I, aV_L, and V_2 to V_6.
    c. LVH. (Notice the very prominent precordial voltage, with V_4 to V_6 recorded at one-half standardization.)

158. Paroxysmal atrial tachycardia (PAT) with 2:1 AV block. Notice the P waves sitting on the T waves. (This arrhythmia is often, but not always, associated with digitalis toxicity.)
159. a. Prior inferior wall MI.
    b. Probable left atrial abnormality.
    c. Nonspecific ST-T changes in V_4 to V_6 (consistent with ischemia or other causes).
160. Atrial flutter with 2:1 conduction (block). Flutter waves at a rate of about 300/min *(arrows)*.

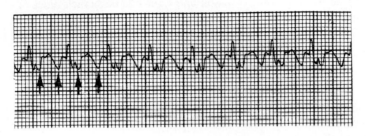

161. a. First-degree AV block.
    b. Right axis deviation. (Notice that the R wave in III is greater than in II.)
    c. Right ventricular hypertrophy with strain (with a tall R wave in V_1 and T wave inversions in the right chest leads.)
162. AV junctional rhythm (retrograde P waves following the QRS).
163. Acute pericarditis. (Notice the diffuse ST elevations in I, II, aV_F, and V_4 to V_6. This pattern differs from the ST elevations of acute MI, which usually are more localized [anterior or inferior] with reciprocal changes. The pattern also differs from that of normal-variant "early repolarization" [Fig. 10-14], which does not usually produce such marked ST elevations in V_5 and V_6 as are seen here. With normal-variant early repolarization, the ST elevations are usually most prominent in V_3 and V_4. Notice also the subtle PR changes [Fig. 10-11].)
164. Sinus tachycardia and P pulmonale (right atrial enlargement).
165. Atrial flutter with variable block.
166. b. Hyperkalemia. (There is widening of the QRS with peaking of the T waves and loss of the P waves [junctional rhythm].)
167. Severe hyperkalemia. The serum potassium was markedly elevated (8.1 mEq/L), and the ECG showed tall peaked T waves. (ST elevations in V_1 and V_2 may also be seen in this setting.) By the next day the serum potassium was normal (4.4 mEq/L).
168. Sinus rhythm with frequent multifocal atrial premature beats (APBs) at the end of the strip. This type of rhythm may lead to sustained multifocal atrial tachycardia (MAT) or atrial fibrillation.
169. Left bundle branch block.
170. Wandering atrial pacemaker. (Notice the subtle change in P waves.)
171. Accelerated idioventricular rhythm (AIVR).
172. The ST-T changes ("scooping") are consistent with digitalis effect, and the rhythm is atrial bigeminy.

173. Sinus rhythm with 2:1 AV block. Because the QRS is of normal duration here, this arrhythmia probably represents a Mobitz type I (Wenckebach) block and not a Mobitz type II block, which is often associated with a wide QRS. (See page 193.)

174. Sinus rhythm with AV Wenckebach. Nonconducted P waves are present on the T wave of the third and eighth QRS-T complexes. AV Wenckebach may be caused by a variety of factors, including drug toxicity (for example, digitalis, beta blockers, and, in this case, verapamil).

175. Evolving pattern of anterior wall infarction and right bundle branch block. Left atrial abnormality is also seen (V_1).

176. Atrial flutter with spontaneous conversion to sinus rhythm. Initially there is atrial flutter with 2:1 conduction. The degree of block increases just before conversion.

177. Atrial fibrillation may lead to left atrial thrombus formation and eventual embolization. An embolic-type cerebrovascular accident is therefore suggested. (Notice that with atrial fibrillation, fibrillatory waves may be hard to detect. The subtle changes in QRS complexes here from one beat to the next may reflect variability in ventricular conduction due to the fast rate.)

178. Complete heart block. Notice the independence of atrial (sinus) P wave activity (with a rate of about 90/min) and ventricular (QRS) complexes (at a rate of about 30/min). The combination of high-degree heart block and syncope is sometimes referred to as the Stokes-Adams syndrome. (This patient was treated with a permanent pacemaker.)

179. Paroxysmal atrial fibrillation.

180. Sinus rhythm, left axis deviation, and an intraventricular conduction delay (QRS duration = 0.12 sec). The major abnormality is extensive anterior wall infarction with pathologic Q waves in aV_L and V_1 to V_6. In addition, the ST segments are elevated in these leads. Persistent ST elevations following infarction suggest a *ventricular aneurysm,* which was the cause of the patient's heart failure in this case.

181. The ECG shows right bundle branch block and right axis deviation. This pattern, given the patient's history and physical examination findings, is most suggestive of an atrial septal defect (p. 233).

182. Wolff-Parkinson-White (WPW) pattern. The triad of short PR interval, wide QRS, and slurring of the QRS upstroke (delta wave) is best seen in II, III, aV_F, and V_4 to V_6. WPW is often associated with supraventricular tachycardias (in particular, a type of reentrant PSVT), which may have been the source of this patient's chief complaint of palpitations.

183. The classic pattern of *torsade de pointes,* a form of ventricular tachycardia characterized by oscillations in QRS amplitude and axis in the same lead. This potentially fatal arrhythmia is usually seen in the setting of abnormally prolonged ventricular repolarization, evidenced by long QT intervals or prominent U waves. Drugs such as quinidine may cause the arrhythmia (quinidine syncope). (See page 188 for other causes.)

184. Intermittent left bundle branch block. The first four beats are conducted with a left bundle branch block pattern, the last four with a normal QRS. In this case the bundle branch block was *rate related.* When the heart rate exceeded a critical value, the bundle branch block appeared. (Notice that all the beats are preceded by a P wave with a constant PR interval. Therefore this could *not* be accelerated idioventricular rhythm.)

185. There is underlying sinus bradycardia with a 2.4-second pause following the third beat. This pause is almost exactly twice the underlying PP interval. Therefore the patient probably has

2:1 SA block. Unlike 2:1 AV block (in which a P wave is not followed by a QRS), 2:1 SA block causes an entire P-QRS-T cycle to be "dropped." This patient had "sick sinus syndrome" and required a permanent pacemaker.

186. c.

187. Long QT (about 0.53 second) at a heart rate of 70/min. The patient had severe hypocalcemia.

188. b. The atrial rate is about 300/min, which is diagnostic of flutter.

189. e. Notice the wide QRS complexes with absent P waves.

190. Sinus rhythm with AV Wenckebach.

191. A dual-chamber pacemaker. Notice the repeating sequence of atrial pacemaker spike, P wave, ventricular pacemaker spike, and wide QRS.

192. The first part of the rhythm strip shows a run of paroxysmal supraventricular tachycardia (PSVT), probably due to AV nodal reentry given the absence of visible P waves. The tachyarrhythmia spontaneously breaks with the resumption of sinus bradycardia, raising the question of a brady-tachy variant of the "sick sinus syndrome."

193. The arrow points to a nonconducted (blocked) atrial premature beat (blocked APB). In fact, each normal beat here is followed by a subtle blocked APB; therefore the rhythm is sinus with atrial bigeminy and blocked APBs. The APBs are not conducted to the ventricles in this case because they come so soon after the previous beat that the AV node is still refractory.

194. Wolff-Parkinson-White pattern (indicated by a short PR interval, widened QRS, and notching or slurring at the beginning of the QRS [delta wave]). It is best seen here in lead II. The anatomic substrate is an atrioventricular bypass tract that preexcites the ventricles. Such patients are especially prone to the development of paroxysmal supraventricular tachycardia (PSVT) associated with reentry involving the bypass tract.

195. Yes. The peaked P waves and right axis deviation are consistent with right atrial and right ventricle overload due to pulmonary hypertension. Sinus tachycardia, delayed precordial transition zone, and nonspecific ST-T changes are also present.

196. Sinus rhythm with alternating 2:1 and 3:1 second-degree AV block. This type of conduction disturbance with multiple nonconducted P waves is sometimes referred to as *advanced second-degree block*. The patient had a pacemaker implanted.

197. Narrow-complex tachycardia with a ventricular rate of about 160/min. Notice the subtle atrial waves at twice that rate (e.g., in aV_L and V_1) with a sawtooth appearance in II; therefore this is atrial flutter with 2:1 conduction (block). It is commonly mistaken for sinus tachycardia or atrial tachycardia.

198. Sinus rhythm with first-degree AV block and left atrial abnormality. The major finding is diffuse but prominent ST depressions (I, II, aV_L, aV_F, V_2 to V_6) consistent with severe subendocardial ischemia. (Lead aV_R shows ST elevations.)

199. Sinus rhythm with prominent Q waves, ST elevations, and T wave inversions in II, III, and aV_F as well as T wave inversions in V_3 to V_6. There is reduced R wave amplitude in V_5 and V_6 with relatively tall R waves in V_1 and V_2. These findings are consistent with a recent extensive infero-postero-lateral/apical MI.

200. Sinus rhythm with ST segment depressions (consistent with ischemia, digitalis, etc.) followed abruptly by ventricular fibrillation initiated by an R-on-T type of VPB.

Bibliography

Chapters 1 to 7
BASIC CONCEPTS AND PATTERNS

Berne RM, Levy MN: *Cardiovascular physiology,* ed 6, St Louis, 1992, Mosby.

Burch GE, dePasquale NP: *A history of electrocardiography,* Chicago, 1964, Year Book Medical Publishers.

Dunn MI, Lipman BS: *Lipman-Massie clinical electrocardiography,* ed 8, Chicago, 1989, Year Book Medical Publishers.

Goldberger E: *Unipolar lead electrocardiography and vectorcardiography,* ed 3, Philadelphia, 1953, Lea & Febiger.

Goldman MJ: *Principles of clinical electrocardiography,* ed 12, Los Altos Calif, 1986, Lange Medical Publications.

Marriott HJC: *Principles of clinical electrocardiography,* ed 7, Baltimore, 1983, Williams & Wilkins.

Mirvis DM: *Electrocardiography: a physiologic approach,* St Louis, 1993, Mosby.

Chapters 8 and 9
MYOCARDIAL ISCHEMIA AND INFARCTION

Froelicher VF: *Exercise and the heart,* ed 2, Chicago, 1987, Year Book Medical Publishers.

Goldberger AL: *Myocardial infarction: electrocardiographic differential diagnosis,* ed 4, St Louis, 1991, Mosby.

Schamroth L: *The electrocardiology of coronary artery disease,* Oxford, 1975, Blackwell Scientific Publications.

Chapter 10
MISCELLANEOUS PATTERNS

Chou TC: *Electrocardiography in clinical practice,* ed 2, Orlando Fla, 1986, Grune & Stratton.

Goldberger A: A specific ECG triad associated with congestive heart failure, *PACE* 5:593, 1982.

Park MK, Guntheroth WG: *How to read pediatric ECGs,* ed 2, St Louis, 1987, Mosby.

Spodick DH: Electrocardiographic responses to pulmonary embolism, *Am J Cardiol* 30:695, 1972.

Surawicz B: Relationship between electrocardiogram and electrolytes, *Am Heart J* 73:814, 1967.

Chapter 11 to 21
ARRHYTHMIAS, CONDUCTION DISTURBANCES, PACEMAKERS
General References

Josephson ME: *Clinical cardiac electrophysiology,* ed 2, Philadelphia, 1992, Lea & Febiger.

Kastor JA: *Arrhythmias,* Philadelphia, 1994, WB Saunders.

Waldo AL, Touboul P (eds): *Atrial arrhythmias: current concepts and management,* St Louis, 1989, Mosby.

Zipes D: Cardiac arrhythmias. In Braunwald EB (ed): *Heart disease: a textbook of cardiovascular medicine,* ed 4, Philadelphia, 1992, WB Saunders.

Selected Additional References on Specific Topics
Supraventricular tachycardias

Josephson ME, Wellens HJJ: Differential diagnosis of supraventricular tachycardia, *Cardiol Clin,* vol 8, August 1990.

Atrial fibrillation

Falk RH, Podrid PJ: *Atrial fibrillation: mechanisms and management,* New York, 1992, Raven Press.

Ventricular arrhythmias

Akhtar M: Clinical spectrum of ventricular tachycardia, *Circulation* 82:1561, 1990.

rhythmia Suppression Trial (CAST): Increased
due to encainide or flecainide in a randomized
arrhythmia suppression after myocardial infarc-
, *N Engl J Med* 321:406, 1989.

Roden DM, et al: Incidence and clinical features of the
quinidine-associated long QT syndrome: implications for
patient care, *Am Heart J* 111:1088, 1986.

Ben-David J, Zipes DP: Torsades de pointes and proar-
rhythmia, *Lancet* 341:1578, 1993.

Digitalis toxicity

Kelly RA, Smith TW: Recognition and management of digitalis toxicity, *Am J Cardiol* 69:108G, 1992.

Smith TW, et al: Digitalis glycosides: mechanisms and
manifestations of toxicity, *Prog Cardiovasc Dis* 26:413,
1984.

Cardiac arrest

Emergency Cardiac Care Committee and Subcommittees,
American Heart Association: Guidelines for cardiopul-
monary resuscitation and emergency cardiac care. I to
IX, *JAMA* 268:2171, 1992.

Grauer K, Cavallaro D: *ACLS Volume II: a comprehensive
review,* ed 3, St Louis, 1993, Mosby.

Jaffee AS (ed): *Textbook of advanced cardiac life support,*
Dallas, 1987, American Heart Association.

Josephson ME (ed): *Sudden cardiac death,* Oxford, 1993,
Blackwell Scientific Publications.

Niemann JT: Cardiopulmonary resuscitation, *N Engl J Med*
327:1075, 1992.

Pacemakers

Moses HW, et al: *A practical guide to cardiac pacing,*
Boston, ed 3, 1991, Little Brown.

Zipes D, Duffin EG: Cardiac pacemakers. In Braunwald E
(ed): *Heart disease: a textbook of cardiovascular medicine,* ed 4, Philadelphia, 1992, WB Saunders.

Index

---

n indicates footnote

n indicates footnote

n indicates footnote